Latino Farmworkers in the Eastern United States

Thomas A. Arcury • Sara A. Quandt
Editors

Latino Farmworkers in the Eastern United States

Health, Safety and Justice

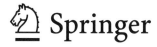 Springer

Editors

Thomas A. Arcury, Ph.D.
Department of Family
and Community Medicine
Wake Forest University School of Medicine
Winston-Salem, NC 27157
USA

Sara A. Quandt, Ph.D.
Department of Epidemiology and Prevention
Division of Public Health Sciences
Wake Forest University School of Medicine
Winston-Salem, NC 27157
USA

ISBN: 978-0-387-88346-5   e-ISBN: 978-0-387-88347-2
DOI: 10.1007/978-0-387-88347-2

Library of Congress Control Number: 2008942080

Printed on acid-free paper

springer.com

Contents

Contributors

Thomas A. Arcury, Ph.D., is a Professor and Vice Chair for Research in the Department of Family and Community Medicine, Wake Forest University School of Medicine, Winston-Salem, NC. He received his doctoral degree in cultural anthropology from the University of Kentucky in 1983 and completed a postdoctoral fellowship in health services research at the Cecil G. Sheps Center for Health Services Research, University of North Carolina, Chapel Hill, in 1996. Dr. Arcury is a medical anthropologist and public health scientist with a research program focused on improving the health of rural and minority populations. Since 1996, he has collaborated in a program of community-based participatory research with immigrant farmworkers and poultry processing workers and their families focused on occupational and environmental health and justice. Although much of his research with farmworkers has focused on pesticide exposure, he has also directed projects examining skin disease and green tobacco sickness. He has authored over 200 refereed articles, and he has participated in the development of diverse educational materials intended to return research results to immigrant worker communities. He has also used research results to effect policy change. Dr. Arcury's contributions have been recognized by the National Institute for Occupational Safety and Health with the 2006 National Occupational Research Agenda (NORA) Innovative Research Award for Worker Health and Safety (with Sara A. Quandt), the National Rural Health Association with the 2004 Outstanding Researcher Award, the Washington Association for the Practice of Anthropology with the 2003 Praxis Award (with Sara A. Quandt). He received the 2007 Mid-Career Investigator in Clinical Sciences Award of Wake Forest University School of Medicine.

Joseph G. Grzywacz, Ph.D., is an Associate Professor of Family and Community Medicine, Wake Forest University School of Medicine, Winston-Salem, NC. Dr. Grzywacz is an interdisciplinary social scientist with doctoral training in adult development and family studies (University of Wisconsin), and postdoctoral training in the social ecology of adult health (University of California, Irvine). Grzywacz's research focuses with primarily on adults' daily work and family lives and how the challenge of combining work and family affects physical and mental health. Dr. Grzywacz has published several papers focused on different domains of Latino farmworkers' mental health including depression, alcohol use and abuse, anxiety, as well as stressors confronted by farmworkers and their families. Grzywacz provides ongoing consultation to the National Institute for Occupational Safety and Health (NIOSH) on Latino farmworker mental health.

Antonio J. Marín, M.A., is a Research Associate in the Department of Family and Community Medicine, Wake Forest University School of Medicine, Winston-Salem, NC. He has collaborated on several research projects related to farmworkers, including projects focused on occupational skin disease and on pesticide exposure. He currently serves as the project manager for an environmental justice project with Latino poultry processing workers in North Carolina. Mr. Marín has worked extensively with lay health promoters as a means of increasing knowledge of environmental and occupational health and of workers' rights among immigrant workers with limited literacy. Marín is a native of Venezuela. He has been active as a community organizer with Latinos in North Carolina for the past decade.

John J. May, M.D., is a graduate of the University of Notre Dame and Case Western Reserve School of Medicine. He trained in internal medicine at the Mary Imogene Bassett Hospital in Cooperstown, New York, and the University of Colorado Medical Center, Denver, CO. Dr. May is a specialist in pulmonary medicine, having completed a fellowship at the University of Colorado. In addition to his pulmonary practice at Bassett Hospital in Cooperstown, Dr. May began seeing patients with various agricultural occupational health problems over two decades ago. He is a cofounder and director of the New York Center for Agricultural Medicine and Health, which is one of the national centers designated by the National Institute for Occupational Safety and Health. May has published widely in research areas that include respiratory, musculoskeletal, hearing, and other disorders affecting both family farmers and farmworkers in the northeastern United States. A particular interest is the application of community-based intervention methods in addressing occupational health challenges for migrant farmworkers. Dr. May now serves as the director of the Bassett Research Institute in Cooperstown, New York.

Sara A. Quandt, Ph.D., is a Professor in the Department of Epidemiology and Prevention, Division of Public Health Sciences, and in the Department of Family and Community Medicine, Wake Forest University School of Medicine, Winston-Salem, NC. She is an Adjunct Professor of Anthropology and an affiliate of the Maya Angelou Center for Health Equity at Wake Forest. Dr. Quandt was trained in medical anthropology and human nutrition at Michigan State University. Her research focuses on health disparities in rural and minority communities. Quandt and colleagues have conducted basic research on pesticide exposure among farmworker families; developed, tested, and implemented pesticide safety interventions; and initiated policy-relevant research at the request of the farmworker and medical communities in food insecurity, green tobacco sickness, mental health, housing, oral health, and skin disease. She serves on the Health and Safety Advisory Committee of East Coast Migrant Head Start Program and is on the External Advisory Committee of the Pacific Northwest Agricultural Safety and Health Center at the University of Washington. She was corecipient with Thomas A. Arcury of the 2006 National Occupational Research Agenda (NORA) Innovative Research Award for Worker Health and Safety for work on reducing the impact of green tobacco sickness among Latino farmworkers. She received the Outstanding Rural Health Researcher Award of the National Rural Health Association in 2007.

Scott D. Rhodes, Ph.D., M.P.H., C.H.E.S., is an Associate Professor in the Department of Social Sciences and Health Policy, Division of Public Health Sciences, and in the Section on Infectious Diseases, Department of Internal Medicine; and is an affiliate faculty of the Maya Angelou Center for Health Equity, at Wake Forest University School of Medicine, Winston-Salem, NC. Dr. Rhodes' research explores sexual health, HIV, and sexually transmitted disease (STD) prevention, obesity prevention, and other health disparities among vulnerable communities. Dr. Rhodes has extensive research experience with Latino immigrant communities; self-identifying gay and bisexual men and men who have sex with men (MSM); urban African American adolescents; persons living with HIV/AIDS; and men of color. He has broad experience in the design, implementation, and evaluation of multiple-level interventions; community-based participatory research (CBPR); exploratory evaluation; the application of behavioral theory; lay health advisor interventions; sociocultural determinants of health; and Internet research.

Quirina Vallejos, M.P.H., is a Research Associate in the Department of Family and Community Medicine, Wake Forest University School of Medicine, Winston-Salem, NC. Ms. Vallejos received a B.A. in Spanish and Latin American Studies at Duke University, and M.P.H. in Community Health Education at the University of North Carolina at Greensboro. Ms. Vallejos is the project manager for two research projects and two educational intervention projects that address the topics of skin disease, pesticide exposure, and environmental tobacco smoke among Latino farmworkers. She is also the Principal Investigator of a US Environmental Protection Agency-funded project to educate Latino parents about lead poisoning testing and prevention. She has served for a year on the housing subcommittee of the Farmworker Advocacy Network, a network of organizations that advocates for improved living and working conditions of migrant and seasonal farmworkers and their families in North Carolina.

Melinda F. Wiggins, M.T.S., is the Executive Director of Student Action with Farmworkers (SAF), a nonprofit organization that brings students and farmworkers together to learn about each other's lives, share resources and skills, improve conditions for farmworkers, and build diverse coalitions working for social change (www.saf-unite.org). Ms. Wiggins is the granddaughter of sharecroppers. She grew up in a rural farming community in the Mississippi Delta. She moved to North Carolina in 1992 to pursue a Masters of Theological Studies at Duke University. Before starting as the Director of SAF in 1996, she coordinated SAF's Into the Fields summer internship program for several years. She first joined the farmworker movement as a SAF intern with the Episcopal Farmworker Ministry during the summer of 1993. Wiggins is involved with many social and economic justice organizations, including the Adelante Education Coalition, Farmworker Advocacy

Network, Farmworker Ministry Committee, and Housing Development Corporation. She coedited *The Human Cost of Food: Farmworkers' Lives, Labor and Advocacy*, published by University of Texas Press in 2002.

Chapter 1
The Health and Safety of Farmworkers in the Eastern United States: A Need to Focus on Social Justice

Thomas A. Arcury and Sara A. Quandt

Abstract This chapter provides the fundamental argument of why the health and safety of farmworkers in the eastern US is a matter of social justice. The organization of the chapters in the volume is outlined, and definitions of common terms (e.g., social justice, eastern US) and conventions (e.g., use of the term Latino/Hispanic) are presented. An overview of each chapter is provided. Finally, acknowledgments for the Third Wake Forest University School of Medicine Farmworker Health Research Workshop are presented.

1.1 A Focus on Social Justice

The health and safety of farmworkers in the eastern United States (US) is a matter of social justice. Our definition of social justice is succinct. Social justice is the process that seeks fairness or equity in the distribution of social burdens and resources across all social groups, and provides all people the opportunity to realize their full potential. For farmworkers, social justice includes working and living in environments in which health and safety hazards are addressed, being paid a living wage, living in communities free of discrimination, and having access to health, education, and social services.

The eastern US includes 22 states from Maine to Florida, and from the Atlantic Coast to Ohio, Kentucky, Tennessee, and Mississippi. Through the early 1990s, farmworkers in this region included African Americans, Afro-Caribbeans, Latino/Hispanics, as well as rural whites from regions such as Appalachia. Since 1990, farmworkers in the eastern US have become overwhelmingly Latino/Hispanic. The eastern US differs from the other major regions in which large numbers of farmworkers are employed, such as the West Coast and Southwest, and Texas and the Midwest. The eastern US does not have the historically large rural Latino/Hispanic population as do these other regions, and therefore, Latino/Hispanics in the eastern US do not have the same levels of community organizations as do farmworkers with bases in California, Arizona, New Mexico, and Texas.

T.A. Arcury and S.A. Quandt (eds.), *Latino Farmworkers in Eastern United States*,
DOI: 10.1007/978-0-387-88347-2_1, © Springer Science+Business Media, LLC 2009

Similar to farmworkers everywhere, those across the eastern US do physical and strenuous labor that puts them at risk for numerous occupational injuries and illnesses. Many are separated from family for periods of 3–9 months each year. This separation places them at special risks, especially for hazards of mental illness and infectious disease. Many farmworkers have the fortune of having their family live with them; these include many farmworkers who are seasonally employed but who do not migrate, and some farmworkers who do migrate. The family members of these farmworkers are exposed to many of the occupational injuries and illnesses of the farmworkers, including living in substandard housing and being exposed to toxic agents such as pesticides.

Although farmworkers and the members of their families experience high levels of physical and mental injury and illness, they have poor access to health services (Alderete et al. 2000; Arcury and Quandt 2007; Villarejo 2003). Most farmworkers have incomes that place them near or below poverty. Farmworker wages seldom exceed minimum wage, and at times fall below minimum wage. Together with little income to pay for health care, few (5–11%) farmworkers have health insurance (Rosenbaum and Shin 2005). Programs to address farmworker health disparities are limited. Community and migrant clinics are supported with federal and state funds, but the number of clinics and the services provided by these clinics cannot meet the needs of the farmworker population in the eastern US.

All agricultural workers, but especially migrant and seasonal farmworkers, have fewer protections than do other workers in the US. Investigators have consistently documented the limited regulatory protection for farm labor (President's Commission on Migratory Labor 1951; Mitchell and Gurske 1956; General Accounting Office 2000; Human Rights Watch 2000).

> [the US] depend[s] on misfortune to build up our force of migratory workers and when the supply is low because there is not enough misfortune at home, we rely on misfortune abroad to replenish the supply (President's Commission on Migratory Labor 1951)

Occupational health and safety are relatively unregulated in US agriculture. Most Latino/Hispanic farmworkers lack knowledge of English and of the safety regulations that do exist. They seldom receive safety training that is required. Farmworkers often work in the face of unsafe conditions because they fear the loss of work and the income to provide for their families. Many farmworkers do not have documentation; they will not report unsafe work or employers who do not follow regulations for fear of retaliation. Even farmworkers with documents often do not want to deal with government representatives because of fear of harassment in an anti-immigrant environment.

Although farmworkers are often discussed, and many groups are engaged in efforts to improve the working conditions and health of farmworkers, little research documents the actual occupational health, living conditions, or social justice experienced by this population. For example, four of the nine Centers for Agricultural Disease and Injury Research, Education, and Prevention supported by cooperative agreements with the National Institute of Occupational Safety and Health have been located in the eastern US. However, only one of these four centers, the Northeast Center for Agricultural and Occupational Health, has a consistent program of research and outreach addressing the health and safety of migrant and seasonal farmworkers and their families. With these potential resources, the limited documentation of occupational injury and illness and intervention to address this injury and illness among farmworkers in the eastern US is evidence of the lack of concern for justice in this region. Without information, critical occupational health and safety programs for farmworkers cannot be implemented, workable and needed occupational safety regulations cannot be drafted, and the level of health care needed for farmworkers cannot be judged.

Farmworker social, occupational, and environmental injustice results from the intersection of high risk among workers and the members of their families, low return for the work that they perform, few regulatory protections and limited services, the experience of discrimination and harassment, and limited documentation of injury and illness. The goal of this volume is to integrate what is known about the health and safety of farmworkers in the eastern US in an effort to inform the process of achieving social justice for farmworkers.

1.2   Organization of the Chapters

The chapters in this volume are organized to integrate what is known about the health and safety of farmworkers in the eastern US and recommend processes to improve social justice for farmworkers. The first chapters provide information on the risks for farmworkers and their families. These chapters outline the different dimensions of the context in which farmworkers labor and live in the eastern US. They also describe the characteristics and quality of the housing in which farmworkers live. The following chapters review different aspects of health and safety for farmworkers. These include occupational injuries, pesticide exposure, infectious diseases, mental health, and the health of children and women. The final chapters provide information about efforts to advocate for social justice for farmworkers and make recommendations for approaches to address social justice for farmworkers.

Each chapter provides a review of current knowledge of its focal topic, whether housing, infectious disease, or mental health. Each also indicates the gaps in current knowledge. Finally, each chapter provides recommendations for addressing justice that will lead to improved health and safety for farmworkers and their families.

1.3   Definitions and Conventions

The language used in research and advocacy often applies several meanings to the same word. This often results in misunderstanding and conflict. Significant consideration has been given to the specific words and concepts used across this volume, as well as the definitions of these words and concepts.

We have presented our definition for the concept of social justice. The region on which this volume focuses, the eastern US, has been defined and the reasons for this regional focus have been stated. We call this region the eastern US, rather than the Eastern Migrant Stream. Many service agencies and publications refer to the Eastern Migrant Stream. However, a minority of the farmworkers in the eastern US migrate from place to place like a stream flowing toward the crops that need to be harvested. A substantial number of farmworkers in the eastern US do migrate to do farm work, but they generally move to one area and remain there for the season. We use the single word "farmworker" throughout this volume. This convention has no particular conceptual foundation. Rather it is based on what the authors have always used.

The term *Latino/Hispanic* is cumbersome. We recognize that the peoples from Spanish- and Portuguese-speaking nations in North and South America reflect diverse and rich cultures and histories. We further recognize that many people from these nations do not speak Spanish, Portuguese, or any other European-based language; rather, they are Indigenous people who speak their own language. No one term can capture all of this diversity. We also recognize that any single term which we select could be considered offensive by some individuals for whom it is used. Faced with selecting a term that would allow us to somewhat succinctly refer to the geographic and cultural background of most farmworkers, we selected *Latino/Hispanic* because it reflects the regulatory realities with which we must work. According to the US government, as stated in the US Office of Management and Budget's Race and Ethnic Standards for Federal Statistics and Administrative Reporting that are set forth in Statistical Policy Directive No. 15, revised October 30, 1997, all residents of the US are of two ethnicities: "Hispanic or Latino" and "Not Hispanic or Latino." The five minimum categories for race are American Indian or Alaska Native, Asian, Black or African American, Native Hawaiian or Other Pacific Islander, and White.

1.4   The Chapters

In addition to this Introduction, this volume has nine chapters. Chapters 2 and 3 discuss the exposures that affect the health, safety, and justice experienced by farmworkers and their families in the eastern US. Chapters 4 through 8 review specific areas of farmworker health, safety, and justice; occupational injuries and illness, pesticide exposure, infectious disease, mental health, and the health of children and women. Chapter 9 reviews ongoing efforts by advocates to improve justice in the area of health and safety for farmworkers. The final chapter proposes an agenda to improve justice in health and safety for farmworkers.

The context for farmworkers in the eastern US affects the health, safety, and justice they experience. This context, which includes geographic, agricultural, demographic, cultural, and political dimensions, has changed dramatically over the past 50 years. In the second chapter, "Latino/Hispanic Farmworkers and Farm

Work in the Eastern United States: The Context for Health, Safety and Justice," Thomas A. Arcury and Antonio J. Marín discuss the context in which farmworkers in the eastern US labor and live. Each of these dimensions affects the health, safety, and justice farmworkers experience. Farmworkers include individuals who are involved in agricultural production, including planting, cultivating, harvesting, and processing crops for sale, and caring for animals. They include seasonal farmworkers, individuals whose principal employment is in agriculture on a seasonal basis, and migrant farmworkers, seasonal farmworkers who, for purposes of employment, establish a temporary home. Although farmworkers in the eastern US are overwhelmingly Latino/Hispanic, they vary in ethnic composition (Latino/Hispanic, Indigenous, non-Latino/Hispanic) and migration status.

Agriculture involving farmworkers in the eastern US is concentrated in production that requires hand labor. Characteristic crops for which farmworkers in the eastern US are employed include apples, peaches and citrus fruit, berries, vegetables, mushrooms, Christmas trees, and tobacco. This agriculture is changing, with more farmworkers moving into activities such as dairy work. Farmers, as well as farmworkers, have shared beliefs and behaviors that affect farmworker exposure to health and safety hazards and access to health care, often to the detriment of farmworkers. Finally, the political context within the US, with its biases toward protecting the "family farm" and against immigrants, as well as the impressive financial resources of the agricultural industry in contrast to the limited resources of farmworker organizations and advocates, circumscribes changes in policy and regulation that would protect farmworker health, safety, and justice.

Information needed to document each dimension of the context for farmworkers in the eastern US is often unavailable, making it difficult to understand who farmworkers are, their number, their personal characteristics, their exposures and health status, and how to best work toward justice for farmworkers and their families in the eastern US. Recommendations to improve health, safety, and justice include more complete and consistent reporting by state agencies of information they collect for farmworkers in their states, and better documentation and reporting of study design by researchers.

Houses at once can be a place of safety and rest, and an important source of exposure to environmental hazards for farmworkers and their families. In the third chapter, "The Condition of Farmworker Housing in the Eastern United States," Quirina M. Vallejos, Sara A. Quandt, and Thomas A. Arcury summarize the limited research documenting the condition of farmworker housing in the eastern US. Farmworker housing in the eastern US, whether employer-provided or obtained in the private market, is generally crowded, in disrepair, and lacking basic facilities. The quality of this housing places farmworkers at risk for a variety of illnesses and injuries. The experiences of farmworkers with housing in the eastern US are similar to farmworkers across the US. Farmworker housing seldom meets the minimum standards for housing established by the US Department of Housing and Human Development. Even though housing standards for farmworkers are minimal, current regulations are often not enforced. Adequate housing has been recognized as a basic human right by the United Nations (Office of the High Commissioner for

Human Rights 2008); therefore, the deplorable condition of most farmworker housing in the eastern US represents a social injustice. The authors present several recommendations to address farmworker housing, including making temporary labor camp standards more stringent and enforcing these standards through pre- and postoccupancy inspection, and providing incentive programs to employers to improve the housing that they provide.

John J. May describes key occupational health challenges encountered by farmworkers in the eastern US in the fourth chapter, "Occupational Injury and Illness in Farmworkers in the Eastern United States." May argues that agricultural work exposes farmworkers to risks for numerous occupational injuries, yet little has been done to document the injuries experienced by farmworkers or to provide sufficient health care when farmworkers experience occupational injuries and illness. The lack of appropriate support available to farmworkers and to health professionals providing their care is indicative of the lack of respect and justice our society affords these essential workers. May describes the causes and symptoms for occupational health problems common to farmworkers, including heat stress, musculoskeletal injuries, skin disease, hearing loss, eye injury, and transportation-related injuries. He also discusses patterns of illness and injury for farmworkers that are common to orchard work, tobacco production, dairy farming, and vegetable and berry production, all important commodities in the eastern US. Importantly, May discusses community-based approaches for designing changes in tools used by farmworkers in agricultural production that can reduce their occupational injuries. He concludes with a list of recommended changes in the provision of health care for farmworkers, the organization of work, and procedures to redesign tools that will reduce injury and improve justice for farmworkers.

The health effects of pesticide exposure for farmworkers and their families have been a major concern for several decades. The exposure of farmworkers to pesticides, the lack of knowledge and control that farmworkers have about their pesticide exposure, and the potential health effects of this exposure make pesticides a major focus for farmworker social and environment justice. Thomas A. Arcury and Sara A. Quandt review the current state of research on farmworker pesticide exposure in the eastern US in Chapter 5. They lay the ground work for this review by presenting a definition for pesticides and outlining why pesticide exposure is an important health concern. Pesticides are not limited to insecticides, but include any substance used to control any pest. Arcury and Quandt provide a model of the different pathways through which farmworkers and their family members are exposed to pesticides at work and at home. They review the US Environmental Protection Agency and Occupational Safety and Health Administration pesticide, field sanitation, and housing regulations meant to protect farmworkers from pesticide exposure. These regulations provide very few protections, and current evaluations show that the enforcement of these regulations in the eastern US is very limited.

Research has examined several domains of farmworker pesticide exposure. Farmworker and farmer beliefs and misconceptions about farmworker pesticides can result in increased exposure for farmworkers. Similarly, several farmworker behaviors place them at increased risk of exposure. Although a growing body of research documents farmworker and farmer pesticide beliefs and safety behaviors, almost no research in the eastern US has measured actual farmworker pesticide exposure. Further, almost no research has measured actual health effects of farmworker pesticide exposure. These gaps in our knowledge of actual biological measures of exposure and of health outcome make it impossible to delineate and prevent the specific routes of pesticide exposure for this population. Arcury and Quandt make several specific recommendations for improving information about farmworker pesticide exposure, including better surveillance of exposure using biomarkers and documentation of health effects of pesticide exposure. They also argue that immediate changes are needed to better protect farmworkers and their families from pesticide exposure, including the expansion of pesticide safety regulations and improved enforcement of these regulations.

Farmworkers are disproportionately affected by the intersecting epidemics of tuberculosis, sexually transmitted diseases, and HIV. Scott D. Rhodes applies his expertise gained from research in preventing HIV among Latino/Hispanic immigrants to describe the prevalence and risk factors for major infectious diseases among farmworkers in the sixth chapter, "Tuberculosis, Sexually Transmitted Diseases, HIV, and Other Infections among Farmworkers in the Eastern United States." Rhodes reviews the epidemiology of tuberculosis, sexually transmitted diseases, and HIV among farmworkers and explores the risks facing farmworkers. Factors that increase the risk for infectious diseases among farmworkers in the eastern US fall into three domains: intrapersonal factors such as knowledge of infectious diseases and available services; cultural and social factors reflecting gender role socialization and use of traditional healers; and the immigrant and farmworker experience, including substandard housing, barriers to services, and loneliness. Furthermore, farmworkers tend to be politically, socially, and economically disenfranchised, which contributes to their increased vulnerability to infectious diseases. Current interventions, even when designed for Latino/Hispanic communities, do not address the needs of immigrant worker communities. With little data to document the risk and infection rates among farmworkers and with no current intervention programs available, Rhodes argues that efforts must be made to strengthen our understanding of needs and the development of effective multilevel strategies to intervene upon the health needs of this particularly vulnerable population. Rhodes uses his own work, which uses a community-based participatory design, in immigrant Latino/Hispanic communities to illustrate effective programs to reduce infectious risk factors and rates.

Occupational health is too often focused on physical injuries and illnesses while ignoring the effects that work can have on mental health. Joseph G. Grzywacz examines the association of social justice with the mental health of farmworkers in Chapter 7, "Mental Health among Farmworkers in the Eastern United States." Grzywacz argues that farmworkers' mental health is affected by a variety of structural and social factors, including the absence of fixed-term permanent employment, poverty-level wages, separation from family and community for extended periods of time, and hostile attitudes toward immigrants. Although little research documents the mental health of farmworkers, particularly in the eastern US, the available evidence suggests that 20–50% of farmworkers have poor mental health as indicated by elevated symptoms of depression or anxiety, frequent heavy alcohol consumption, or recent experiences of lay-defined illnesses such as susto or nervios.

Grzywacz provides a conceptual framework for understanding that poor mental health among farmworkers is a social injustice, showing that farmworkers experience unequal treatment of poor mental health, unequal exposures to risks for poor mental health, unequal access to care for poor mental health, and unequal voice in effecting change. He argues that research can help effect solutions to the social injustice of farmworker mental health through the systematic documentation of changes in mental health among farmworkers, providing better measures of mental health, and informing processes for improving the delivery of mental health services. Finally, he discusses how solutions to the social injustice of farmworker mental health needs to begin with making mental health services accessible for farmworkers, and redesigning farmworker jobs to ensure the provision of a livable wage and basic human rights.

Although the majority of farmworkers are men, children and women are often present in farmworker communities as farmworkers themselves or as dependents. Children and women are also at risk of health effects from farm work. Sara A. Quandt summarizes research on the health of women and children in farmworker communities in the eastern US in Chap. 8, "Health of Children and Women in the Farmworker Community in the Eastern United States." As in other domains of farmworker social justice, the research on health issues for children and women in farmworker communities in the eastern US is very limited, making it difficult to fully document the extent of most health and safety concerns. The research on children in farmworker communities indicates that they have limited access to care and significant unmet health needs. Obesity and food security are concerns. The environment poses significant risks, including exposure to pesticides and lead. Women lack access to reproductive health services. Mental health and sexual harassment for women in farmworker communities are important social justice problems. For children and women, access to linguistically and culturally appropriate health care is limited, further amplifying difficulties in attaining health, safety, and justice.

Achieving health, safety, and justice for farmworkers will require advocacy and intervention. Melinda F. Wiggins provides a list of specific changes for which advocates are working that will move farmworkers closer to social justice. In Chapter 9, "Farm Labor and the Struggle for Justice in the Eastern United States Fields," Wiggins provides a historical context for farmworker advocacy. She notes that most farm work has been done by people of color who experience labor abuses and who lack the power to make systemic change in the agricultural system. She documents that farmworkers suffer from "agricultural exceptionalism," the practice of excluding farmworkers from legal protections benefiting other workers. The agricultural industry has resisted changes to this system. Farmworkers, who are a primarily migrant, undocumented, and disenfranchised population, have not been able to develop organizations to foster needed changes in this system.

Wiggins also highlights major efforts of farmworkers to organize and provides a history of farmworker advocacy, giving examples of current national (Farmworker Justice) and state-specific (Justice for Farmworkers Coalition in New York, Farmworker Advocacy Network in North Carolina) farmworker advocacy organizations. Wiggins also considers the potential of community–academic alliances to further farmworker advocacy, focusing specifically on community-based participatory research. Some of the specific changes she suggests for achieving farmworker justice include the provision of public and private resources for organizations supporting farmworkers; the formation of stronger collaborations among farmworker service agencies, advocacy organizations, and labor unions; changes in state labor, health, and safety legislation so that farmworkers have the same coverage as all other employees; and enactment of a guestworker program that is worker-friendly.

Farmworkers experience high levels of injury and illness that reflects the lack of social justice afforded to this community. In the final chapter, Thomas A. Arcury, Melinda Wiggins, and Sara A. Quandt outline an agenda for farmworker justice. Arcury, Wiggins, and Quandt summarize three themes that are common across the chapters in this volume. Information about farmworkers in the eastern US, including their numbers, personal characteristics, environmental exposure, health status, and occupational injuries, is severely lacking. Although information about farmworkers is limited, all of the existing information documents grave concerns for farmworker health and justice. Much of the injustice experienced by farmworkers is a consequence of antiquated agricultural labor policy that pretends that most farm labor is provided by family members and not by hired workers. Arcury, Wiggins, and Quandt also summarize three positive trends toward farmworker justice that are documented across the chapters. The efforts of local, regional, and national farmworker advocacy organizations have begun to improve policies that affect farmworker health, safety, and justice. Labor organizations have begun to make progress in the eastern US. Community-based participatory research uniting academic scientists and farmworker organizations has expanded in the eastern US. These collaborations are proving successful in developing health interventions that reduce farmworker injury and illness, and provide data needed to change policy. Finally, the agenda for farmworker justice proposed by Arcury, Wiggins, and Quandt has three arms. First, efforts must be made to change the perspective of the American consumer about the human cost of producing the food that they eat. Greater demand by the American consumer for fair labor practices is essential to creating a safe and equitable work place for farmworkers. Second, research needs to systematically document the characteristics of farmworkers in the eastern US, the conditions of farm work, and of the injuries and illnesses experienced by farmworkers. This documentation will provide information needed to develop targeted policy and programs to improve safety and justice. Third, specific changes in policy and regulation will be needed to improve the lives of farmworkers, including improving farm labor laws, increasing enforcement of the laws, and increasing support and protection for workers who organize.

1.5   Acknowledgments

This volume results from the Third Wake Forest University School of Medicine Farmworker Health Research Workshop. The First Wake Forest University School of Medicine Farmworker Health Research Workshop took place at the 1999 American Public Health Association annual meeting. This 1-day workshop, "Farmworkers and Pesticides: Community-Based Research," brought together scientists, community-based organization members, and agency representatives currently involved in collaborative environmental health research on farmworker pesticide exposure to continue the development of common organizational frameworks and research methods to promote effective community-based prevention research (Arcury et al. 2000; Arcury and Quandt 2001). The Second Wake Forest University School of Medicine Farmworker Health Research Workshop was convened at the Graylyn International Conference Center, Wake Forest University, Winston-Salem, North Carolina, on September 30, 2004. For this one-and-a-half-day "Farmworker Pesticide Exposure Comparable Data Conference" a group of 25 scientists met to document the methodologic problems faced in farmworker pesticide exposure research and develop consensus on how these methodologic problems can be addressed (Arcury et al. 2006).

The work of the Third Wake Forest University School of Medicine Farmworker Health Research Workshop was completed over an 11-month period from September 2007 through July 2008. The participants in this third workshop included activists, health-care providers, health educators, and researchers who have each spent 5–20 years addressing the health of agricultural workers. Each of the chapters in this volume has one or two authors listed. Although authors are ultimately responsible for the chapters with their by-lines, writing for this entire volume has been a collaborative effort. The writing was completed in three periods, and in each period all authors were provided with comment and suggestion from all other authors.

From September 2007 through April 2008, authors developed their chapters, writing abstracts, outlines, and, finally, the actual chapters. The authors met several times via conference call to review and discuss the work on each chapter. In early May 2008, drafts of all of the chapters were distributed to all of the authors. All authors read and prepared comments on each chapter. The authors attended a 1-week (May 9 through 13) workshop at *Tenuta di Spannocchia*, located outside Siena, Italy (Fig. 1.1). At this workshop each chapter was discussed in detail and authors made suggestions for revision (Fig. 1.2). Having an understanding of all of the chapters, authors made decisions to move sections among some of the chapters (Fig. 1.3). All of the authors left this workshop with directions for revision (Fig. 1.4). During the remainder of May and through June, the authors completed revisions of their chapters and submitted them again for final comments and suggestions from the entire group. Finally, content- and copyediting were completed in July.

Support of the work to develop the chapters in this volume was provided in part by grants R01 ES08739, Community Participatory Approach to Measuring

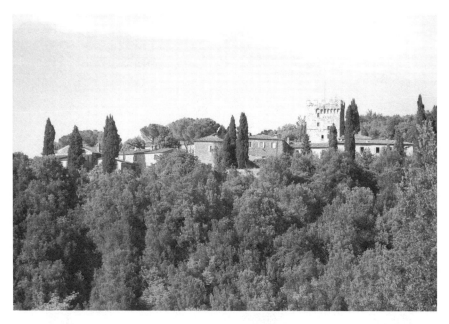

Fig. 1.1 *Tenuta di Spannocchia*, site of the Third Wake Forest University School of Medicine Farmworker Health Research Workshop. Copyright, Thomas A. Arcury

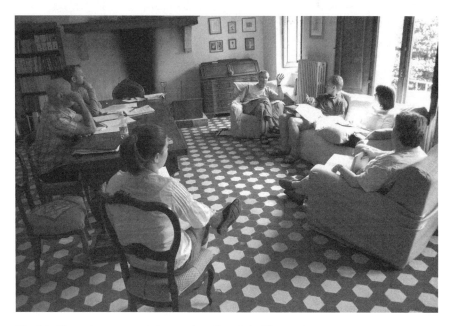

Fig. 1.2 The authors at a workshop session. Copyright, Thomas A. Arcury

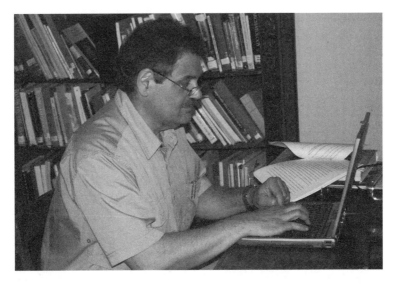

Fig. 1.3 Thomas A. Arcury revising a chapter. Copyright, Thomas A. Arcury

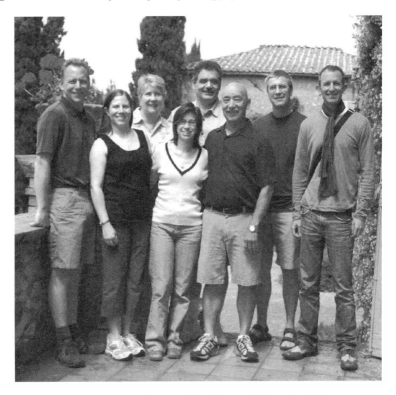

Fig. 1.4 The authors at *Tenuta di Spannocchia*: (left to right) Joseph G. Grzywacz, Quirina M. Vallejos, Sara A. Quandt, Melinda F. Wiggins, Thomas A. Arcury, Antonio J. Marín, John J. May, Scott D. Rhodes. Copyright, Thomas A. Arcury

Farmworker Pesticide Exposure: PACE3, and R01 ES012358, Occupational Skin Disease among Minority Farmworkers from the National Institute of Environmental Health Sciences. The support of the National Institute of Environmental Health Sciences is greatly appreciated. Chapter 6 was funded in part by a cooperative agreement (TS-1023) from the Centers for Disease Control and Prevention (CDC) through the Association for Prevention Teaching and Research; a grant (R21 HD049282) from the National Institute for Child Health and Human Development; and a supplement (02885-08) from the CDC through the Communicable Disease Branch, North Carolina.

The authors received support from numerous people that ensured the success of the conference. We extend our thanks to them all. Claudine Curran and Sharon Coleman negotiated travel arrangements that ensured a productive conference. The staff of *Tenuta di Spannocchia* handled all local conference arrangements and provided opportunities for the authors to examine the history and structure of Italian agricultural labor as a contrast with American agriculture.The completion of this volume was aided by Alice Arcury-Quandt and Teresa Kohrman, who copyedited and formatted multiple versions of each chapter. Janine Tillett, M.S.L.S., David Stewart, M.S.L.S., Rochelle Kramer, M.L.S., and Molly Keener, M.L.I.S., of Coy Carpenter Library of Wake Forest University School of Medicine verified citations. We thank them for their assistance, patience, and attention to detail.Several specific chapters enlisted the assistance of others. Carol Brooke, J.D., M.P.H., of the NC Justice Center reviewed Chapters 2 and 9, providing valuable insights into the regulations concerning farmworker housing. Amit Verma, M.P.H., and Mark R. Schulz, Ph.D., analyzed additional data for Chapter 3, and Jacqueline M. Burnell assisted with editing that chapter. Karen Klein, M.A., E.L.S., of the Research Support Core at Wake Forest University School of Medicine, provided editorial assistance with Chapter 6. Jeannie Economos, Joan Flocks, J.D., and Reverend Richard Witt provided their insights in interviews conducted for Chapter 9, and Dave DeVito, Flocks, and Tony Macias read and commented on the chapter.

References

Alderete E, Vega WA, Kolody B et al. (2000) Lifetime prevalence of and risk factors for psychiatric disorders among Mexican migrant farmworkers in California. Am J Public Health 90:608–614

Arcury TA, Quandt SA (eds) (2001) Migrant and seasonal farmworkers and pesticides: community-based approaches to measuring risks and reducing exposure. Environ Health Perspect 109(Suppl 3):427–473

Arcury TA, Quandt SA (2007) Delivery of health services to migrant and seasonal farmworkers. Ann Rev Public Health 28:345–363

Arcury TA, Quandt SA, McCauley L (2000) Farmworkers and pesticides: community-based research. Environ Health Perspect 108(8):787–792

Arcury TA, Quandt SA, Barr DB et al. (eds) (2006) Farmworker exposure to pesticides: methodological issues for the collection of comparable data. Environ Health Perspect 114:923–968

General Accounting Office (2000) Pesticides: improvements needed to ensure the safety of farmworkers and their children. GAO/RCED-00-40. General Accounting Office, Washington

Human Rights Watch (2000). Fingers to the bone: US failure to protect child farmworkers. Human Rights Watch, New York

Mitchell JP, Gurske PE (1956) Status of agricultural workers under state and federal labor laws. US Department of Labor, Bureau of Labor Standards, Washington

Office of the High Commissioner for Human Rights (2008) Fact sheet no. 21, the human right to adequate housing. http://www.unhchr.ch/html/menu6/2/fs21.htm. Cited 7 Feb. 2008

President's Commission on Migratory Labor (1951) Migratory labor in American agriculture: report of the president's Commission on Migratory Labor. US Government Printing Office, Washington

Rosenbaum S, Shin P (2005) Migrant and seasonal farmworkers: health insurance coverage and access to care. The Kiser Commission on Medicaid and the Uninsured. The Henry J Kiser Family Foundation, Washington

Villarejo D (2003) The health of U.S. hired farm workers. Annu Rev Public Health 24:175–193

Chapter 2
Latino/Hispanic Farmworkers and Farm Work in the Eastern United States: The Context for Health, Safety, and Justice

Thomas A. Arcury and Antonio J. Marín

Abstract The context in which farmworkers in the eastern United States (US) labor and live affects their health and safety, and the process of achieving justice. This context includes geographic, agricultural, demographic, cultural, and political dimensions, with each of these dimensions experiencing considerable change in the past 50 years. This chapter provides an overview of the context for farmworkers in the eastern US, and defines who is a farmworker for this volume. Although farmworkers in the eastern US became a largely Latino/Hispanic population in the early 1990s, this population continues to be varied in ethnic composition (Latino/Hispanic, Indigenous, non-Latino/Hispanic) and migration status. The information needed to document each dimension of the context for farmworkers in the eastern US is often unavailable. The lack of information makes it difficult to understand who farmworkers are, their number, their personal characteristics, their exposures and health status, and how best to work toward justice for farmworkers and their families. Recommendations to improve health, safety, and justice include more complete and consistent reporting by state agencies of information they collect for farmworkers in their states, and better documentation and reporting of study design by researchers. This information will provide a foundation for understanding diversity in the health and safety of farmworkers, and help direct efforts needed to improve social justice.

2.1 Introduction

Understanding the health and safety of farmworkers in the eastern United States (US) and addressing justice for farmworkers require familiarity with the context in which these farmworkers labor and live. This context has geographic, agricultural, demographic, cultural, and political dimensions. Each of these dimensions has undergone considerable change in the past 50 years, and each dimension continues to change.

The information needed to document each dimension of the context in which farmworkers labor and live is often unavailable. The limited information makes it

T.A. Arcury and S.A. Quandt (eds.), *Latino Farmworkers in Eastern United States*,
DOI: 10.1007/978-0-387-88347-2_2, © Springer Science+Business Media, LLC 2009

difficult to understand who farmworkers are, the number of farmworkers in the eastern US, the personal characteristics of farmworkers, the exposures and health status of farmworkers, and how best to work toward justice for farmworkers and their families. For this chapter, and for this volume, information from multiple sources was culled to document health, safety, and justice for farmworkers. Sometimes the information gathered about farmworkers appears contradictory. The reasons for apparent contradictions are several. Farmworkers in various sections of the eastern US are diverse, those recording information about farmworkers use different methods, regulations defining "farmworker" differ among agencies and among states, and the types and quality of information vary among states and among agencies. This chapter, and this entire volume, presents and integrates all of the available information for farmworkers in the eastern US. Seemingly contradictory evidence is reported and discussed in an effort to document limitations of available information. An essential first step in promoting farmworker justice is clearly assessing what is known.

2.2 Farmworkers Defined

We focus on seasonal and migrant farmworkers in this volume. The definition of who is considered a farmworker varies among analysts and for different programs and regulations. Factors included in defining farmworkers and their eligibility for services include different agricultural commodities (crops, dairy, poultry, livestock) and sectors (materials processing, fisheries, forestry) in which an individual might work, migration statuses (e.g., family moved to seek farm work, change residence from one school district to another, establish temporary abode), their ages, income requirements (e.g., none, income less than poverty while engaged in farm work), and eligibility periods (e.g., employed in farm work in the last 24 months, the last 36 months, 12 of the last 24 months).

In this volume farmworkers include individuals who are involved in agricultural production, with agricultural production including planting, cultivating, harvesting, and processing crops for sale, and caring for animals. Nonfood commodities such as tobacco, Christmas trees, sod, flowers, and ornamental plants are included as agricultural crops. Agricultural work excludes manufacturing activities, such as preserving fruits and vegetables, working in grain storage, slaughtering or butchering of livestock and poultry, or making cheese and cooking food. *Seasonal farmworkers* are individuals whose principal employment is in agriculture on a seasonal basis. They do not change residence in order to work in agriculture. *Migrant farmworkers* are individuals whose principal employment is in agriculture on a seasonal basis, and who, for purposes of employment, establish a temporary home. The migration may be from place to place within a state, interstate, or international.

The National Agricultural Workers Survey (NAWS) differentiates six types of farmworkers (Carroll et al. 2005). The nonmigrant worker is equivalent to what we refer here to as a seasonal farmworker; in 2002, nationally the NAWS estimates indicate that 58% of farmworkers were nonmigrant. Migrants can be foreign-born newcomers (a foreign-born farmworker who has traveled to the US for the first time), international shuttle farmworkers (travel from permanent homes in a foreign country to the US for employment but work only within a 75-mile radius of that location), domestic shuttle farmworkers (have permanent residences in the US but travel 75 miles or more to do farm work in a single location and work only within a 75-mile radius of that location), international follow-the-crop farmworkers (travel to multiple US farm locations for work from permanent homes in a foreign country), and domestic follow-the-crop farmworkers (travel to multiple US farm locations for work from permanent homes in the US). The follow-the-crop farmworker most closely resembles the classic image of a migrant farmworker who moves in one of the "migrant streams" from south to north as crops ripen for harvest. In 2002, national estimates based on the NAWS indicate that 13% of farmworkers were foreign-born newcomers, 57% were nonmigrant or settled, 8% were follow-the-crop migrants, and 18% were shuttle migrants. Estimates for farmworkers in the eastern US based on 2002 NAWS data show that 13% were foreign-born newcomers, 57% were nonmigrant, 13% were follow-the-crop migrants, and 17% were shuttle migrants (Fig. 2.1).

We include the families of farmworkers in our discussions for this volume. The spouses, children, and other family members who live with farmworkers are often exposed to the same health risks as are the farmworkers. Often these family members, spouse and children, are employed in farm work (see Chap. 8). They live in the same housing (see Chap. 3), are exposed to agricultural and residential pesticides (see Chap. 5), encounter similar levels of health care (Arcury and Quandt 2007), and are confronted by similar stressors and hardships (see Chap. 7).

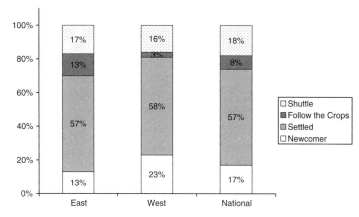

Fig. 2.1   Type of farmworker by geographic region
2002 National Agricultural Workers' Survey (NAWS) (Aguirre International 2005a–c)

The NAWS does not include farmworkers with H2A visas in its estimates. An H2A visa allows an individual to enter the US to work in agriculture for a specified period of time for a particular farmer, who is obligated to provide an average of 35 h of work per week, a specific hourly wage, inspected housing, and to meet all safety requirements, including Worker Protection Standard training (US Environmental Protection Agency 1995). Almost all farmworkers with H2A visas are international shuttle migrants. A few are international follow-the-crop migrants; for example, some farmworkers with H2A visas spend much of the agricultural season in eastern North Carolina cultivating and harvesting tobacco, but then travel several hundred miles to western North Carolina to harvest Christmas trees in October and November. A large number of farmworkers with H2A visas work in North Carolina each year, with 8,730 present in 2007.

2.3   Geographic Context

The eastern US considered in this volume includes 22 states. This includes the southeastern states bordering the Gulf of Mexico and Atlantic Ocean (Florida, Georgia, Alabama, Mississippi, South Carolina, North Carolina, and Virginia), the mid-Atlantic states (Maryland, Pennsylvania, Delaware, and New Jersey), interior states (Tennessee, Kentucky, West Virginia, and Ohio), and New England (New York, Massachusetts, Connecticut, Rhode Island, New Hampshire, Vermont, and Maine). This region is considered the "Eastern Migrant Stream." However, the 2004 NAWS finds that only 13% of farmworkers in the eastern US are follow-the-crop migrants. Therefore, the idea of a stream of migrant farmworkers flowing from Florida and Texas, through the South, into the Mid-Atlantic and on into New England as crops ripen, while romantic, is probably no longer accurate.

Little information actually documents the movement of farmworkers during an agricultural season. Quandt et al. (2002) used information from several studies in North Carolina to document the movement of farmworkers during an agricultural season. The farmworkers included in these studies were migrant farmworkers living in camps during the summer. Approximately one third of the workers moved during the course of the summer, with work availability and work-related illness being the major causes of their moving from a camp. Workers who migrated often returned to a camp that they left when more work became available.

2.4   Agricultural Context

Agriculture in the eastern US is diverse and changing. The agriculture that involves farmworkers is concentrated in those commodities, crops and animals, that require hand labor – animal care, or planting, cultivating, and harvesting crops. Some crops that historically required hand labor, such as cotton, have become completely mechanized. Mechanization remains limited for other crops, such as tobacco and most vegetables.

2.4.1 From Family Farm to Commercial Agriculture

Historically, family farms characterized most of the agriculture in the US. A family farm is an operation for which family members provide most of the management, labor, and capital. Although most farms in the eastern US remain family operations, much of the agricultural production is provided by commercial farms. The number of farms in the US has declined, from more than 5.3 million in 1950, to 2.1 million in 2002. Among family farms, the average age of the principal operator continues to increase, while the number of family members living and working on farms continues to decline. The average age of a principal farm operator was 55.3 years in 2002, up from 51.7 years in 1974. All of these processes are characteristic of the eastern US.

The decline in the number of family farms and the number of family members working on farms has resulted in greater levels of commercial agriculture, and a greater need for hired farm labor. This demand for hired farm labor affects family farms as well as commercial farms. It affects all forms of agriculture, animal and dairy production, as well as crop production. However, although agriculture is becoming more commercial and less family in nature, the laws regulating agricultural labor remain based on the model of the family farm. Referred to as "agricultural exceptionalism" (see Chap. 9), these labor regulations limit the requirements of safety regulations, workers' compensation, health insurance, and overtime pay for farmworkers, while allowing workers as young as 14 years of age to work in the fields.

2.4.2 The Risk and Safety Culture of American Farmers

American farmers have their own culture, a set of generally shared beliefs and values that affect the health, safety, and justice for farmworkers. A series of recent in-depth interviews with small crop and livestock farmers in the Northeast helps to describe the farm community's view of occupational hazards (Sorensen et al. 2008). Farmers do not view "risk" as undesirable. They have observed generations accepting risk as inherent to their way of life. Many risk their entire fortune with each spring's planting. Thus as a group they have a remarkably high tolerance for risk, believing that most things will work out in the end. While farmers readily acknowledge the dangers inherent in farming, they often adopt an optimistic bias (Weinstein 1988, 1989) with regard to hazard. Their experience with risk over the years leads them to believe that they have sufficient knowledge, experience, and skill to be exempted from agriculture's dangers. Near-misses may only serve to reinforce this view. Most farmers place considerably greater priority on the efficient production of food and fiber than upon safety. As businessmen, they see most safety measures as contributing little to their efficiency and productivity. This most certainly applies to their personal safety, but unfortunately tends to carry over to safety in general. At the same time, these farmers express considerable concern regarding the safety of spouses, children, and employees. This attitude is reflected in decisions to personally undertake the most risky tasks and in the resultant elevated rates of injuries to farmers when compared to employees on small family farms (Pratt et al. 1992).

In studies among California farmworkers and farm owners, Grieshop and colleagues explored concepts related to the "locus of control" over safety and workplace injury. There was a powerful and pervasive belief among the farmworkers that injury and illness were under an external control, external to both the worker and the farm owner. These workers valued prevention efforts, but believed equally in accepting the inherent dangers of the job and trusting in their ability to react or cope with hazards that arise. In contrast, farm owners viewed injury prevention as under internal control rather than in the hands of luck or fate. These farmers were convinced that prevention was far preferable to acceptance of risk (Grieshop et al. 1996).

The farmer's high tolerance of risk, denial of susceptibility, and skepticism regarding safety measures may contribute significantly to the problems encountered by some farmworkers. In some cases, exposure of these workers to heat, chemical, ergonomic, and other hazards may be deliberate and malignant (Salazar et al. 2005), while in others it may simply reflect an extension of the owner's personal approach to risk and prevention. Unfortunately, the considerable power imbalance inherent in the grower–farmworker relationship can amplify the risk encountered by these workers. This problem may be further exacerbated by the priorities and beliefs of the farmworkers. Farmworkers' perception of being in the hands of fate and their recognition of the extreme power imbalance both significantly reduce the likelihood of their objecting to observed hazards in the workplace. Many of these workers face an economic imperative to maximize work hours and weekly income. For many workers physical work is inextricably linked to physical pain and musculoskeletal strain. The farmworkers' view that musculoskeletal injury is "just part of the job" contrasts notably with the health professional's view that "work shouldn't make you sick." The effects of these farmer values on health and safety for farmworkers are particularly seen in the discussion of farmworker injury and illness (see Chap. 4) and farmworker exposure to pesticides (see Chap. 5).

2.4.3 Regional Crops in the Eastern US with Farmworker Involvement

Production of many agricultural commodities in the eastern US requires the hand labor of farmworkers for planting, cultivating, and harvesting. These commodities include fruits, such as apples, berries, citrus, melons, and peaches, and vegetables, including cucumbers, mushrooms, sweet potatoes, and tomatoes, as well as nonfood commodities, such as Christmas trees, ferns, and tobacco. Table 2.1 provides information on some agricultural commodities that particularly involve farmworkers in the eastern US. Review of the farms and acreage devoted to these different commodities documents the variability in the work performed by farmworkers in the eastern US. For example, while cucumbers are produced in all the states, a large number of farms and a large amount of acreage are devoted to the production of cucumbers in the southeastern states. Within the states producing cucumbers, North Carolina stands out for the large proportion of acres (11,295 of 16,396 acres, 69%) that is harvested for processing (making pickles). Pennsylvania has by far the greatest need for workers to pick mushrooms. Maine leads the region in acres devoted to berries. North Carolina and Kentucky have the greatest acres in tobacco.

The process of planting, cultivating, and harvesting different agricultural commodities places farmworkers at risk for different injuries and illnesses (see Chaps. 4 and 5). For example, pesticides, including fungicides, herbicides, and insecticides, are applied to all of these commodities; however, the toxicity of pesticides used for each commodity differs. Picking some fruits and vegetables, such as berries, cucumbers, and sweet potatoes, requires bending and lifting. Harvesting orchard fruits includes risks for falls and eye injuries. Tobacco harvesting exposes workers to nicotine and nicotine poisoning (called green tobacco sickness). Harvesting mushrooms requires work in humid environments with high levels of molds.

2.4.4 Livestock and Poultry

The number of Latino/Hispanic immigrants working in livestock and poultry production, as well as in seafood processing, such as crab picking, is increasing. For example, in the Northeast, Latino/Hispanic immigrants are being hired to work on dairy farms (Earle-Richardson and May 2002; Stack et al. 2006). Individuals working in livestock and poultry production are often full-time, long-term employees, and do not fit the definition of migrant and seasonal farmworker. Many working in seafood processing are seasonal workers, often with H2B visas; these workers face many of the same problems of health, safety, and justice as do farmworkers. While the shortage of labor in seafood processing has been discussed, little research has addressed the occupational health of these workers (Brown 2008).

The number of concentrated animal feeding operations (CAFOs) for poultry and hogs, particularly in the Southeast, has grown substantially since 1990 (Table 2.2). The potential health effects of CAFOs for workers and on the surrounding communities continue to be documented (Kirkhorn and Schenker 2002; Mirabelli et al. 2006; Tajik et al. 2008). Little research has considered the ethnicity or immigration status of workers in these operations. However, observations of workers in North Carolina indicate that many are Latino/Hispanic immigrants. In the poultry industry, many of those who collect eggs are Latino/Hispanic, and many of those "catching" chickens in poultry houses for shipment to processing plants are Latino/Hispanic.

Table 2.1 Number of farms for selected crops produced in the eastern United States, 2002

State	Cucumbers		Mushrooms		Peaches		Berries		Tobacco		Christmas trees	
	Farms	Acres	Farms	Square feet	Farms	Acres	Farms	Acres	Farms	Acres	Farms	Trees harvested
Alabama	232	1,925	2	N/A[a]	379	4,042	272	589	8	199	99	35,670
Connecticut	119	373	3	N/A	139	464	230	619	80	1,925	495	133,861
Delaware	27	4,109	3	N/A	16	221	53	134	0	0	64	16,183
Florida	262	17,984	13	N/A	111	432	627	8,389	115	3,851	87	15,320
Georgia	235	12,604	0	0	304	13,242	523	4,822	822	25,060	253	80,952
Kentucky	280	146	19	61,446	320	602	357	393	29,237	110,734	230	56,473
Maine	170	135	5	N/A	70	29	784	23,979	0	0	335	164,406
Maryland	146	3,552	7	N/A	229	1,229	228	461	159	1,162	263	99,183
Massachusetts	175	1,336	4	N/A	198	426	890	15,976	50	1,113	408	72,522
Mississippi	35	40	1	N/A	184	656	293	1,408	7	158	163	39,594
New Hampshire	72	47	2	N/A	79	120	203	543	0	0	234	107,725
New Jersey	242	3,476	4	133,560	315	8,113	561	12,565	0	0	1,167	132,458
New York	368	3,265	15	332,086	496	2,364	971	2,916	1	N/A	1,648	618,917
North Carolina	686	16,396	11	98,179	327	1,496	605	6,213	7,850	167,677	1,528	2,915,507
Ohio	294	2,606	11	23,179	638	1,582	772	1,555	1,845	5,764	1,105	372,957
Pennsylvania	375	670	102	18,966,736	1,021	5,756	1,555	2,395	897	5,470	2,164	1,724,419
Rhode Island	23	15	0	0	34	47	60	254	0	0	83	23,085
South Carolina	267	4,858	5	113,456	380	15,069	234	701	873	30,241	181	38,871
Tennessee	113	116	8	N/A	149	734	340	603	8,206	35,960	186	149,770
Vermont	51	52	4	N/A	29	32	207	471	0	0	359	151,249
Virginia	322	2,069	12	61,790	451	2,029	369	728	4,184	30,308	767	507,791
West Virginia	59	31	13	87,024	207	1,329	153	134	544	1,373	351	60,098

2002 Census of Agriculture, Vol. 1, Chap. 2: US State Level Data. http://www.nass.usda.gov/census/census02/volume1/us/index2.htm
[a] Data suppressed in original source

Table 2.2 Number of farms producing selected livestock and poultry in the eastern United States, 2002

State	No. of farms		
	Hogs and pigs	Milk cows	Any poultry
Alabama	561	223	4,417
Connecticut	176	310	683
Delaware	86	96	697
Florida	1,090	923	2,530
Georgia	995	841	4,139
Kentucky	1,220	2,939	3,302
Maine	310	556	1,211
Maryland	379	825	1,639
Massachusetts	250	380	1,030
Mississippi	504	627	4,471
New Hampshire	212	255	711
New Jersey	378	136	1,330
New York	1,490	7,388	3,327
North Carolina	2,332	1,250	6,251
Ohio	4,986	4,754	5,773
Pennsylvania	3,785	9,629	7,043
Rhode Island	51	43	173
South Carolina	736	326	1,959
Tennessee	1,130	1,427	5,066
Vermont	206	1,508	983
Virginia	834	1,580	3,341
West Virginia	717	525	2,278

2002 Census of agriculture, Vol. 1, Chap. 2: US state level data.
http://www.nass.usda.gov/census/census02/volume1/us/us1intro.pdf

2.5   Demographic Context

Agricultural workers in the eastern US once included large numbers of local youth doing farm work as a summer job or working on actual family farms. Migrant and seasonal agricultural workers until recently included substantial numbers of African Americans, Afro-Caribbeans, Native Americans, and Appalachian whites, as well as Latino/Hispanics (Leone and Johnston 1954). Now, although each of these groups still remains involved in seasonal farm work, most farmworkers working in the eastern US are Latino/Hispanic immigrants, with most of Mexican heritage (Carroll et al. 2005). Latino/Hispanics are becoming the largest minority population in the US (Passel and Cohn 2008). In several eastern states, the growth of the Latino/Hispanic population has been extraordinary. For example, the Latino/Hispanic population of Georgia is estimated to have grown from 425,305 persons in 2000 to 625,382 persons in 2005, a 47.0% change; the estimated growth for North Carolina is from 367,390 persons in 2000 to 544,470 persons in 2005, a 48.2% change; and the estimated growth for South Carolina is from 90,263 persons in 2000 to 136,616 persons in 2005, a 51.4% change (Pew Hispanic Center 2008).

2.5.1 Numbers of Farmworkers

The number of farmworkers in the eastern US is not known. No census of farmworkers has ever been conducted. The last estimate of the number of farmworkers in all the states was published in 1990. Larson (2000) prepared estimates for the number of farmworkers in ten states for 2000, including four in the eastern US (Florida, Maryland, Mississippi, and North Carolina). Additional estimates have been prepared for New York and New Jersey (Earle-Richardson et al. 2005; Borjan et al. 2008).

The number of farmworkers in each of the eastern states varies substantially (Table 2.3). The 1990 estimates are very much out-of-date, but they are the only national data available. The 2000 estimates provide information for a few of the states. The 2002 Census of Agriculture provides three different indicators of the number of farmworkers in each state; data on "Farms with Hired Migrant Farm Labor" and "Farms Reporting Only Contract Migrant Farm Labor" were not reported in earlier censuses, and changes in the number of farms cannot be evaluated. Comparing the 2000 migrant and seasonal farmworker estimates with the 1990 estimates indicates a general decline in the number of farmworkers in most eastern states. For example, the estimated number of migrant and seasonal farmworkers in Florida declined from 435,373 in 1990 to 194,817 in 2000, while the number in North Carolina declined from 344,944 to 100,316 in the same period. Estimates for several states do show increases in the number of farmworkers. The estimated number of farmworkers in Mississippi increased from none in 1990 to 10,368 in 2000; the estimated number of farmworkers in Maryland increased from 4,267 to 7,894; and the estimated number in New Jersey increased from 13,522 to 16,762.

The different sources of information about the numbers of farmworkers in the eastern US since 2000 are often contradictory, making estimates of the injuries experienced or the services needed difficult to establish. For example, the 2000 estimate for migrant and seasonal farmworkers in Florida is 194,817, while the US Census of Agriculture reports 68,971 farm employees who worked less than 150 days for 2002. Comparing the 1990 and 2000 estimates for the number of migrant and seasonal farmworkers in New York indicates a greater than 50% decline in the number of farmworkers, from 30,811 to 14,121; however, the US Census of Agriculture reports that in 2002 there were 43,347 farm employees who worked less than 150 days, and 946 farms that hired migrant labor. However, the different sources of information about the numbers of farmworkers for some of the states are often quite similar. The 2000 estimate for North Carolina, for example, places the number of migrant and seasonal farmworkers at 100,316, and the US Census of Agriculture reports 97,138 farm employees who worked less than 150 days for 2002.

Other sources of information are available for some states that estimate the number of farmworkers. For example, the North Carolina Employment Security Commission estimates the number of agricultural workers at "peak season" by county each year. Employment Security Commission staff have made public statements that their estimates are very conservative and probably underestimate the number of farmworkers. For 2007, the published estimates from the North Carolina Employment Security Commission are that 37,610 migrant farmworkers, 25,407 seasonal farmworkers, and

Table 2.3 Indicators of the number of farmworkers in the eastern United States, by State

State	Total MSFW		2002 Census of agriculture[a]		
	1990[b]	2000[c]	Workers working less than 150 days	Farms with hired migrant farm labor	Farms reporting only contract migrant farm labor
Alabama	6,483		25,994	303	57
Connecticut	9,421		7,559	135	7
Delaware	5,397		2,151	70	3
Florida	435,373	194,817	68,971	1,303	453
Georgia	93,604		42,307	858	141
Kentucky	0		99,003	3,311	687
Maine	8,660		13,551	137	14
Maryland	4,267	7,894	10,551	212	11
Massachusetts	7,813		8,265	243	29
Mississippi	0	10,368	23,915	157	113
New Hampshire	726		2,789	41	6
New Jersey	13,522	16,762[d]	13,676	523	43
New York	30,811	14,121[e]	43,347	946	50
North Carolina	344,944	100,316	97,138	3,097	364
Ohio	11,621		54,180	518	108
Pennsylvania	24,711		41,606	745	59
Rhode Island	459		677	26	5
South Carolina	18,560		18,650	469	57
Tennessee	6,571		43,366	1,338	288
Vermont	1,785		4239	129	1
Virginia	15,079		34,367	1,016	159
West Virginia	2,700		8,441	99	17

[a]2002 Census of agriculture, Vol. 1, Chap. 2: US state level data. http://www.nass.usda.gov/census/census02/volume1/us/us1intro.pdf
[b]USOMH (1990)
[c]Larson (2000)
[d]Borjan et al. (2008)
[e]Earle-Richardson et al. (2005)

8,730 farmworkers with H2A visas worked in North Carolina. This same publication reports that 36,465 of the migrant farmworkers were "Spanish."

The conclusion that must be drawn is that no one knows how many farmworkers, migrant or seasonal, work in the eastern states or in the entire nation. Not knowing the number of farmworkers makes addressing health and justice difficult for this population. Analysts cannot calculate rates of injuries or illnesses (see Chap. 4), nor can they know the level of health and other services that must be provided.

2.5.2 Farmworker Personal Characteristics

The 2002 and 2004 National Agricultural Workers Surveys (NAWS) (Carroll et al. 2005; Gabbard 2006) provide the only current information on the personal characteristics of farmworkers across the eastern US, and a comparison of farmworkers in the

Table 2.4 Selected eastern United States and national farmworker demographic characteristics from the 2002 (Carroll et al. 2005) and 2004 (Gabbard 2006) National Agricultural Workers Surveys

Demographic characteristic	Eastern United States	United States
Mean age (years)	33.6	34.1
Female (%)	19	25
Language		
Spanish is primary language (%)	60	78
Able to speak English well (%)	37	25
Able to speak English at all (%)	31	40
Ethnicity		
Foreign born (%)	63	76
Born in Mexico (%)	55	72
Indigenous (2002) (%)		5
Stating not Hispanic or Latino (%)	31	16
Migration status		
Newcomer 2002 (%)	13	17
Nonmigrant 2002 (%)	57	57
Follow the crops 2002 (%)	13	8
Shuttle 2002 (%)	17	18
Migrant 2004 (%)	36	36
Newcomer 2004 (%)	13	14
Weeks employed	32.8	31.9
Average personal income ($)	14,168	
Average family income ($)	18,580	
Percent with families below poverty (%)	26	28

eastern US with national farmworker information (Table 2.4). Farmworkers are relatively young, with an average age of 33.6 years, and most are men. The majority of farmworkers in the eastern US interviewed by the 2004 NAWS spoke Spanish as a primary language (60%), were foreign born (63%), and were born in Mexico (55%). The national farmworker population interviewed for the 2004 NAWS was more Spanish-speaking (78%), foreign born (76%), and Mexico born (72%) than was that of the eastern US. It is important to note that almost one third of the eastern US farmworkers interviewed by the 2004 NAWS indicated that they were not Hispanic or Latino. The NAWS documents the continuing variability of the farm labor force in the eastern US. However, the farmworkers included in the NAWS differ from farmworkers documented by service providers and researchers in the eastern US. The clients most often discussed by service providers and included in research are overwhelmingly Latino/Hispanic. For example, a recent survey of migrant farmworkers in North Carolina found only Latino/Hispanic workers, with few who could speak any English (Arcury et al. 2007).

Farmworkers in the eastern US participating in the 2002 NAWS are similar to all farmworkers in the US in migration status. Most (57%) in the east and nationally are settled. The same percentage in the east and nationally are shuttle migrants. A somewhat smaller percentage in the eastern US are newcomers and a somewhat greater percentage in the eastern US are follow-the-crop migrants than is estimated for the national sample.

The 2004 NAWS participants in the eastern US had an average annual personal income of $14,168, and an average family income of $18,580. The 2004 US Department of Health and Human Services Poverty Guidelines for a single-person family was $9,310, for a two-person family was $12,490, for a three-person family was $15,670, and for a four-person family was $18,850 (US Department of Health and Human Services 2004). This places 30% of farmworkers below the poverty level.

An important characteristic of many farmworkers being recognized by service providers and researchers is their indigenous heritage. Being indigenous indicates that the farmworker is Native American. It also indicates that the individual's primary language is indigenous, such as Mixteco, Quiché, or Zapoteco, rather than Spanish. If these indigenous farmworkers speak Spanish at all, it is as a second language. Five percent of those who participated in the 2002 NAWS identified themselves as indigenous. Typically 20–25% of study participants in North Carolina are indigenous. A project conducted in Oregon has focused on the growing indigenous farmworker community (Farquhar et al. 2008). Being indigenous and speaking an indigenous language limits farmworkers further in accessing health and other services, knowing their rights, and reporting situations in which occupational safety and health regulations are not followed.

2.6   Cultural Context

Although the substantial majority of farmworkers in the eastern US are Latino/Hispanic, the ethnic and cultural backgrounds of farmworkers in the eastern US vary. Almost one third (31%) of farmworkers from the eastern US who participated in the 2004 NAWS reported that they were not Latino/Hispanic (Table 2.4). Recent studies conducted in the Northeast include substantial numbers of Native Americans and Afro-Caribbeans (May et al. 2008; Rabinowitz et al. 2005); recent studies in the Southeast include substantial numbers of African Americans (Gadon et al. 2001).

Most Latino/Hispanic farmworkers in the eastern US are of Mexican heritage. More than half (55%) of farmworkers from the eastern US who participated in the 2004 NAWS reported that they were born in Mexico (Table 2.4). Much of the research among farmworkers that has been conducted between 1995 and 2008 has found that an even greater proportion of farmworkers working in the eastern US were born in Mexico. However, some Latino/Hispanic farmworkers who were born in the US are the children of immigrants from Mexico. Other Latino/Hispanic farmworkers are natives of other Central American counties, such as Guatemala and Honduras, and others are from Caribbean states, including Puerto Rico and the Dominican Republic. Finally, not all Mexican farmworkers are Latino/Hispanic. Many are indigenous people, who, while being from Mexico or Guatemala, do not speak Spanish, or speak Spanish as second language.

Although the ethnic and cultural variations among farmworkers are very difficult to document, most attention to the culture, values, and beliefs of farmworkers has been focused on those who are Latino/Hispanic and who are from Mexico. That all communities have culture, and that the shared beliefs that constitute culture affect behavior should be remembered when discussing the culture of farmworkers and considering how the context of culture affects health, safety, and justice. For example, the culture of American farmers and how beliefs about risk influence the safety behaviors of American farmers are discussed in an earlier section of this chapter.

2.6.1 General Beliefs and Values of Latino/Hispanic Farmworkers

Several aspects of the cultural context of Latino/Hispanic farmworkers have important implications for health, safety, and justice. The most important of these are familism, *personalismo*, and *respeto*. Latino/Hispanic farmworkers are tied strongly to their families, whether the members of their families are with them in the US or remain in a home community elsewhere in the US or in a foreign country (i.e., Mexico). The persons and degrees of relation included as family among Latino/Hispanic farmworkers are greater than those included by most other North Americans. The sense of responsibility to family is also very strong among Latino/Hispanic farmworkers. The majority of Latino/Hispanic farmworkers laboring in the US are doing so to support families in their communities of origin. A key indicator of the sense of responsibility to family among Latino/Hispanic farmworkers is the number of farmworkers, migrant and seasonal, who send remittances to family members in their home communities. The size and number of remittances are important for the survival of family members in the communities of origin and have an important economic development effect in these communities (Grey and Woodrick 2002; Suro et al. 2002; Pew Hispanic Center 2003). For example, Cortina and de la Garza (2004) found that Mexican and El Salvadoran immigrant remittances were intended for food and basic consumption (67%), home building or improvement (5%), education (3%), and health care (9%). With the importance that Latino/Hispanic farmworkers place on sending remittances to their families, they are inclined to continue working in very difficult and dangerous situations and not engage in behaviors (e.g., refusing to work in unsafe conditions or reporting employers to regulatory agencies) that might result in the loss of employment.

Latino/Hispanic farmworkers expect to develop warm, friendly, and personal relationships, and seek this *personalismo* with their employers as well as with their co-workers (Molina et al. 1994). They also expect to be treated with respect and dignity (*respeto y dignidad*) based on their age, gender, and social position, and show this respect and dignity to others (Molina et al. 1994; Lecca et al. 1998). On the basis of these values, Latino/Hispanic farmworkers expect that their employer will protect them; they also are hesitant to disagree with their employer about occupational safety.

Machismo is an often-cited belief among Latino/Hispanics that refers to a strong sense of masculine pride. The degree to which *machismo* actually exists, as well as the degree to which it represents a set of risk behaviors and a chauvinistic attitude toward women, is a matter of debate. However, research with male farmworkers and farmers in Mexico indicates that they are willing to forego occupational safety because they feel that as strong men they are immune to injury and that they should ignore risk (Hunt et al. 1999; Quandt et al. 1998). This attitude appears very similar to that described for American farmers (see Sect. 2.4.2).

2.6.2 Health Values, Beliefs, Behaviors

2.6.2.1 General Health Beliefs

Several general health beliefs among Latino/Hispanic farmworkers have been identified that may affect their health and safety. One is that the locus of health or illness is outside the control of the individual, whether due to supernatural causes or due to God's will. Humoral medicine is a health belief system that is widely held among people native to Mexico and other Latin American countries (Rubel 1960; Weller 1983). Within this system of beliefs, different substances and materials have different humors that make them "hot" or "cold." Depending on the beliefs of individuals, hot and cold may be concrete, referring to actual temperature, or it may be metaphysical, referring to the nature of the substance regardless of its concrete temperature. For example, water is by nature cool (metaphysical), no matter what its temperature (concrete). Mixing substances or conditions that are hot with those that are cold will result in illness. Humoral medicine concepts are part of the health belief systems of many societies; for example, in the US it is widely believed that an individual who goes outside into cold weather with wet hair will get sick.

These general health beliefs may reduce the occupational health and safety of Latino/Hispanic farmworkers by limiting their use of appropriate conventional health services. They also limit workers' demands that employers adhere to occupational safety regulations (Greishop et al. 1996). These general health beliefs also affect the adherence of Latino/Hispanic farmworkers to occupational safety practices. For example, on the basis of humoral medicine beliefs, workers limit washing hands at work and showering immediately after work, because they do not want to get ill from placing their hot body in water which is considered metaphysically cold (Quandt et al. 1998; Flocks et al. 2007). This may lead to increased pesticide dose.

2.6.2.2 Lay Definitions of Illness

Lay-defined illnesses not recognized by biomedicine have been documented in Latin American countries, and among Latino/Hispanic persons living in the US. These include the illnesses *susto*, *nervios*, *empacho*, and *mal de ojo* (Weller and Baer 2001; Weller et al. 1993, 2002, 2008). The use of these lay definitions of illness has been documented among Latino/Hispanic farmworkers in the eastern US (Baer and Bustillo 1993, 1998; Baer and Penzell 1993). Latino/Hispanic farmworkers also bring culturally based lay definitions to biomedically recognized illnesses, including green tobacco sickness (Rao et al. 2002), tuberculosis (Poss 1998), and diabetes (Heuer and Lauch 2006).

Latino/Hispanic farmworkers are similar to all other people in applying lay definitions to illnesses. However, for Latino/Hispanic farmworkers the application of lay definitions to illnesses that result from the work and "lifestyle" of being a farmworker may result in their not seeking needed health care and greater effects of occupational injuries and exposures on their health. For example, Baer and Penzell (1993) document that farmworkers exposed to pesticides in Florida interpreted the resulting symptoms within the framework of lay defined *susto*, and therefore did not seek needed medical care.

2.6.2.3   Self-Treatment vs. Medical Care

Although Latino/Hispanic farmworkers acknowledge the efficacy of conventional medical care, they often limit their use of this care because of the costs (e.g., payment for care, lost time from work), the barriers to obtaining medical care in the US (e.g., hours of operation, transportation, language), and the desire to avoid interactions with authorities (Arcury and Quandt 2007). Farmworkers will often ignore or self-treat injuries and illnesses rather than use medical care. In the case of green tobacco sickness, farmworkers report working sick for the entire season because they do not want to risk losing their jobs and do not know how to effectively treat the illness (Rao et al. 2002). Latino/Hispanic farmworkers report using various traditional and home remedies to treat and prevent illnesses, including herbs, chlorine bleach, milk, and medicine purchased at *tiendas* (small local stores that serve Latino/Hispanic communities in the US) (Poss et al. 2005; Arcury et al. 2006; Mainous et al. 2005, 2008). Much of the self-treatment that farmworkers use is effective; however, it can have serious consequences (Cathcart et al. 2008).

The willingness of Latino/Hispanic farmworkers to self-treat occupational injuries and illness rather than obtain formal medical care increases their risk for continued illness, complications, and long-term health effects. This approach also limits knowledge of the extent of occupational injuries and illnesses experienced by farmworkers (Feldman et al. 2009). Increasing health outreach to farmworkers that provides culturally appropriate treatment recommendations and health education is needed.

2.7   Political Context

The political context for farmworkers in the eastern US is shaped by major political processes, as well as the actions of specific organizations. Immigration reform and international trade agreements are the major political processes shaping the political context of farmworkers. The shape of immigration laws, international trade agreements, occupational safety regulations, and wage and housing policies are affected by national and local political and advocacy organizations.

2.7.1 Political Processes

The loudest political process affecting farmworkers is the rhetoric surrounding immigration reform. Most farmworkers are immigrants, and at least half of all farmworkers are undocumented workers. Many conservative political leaders and organizations describe the presence of the large number of Latino/Hispanic immigrants in the US as an attack on the character of the nation, as well as a source of crime and infectious disease. Immigrant farmworkers are no exception to this characterization. Anti-immigrant sentiment has a long and virulent history in the US, and some anti-immigrant leaders today can only be described as xenophobic and vitriolic in their statements. Other leaders and organizations, including politicians, associations representing agricultural producers, and farmworker advocates, understand the need for the labor of the Latino/Hispanic immigrant farmworkers. They recognize that the survival of an important industry and the economy of many rural communities are dependent on the labor of farmworkers, whether or not they have the needed documents to work in the US.

Several policies have been proposed to address the need for Latino/Hispanic immigrant farmworkers. These include an expansion of the H2A visa program for agricultural workers. An important variant being considered for the expansion of the H2A program is the legislation called *The Agricultural Job Opportunities, Benefits and Security Act* or "AgJOBS." Supported by farmworker advocates and major agricultural employers to address the agricultural immigration crisis, AgJOBS would revise the current H2A temporary foreign agricultural worker program, and allow for "earned legalization" for many undocumented farmworkers and workers with H2A visas.

The second major political process forming the political context for farmworkers is the globalization of agriculture. International treaties, in particular the North American Free Trade Agreement, have facilitated the movement of agricultural commodities across national borders. While such legislation continues to be criticized in the US for allowing low-skill manufacturing jobs to be exported to Mexico, its major effect has been to allow low-cost US agricultural products to be exported to Mexico. The result has been the inability of small Mexican farmers to compete, forcing many of these small farmers to look elsewhere for work. Many Mexicans are coming to do farm work in the US because they cannot make a living as farmers in Mexico.

2.7.2 Political Organizations

Political organizations representing capital and labor do work together to make changes in the political context of Latino/Hispanic farmworkers. An example of such collaboration is the AgJOBS legislation. However, these organizations more often work at cross-purposes. Political organizations representing both capital and labor argue that their goals are to improve the agricultural economy while protecting the health and safety of agricultural workers.

Political organizations representing capital are numerous and well-funded. They include large, international agricultural processors such as ConAgra Foods and Archer Daniels Midland; trade associations for agricultural equipment and chemical industries, such as CropLife America, the major pesticide industry trade organization, and its state affiliates; national and state agricultural commodity groups, such as the International Tobacco Growers Association, North American Strawberry Growers Association, National Christmas Tree Association, and the National Dairy Council; and farmer advocacy groups, such as American Farm Bureau, state Farm Bureau federations, and Cooperative Extension. State Farm Bureau federations, as well as the American Farm Bureau, have their own lobbyists and political action committees for the purpose of effecting agricultural legislation. For example, the New York Farm Bureau Federation has a button for an "e-lobby Center" at the top of its Web site. The Virginia Farm Bureau Federation founded the Virginia AgPAC in 1999.

Political organizations representing capital generally argue that occupational safety regulations are sufficient to protect the health of farmworkers, and that many regulations are not needed because threats to occupational exposures are overstated or because agricultural employers are conscious of the safety of their workers. They further argue that making policies and regulations more stringent, such as greater pesticide safety training, paying farmworkers overtime wages, or improving housing quality requirements, would be detrimental to the "family farm" (see Sect. 2.4.1). Organizations representing capital often work to remove these policies and regulations unless they believe that policies and regulations that protect farmworkers and their families also have an economic benefit for their members.

Political organizations representing farmworkers are neither numerous nor well-funded. Some of these organizations are discussed in Chap. 9. Nationally and regionally, they include unions, such as the United Farm Workers of America and the Farm Labor Organizing Committee, which are active in the eastern US; they also include advocacy groups, such as Farmworker Justice, Inc., and the Southern Poverty Law Center. Many political organizations representing labor are specific to states, such as *El Comité de Apoyo a los Trabajadores Agrícolas* (CATA)/The Farmworker Support Committee in New Jersey and Pennsylvania, the Farmworker Advocacy Network in North Carolina, and Coalition of Immokalee Workers and The Farmworker Association of Florida, Inc., in Florida. These organizations are active in supporting new state and national legislation that promotes health, safety, and justice for farmworkers and their families. For example, Farmworker Justice, Inc., has been a major advocate for national AgJOBS legislation; the North Carolina Farmworker Advocacy Network was a major force in the passage of farmworker housing legislation in 2007. These political organizations also work to amend existing "agricultural exceptionalist" laws that affect farmworker health, safety, and justice (e.g., Harris 2005).

2.8 Summary and Recommendations to Address Health, Safety, and Justice

The context for farmworker health, safety, and justice in the eastern US is complex and changing. This chapter has presented our definition of who we consider to be farmworkers and provided an overview of the geographic, agricultural, demographic, cultural, and political dimensions of the context in which these farmworkers labor and live. Information on farmworkers and their context is inconsistent for the states in the eastern US. Little information is available for several of the dimensions, and different sources are at times contradictory in the information they provide. The lack of clarity in data describing farmworkers hampers our ability to address justice; health problems that are not defined or documented cannot be addressed. The descriptions of farmworkers and their contexts presented in this chapter may be different from the experience of some readers. This argues for a greater effort to document the work and health of all farmworkers. Knowing the actual variability, and the actual needs, of farmworkers in the eastern US will support an approach to justice for all farmworkers.

Farmworkers are individuals who are involved in agricultural production, with agricultural production including planting, cultivating, harvesting, and processing crops for sale, and caring for animals. A major change in the context of farm work has been the increasing proportion of farmworkers in the eastern US who are Latino/Hispanic. This has resulted in a population with beliefs, values, and behaviors that are new to the region, and to those who provide services to the farmworker population. It has also resulted in anti-immigrant political and social rhetoric to be directed toward farmworkers. Another major change in farm work is the continuing decline in the number of "family farms" and the continuing large-scale commercialization in agriculture. This has created opportunities for farmworkers to obtain jobs in sectors of agriculture, such as dairy and poultry production, in which they had not worked previously. These changes also argue for changes in special regulatory protections that have been permitted for agriculture, such as the lack of paying overtime wages and lower ages for workers, to protect the family farm. This agricultural exceptionalism limits the health, safety, and justice for farmworkers.

This review of the context for farmworkers in the eastern US supports two major recommendations. The first recommendation is that state agencies across the region work together to improve the consistency and quality of the information they collect and report about farmworkers. Further, more of the information that agencies have collected about farmworkers in their states needs to be made available. Making the collection of this regulatory information consistent and making existing data available will provide a more complete picture of the commonalities and variation among farmworkers. This information will provide a foundation for understanding the health and safety of farmworkers, and help direct efforts needed to provide social justice for farmworkers.

The second recommendation is that researchers investigating farmworkers in the eastern US better document the populations they study, their procedures for locating and recruiting participants, and their methods for collecting data. This documentation will provide a way to compare the different communities in which research is conducted. Therefore, rather than having results that are inconsistent across studies, a mechanism to appreciate the diversity of farmworkers and differences in their health and safety will be available.

References

Aguirre International (2005a) National Agricultural Workers Study: for public access data 1989–2002. Aguirre International, Burlingame, CA. http://aguirreinternational.com/naws/downloads/National_report_2002.pdf. Cited 8 Aug 2008

Aguirre International (2005b) National Agricultural Workers Study: for public access data, Eastern Area Stream 1989–2002. Aguirre International, Burlingame, CA. http://aguirreinternational.com/naws/downloads/Eastern_report_2002.pdf. Cited 8 Aug 2008

Aguirre International (2005c) National Agricultural Workers Study: for public access data, Western Area Stream 1989–2002. Burlingame, CA: Aguirre International. http://aguirreinternational.com/naws/downloads/Western_report_2002.pdf. Cited 8 Aug 2008

Arcury TA, Quandt SA (2007) Delivery of health services to migrant and seasonal farmworkers. Annu Rev Public Health 28:345–363

Arcury TA, Vallejos QM, Feldman SR et al. (2006) Treating skin disease: self-management behaviors of Latino farmworkers. J Agromedicine 11:27–35

Arcury TA, Feldman SR, Schulz MR et al. (2007) Diagnosed skin diseases among migrant farmworkers in North Carolina: prevalence and risk factors. J Agric Saf Health 13:407–418

Baer RD, Bustillo M (1993) Susto and mal de ojo among Florida farmworkers: EMIC and ETIC perspectives. Med Anthropol Q 7:90–100

Baer RD, Bustillo M (1998) Caida de mollera among children of Mexican migrant workers: implications for the study of folk illnesses. Med Anthropol Q 12:241–249

Baer RD, Penzell D (1993) Research report: susto and pesticide poisoning among Florida farmworkers. Cult Med Psychiatry 17:321–327

Borjan M, Constantino P, Robson MG (2008) New Jersey migrant and seasonal farm workers: enumeration and access to healthcare study. New Solut 18:77–86

Brown MH (March 24, 2008) In visa dispute, businesses face summer worker gap: congressional dispute on visas puts Shore businesses in a bind. Baltimore Sun. http://www.baltimoresun.com/news/nation/bal-te.visas24mar24,0,5974178.story. Cited 8 Jun 2008

Carroll D, Samardick RM, Bernard S et al. (2005) Findings from the National Agricultural Workers Survey (NAWS) 2001–2002: a demographic and employment profile of United States farm workers (Research Report No. 9). US Department of Labor

Cathcart S, Feldman SR, Vallejos Q et al. (2008) Self-treatment of contact dermatitis with bleach in a Latino farmworker. Dermatitis 9:102–104

Cortina J, de la Garza R (2004) Immigrant remitting behavior and its developmental consequences for Mexico and El Salvador. The Tomás Rivera Policy Institute, Los Angeles

Department of Health and Human Services Office of the Secretary (2004) Annual update of the HHS Poverty Guidelines. Federal Register Vol. 69: pp. 7336–7338. http://aspe.hhs.gov/poverty/04fedreg.pdf. Cited 17 Jul 2008

Earle-Richardson G, May JJ (2002) Tienes leche? The changing demographics of the dairy workforce. J Agric Saf Health 8:5–6

Earle-Richardson G, Jenkins PL, Stack S et al. (2005) Estimating farmworker population size in New York State using a minimum labor demand method. J Agric Saf Health 11:335–345

Farquhar S, Samples J, Ventura S et al. (2008) Promoting the occupational health of indigenous farmworkers. J Immigr Minor Health 10:269–280

Feldman AR, Vallejos QM, Quandt SA et al. (2009) Healthcare utilization for skin disease in migrant Latino farmworkers: skin disease is common, but formal healthcare utilization is not. J Rural Health 25:98–103

Flocks J, Monaghan P, Albrecht S et al. (2007) Florida farmworkers' perceptions and lay knowledge of occupational pesticides. J Community Health 32:181–194

Gabbard S (2006) Emerging trends in farmworker demographics: Results from the National Agricultural Workers' Survey. Presentation at the NACHC National Farmworker Health Conference (May), San Antonio, TX

Gadon M, Chierici RM, Rios P (2001) Afro-American migrant farmworkers: a culture in isolation. AIDS Care 3:789–801

Grey MA, Woodrick AC (2002) Unofficial sister cities: meatpacking labor migration between Villachuato, Mexico, and Marshalltown, Iowa. Hum Organ 61:364–376

Grieshop JI, Stiles MC, Villanueva N (1996) Prevention and resiliency: a cross cultural view of farmworkers' and farmers' beliefs about work safety. Hum Organ 55:25–32

Harris C (2005) CATA policy manual: laws affecting the farmworker population and CATA's position. El Comité de Apoyo a los Trabajadores Agrícolas (CATA)/The Farmworker Support Committee, Glassboro, NJ. Available at http://www.cata-farmworkers.org/english%20pages/CATA%20Policy%20Manual.pdf. Cited 15 Jun 2008

Heuer L, Lauch C (2006) Living with diabetes: perceptions of Hispanic migrant farmworkers. J Community Health Nurs 23:49–64

Hunt LM, Ojanguren RT, Schwartz N et al. (1999) Balancing risks and resources: applying pesticides without using protective equipment in southern Mexico. In: Hahn RA (ed) Anthropology and public health: bridging differences in culture and society. Oxford, New York

Kirkhorn SR, Schenker MB (2002) Current health effects of agricultural work: respiratory disease, cancer, reproductive effects, musculoskeletal injuries, and pesticide-related illnesses. Agric Saf Health 8:199–214

Larson AC (2000) Migrant and seasonal farmworker enumeration profiles study. http://www.ncfh.org/00_ns_rc_enumeration.php. Cited 17 Jul 2008

Lecca P, Nunes JV, Quervalu I (1998) Cultural competency in health, social, and human services: directions for the twenty-first century. Garland, New York

Leone LP, Johnston HL (1954) Agricultural migrants and public health. Public Health Rep 69:1–8

Mainous AG III, Cheng AY, Garr RC et al. (2005) Non-prescribed antimicrobial drugs in Latino community, South Carolina. Emerg Infect Dis 11:883–888

Mainous AG III, Diaz VA, Carnemolla M (2008) Factors affecting Latino adults' use of antibiotics for self-medication. J Am Board Fam Med 21:128–134

May J, Hawkes L, Jones A et al. (2008) Evaluation of a community-based effort to reduce blueberry harvesting injury. Am J Ind Med 51:307–315

Mirabelli MC, Wing S, Marshall SW et al. (2006) Asthma symptoms among adolescents who attend public schools that are located near confined swine feeding operations. Pediatrics 18:e66–e75

Molina C, Zambrana RE, Aguirre-Molina M (1994) The influence of culture, class, and environment on health care. In: Molina CW, Aguirre-Molina M (eds) Latino health in the US: A growing challenge. American Public Health Association, Washington

Passel JS, Cohn D (2008) U.S. population projections: 2005–2050. Pew Research Center, Washington

Pew Hispanic Center (2003) Remittance senders and receivers: tracking the transnational channels. Pew Hispanic Center, Washington. http://pewhispanic.org/reports/report.php?ReportID=23. Cited 17 Jul 2008

Pew Hispanic Center (2008) A statistical portrait of Hispanics at mid-decade. Pew Research Center, Washington. http://pewhispanic.org/reports/middecade. Cited 8 Jun 2008

Poss JE (1998) The meanings of tuberculosis for Mexican migrant farmworkers in the United States. Soc Sci Med 47:195–202

Poss J, Pierce R, Prieto V (2005) Herbal remedies used by selected migrant farmworkers in El Paso, Texas. J Rural Health 21:187–191

Pratt DS, Marvel LH, Darrow D et al. (1992) The dangers of dairy farming: the injury experience of 600 workers followed for two years. Am J Indust Med 21:637–650

Quandt SA, Arcury TA, Austin CK et al. (1998) Farmworker and farmer perceptions of farmworker agricultural chemical exposure in North Carolina. Hum Organ 57:359–368

Quandt SA, Preisser JS, Arcury TA (2002) Mobility patterns of migrant farmworkers in North Carolina: implications for occupational health research and policy. Hum Organ 61:21–29

Rabinowitz PM, Sircar KD, Tarabar S et al. (2005) Hearing loss in migrant agricultural workers. J Agromed 10:9–17

Rao P, Quandt SA, Arcury TA (2002) Hispanic farmworker interpretations of green tobacco sickness. J Rural Health 8:503–511

Rubel AJ (1960) Concepts of disease in Mexican-American culture. Am Anthropol 62:795–814

Salazar M, Keifer M, Negrete M et al. (2005) Occupational risk among orchard workers: A descriptive study. Fam Community Health 28:239–252

Sorensen JA, May JJ, Paap K et al. (2008) Encouraging farmers to retrofit tractors: a qualitative analysis of risk perceptions among a group of high-risk farmers in New York. J Agric Saf Health 14:105–117

Stack SG, Jenkins PL, Earle-Richardson G et al. (2006) Spanish-speaking dairy workers in New York, Pennsylvania and Vermont: results from a survey of farm owners. J Agromedicine 11:37–44

Suro R, Bendixen S, Lowell BL et al. (2002) Billions in motion: Latino immigrants, remittances and banking. A report produced in cooperation between the Pew Hispanic Center and the Multilateral Investment Fund. Pew Hispanic Center, Washington. http://idbdocs.iadb.org/wsdocs/getdocument.aspx?docnum=548657. Cited 17 Jul 2008

Tajik M, Muhammad N, Lowman A et al. (2008) Impact of odor from industrial hog operations on daily living activities. New Solut 18:193–205

United States Office of Migrant Health (1990) An atlas of state profiles which estimate number of migrant and seasonal farmworkers and members of their families. US Department of Health and Human Services, Rockville

US Environmental Protection Agency (US-EPA) (1995) Pesticide worker protection standard training (40 CFR Part 170). Federal Register Vol. 60(70): pp. 18554–18555. http://www.epa.gov/oppfead1/safety/workers/PART170.htm. Cited 17 Jul 2008

Weinstein ND (1988) The precaution adoption process. Health Psychol 7:355–386

Weinstein ND (1989) Optimistic biases about personal risks. Science 249:1232–1233

Weller SC (1983) New data on intracultural variability: the hot-cold concept of medicine and illness. Hum Organ 42:249–257

Weller SC, Baer RD (2001) Intra- and intercultural variation in the definition of five illnesses: AIDS, diabetes, the common cold, Empacho, and Mal De Ojo. Cross-Cult Res 35:201–226

Weller SC, Pachter LM, Trotter RT II et al. (1993) Empacho in four Latino groups: a study of intra- and inter-cultural variation in beliefs. Med Anthropol 15:109–136

Weller SC, Baer RD, de Alba Garcia JG et al. (2002) Regional variation in Latino descriptions of susto. Cult Med Psychiatry 26:449–472

Weller SC, Baer RD, de Alba Garcia JG et al. (2008) Susto and nervios: expressions for stress and depression. Cult Med Psychiatry 32:406–420

Chapter 3
The Condition of Farmworker Housing in the Eastern United States

Quirina M. Vallejos, Sara A. Quandt, and Thomas A. Arcury

Abstract This chapter reviews the literature that documents the condition of farmworker housing in the eastern United States. Significant discrepancies exist between farmworkers' and the general population's exposure to hazardous housing conditions. Although documentation of health effects of farmworkers' substandard housing is scarce, research among other populations demonstrates effects farmworkers are likely to experience. Regulations that apply to employer-provided temporary labor camps for farmworkers are deficient compared with standards for the Section 8 Housing Voucher Program. Housing standards for rural private market housing and for employer-provided farmworker housing need to be strengthened and better enforced. Although several programs that provide housing assistance to farmworkers exist, they have the capacity to provide assistance to only a small portion of farmworkers who live in substandard housing. Additional programs and resources are needed to address the housing needs of farmworkers.

3.1 Introduction

Safe and secure housing is a basic human need. In this chapter, we describe the housing of farmworkers in the eastern United States (US), and show that much of this housing has the potential to adversely affect the health and safety of farmworkers and their families. Little information documents farmworker housing in the eastern US or in other regions of the nation. The limited documentation makes it difficult to fully describe the conditions in which farmworkers live and the effects of these living conditions on the health and safety of farmworkers and the members of their families. The deplorable condition of most farmworker housing is an injustice that leads to injury and illness in this population. The lack of information documenting the status of farmworker housing in the eastern US helps to conceal this continuing injustice.

The purpose of this chapter is to review the current documentation of farmworker housing in the eastern US, illustrate how current standards result in unsafe and unjust living conditions for farmworkers, and recommend changes in housing policy that will improve health, safety, and justice for farmworkers. This review

T.A. Arcury and S.A. Quandt (eds.), *Latino Farmworkers in Eastern United States*,
DOI: 10.1007/978-0-387-88347-2_3, © Springer Science + Business Media, LLC 2009

begins with an explanation of why housing is important and why inadequate housing is a concern for farmworker health, safety, and justice. The research that has addressed farmworker housing in the eastern US is reviewed, and limitations of this research literature are summarized. Housing conditions experienced by farmworkers in the eastern US, as documented by the limited research, are described and variability in farmworker housing conditions is documented. Farmworker housing conditions in the eastern US are compared to national farmworker housing data. The potential health effects of the substandard housing in which farmworkers live are discussed.

The discussion of farmworker housing standards and policy includes three topics. Farmworker housing in the eastern US is compared to established housing standards. The effectiveness of migrant housing regulations is reviewed. Programs that could assist farmworkers with housing are discussed. Finally, recommendations to improve farmworker housing are presented.

3.2 Farmworker Housing and Social Justice

Farmworkers in the eastern US, and across the entire nation, experience poor housing conditions (Holden 2000; HAC 2001). Despite the existence of temporary labor camp standards that are enforced by the Occupational Safety and Health Administration (OSHA), many farmworkers live in housing that is substandard and unsanitary. It is crowded, is not structurally sound, has faulty electrical systems or no electrical service, has faulty plumbing or no plumbing, lacks facilities for food storage and preparation, and contains biological (e.g., mold, insects) and chemical (e.g., pesticides, lead) toxicants. This substandard and unsanitary housing contributes to poor health for farmworkers and their families. A few programs exist aimed at facilitating improvements of farmworker housing conditions, but these are insufficient to adequately address the problem of farmworkers' routine exposure to substandard housing conditions. Evidence suggests these disparities in housing conditions may be leading to health disparities for this minority, low-income population.

The United Nations' International Bill of Rights recognizes adequate, affordable housing as a basic human right (Office of the High Commissioner for Human Rights 2008). The importance of adequate housing for ensuring access to drinking water, adequate sanitation, and an adequate standard of living demonstrates why housing is considered a human right. Because housing is an internationally recognized human right, nations are obliged to guarantee the right of adequate housing.

Housing and health are inextricably linked. Healthy housing is necessary for health maintenance. According to the Healthy Housing Reference Manual (CDC and HUD 2006), housing should provide protection from the elements and provide a thermal environment that facilitates maintenance of body temperature, an atmosphere of reasonable chemical purity, adequate natural and artificial illumination, protection from excessive noise, and adequate space for play and exercise. Healthy housing should also promote psychological health by providing adequate privacy for individuals, opportunities for normal family and community life, and facilities for maintenance of cleanliness of dwelling and persons. Housing should also serve the function of protecting residents from disease by providing a sanitary water supply, toilet facilities that prevent sewage contaminating the interior of the dwelling, facilities for preserving food, and sufficient space to limit risk of contact infection. In addition, housing should protect inhabitants from injury through proper maintenance of stairs and floors, from fire through proper maintenance of a fire alarm and electrical systems, and from toxic gases through proper maintenance of temperature control systems (CDC and HUD 2006).

The state of farmworker housing is a social injustice. The remainder of this chapter documents that, although housing is a basic human right, the housing of farmworkers is deficient in many ways. Few regulations are in place to ensure adequate housing for farmworkers and these regulations are poorly enforced. This inadequate housing has important ramifications for farmworker health and safety.

3.3   Research Documenting Farmworker Housing Conditions in the Eastern US

Few studies of farmworker housing have been completed anywhere in the US. Studies conducted in the eastern US are even more limited. There are four relevant studies, with one providing regional data (Holden 2000) and the other three focused on farmworker housing in North Carolina (Early et al. 2006; Gentry et al. 2007; Arcury unpublished data). Two policy reports have been issued on farmworker housing in the eastern US in recent years, but neither of these contains primary housing data (Flocks and Burns 2006; Rural Opportunities, Inc. 2000).

Each of the four studies of farmworker housing in the eastern US used different data collection methods, sampled from different components of the farmworker population, and investigated different aspects of farmworker housing. A review of the research designs and methods for each of these studies and a summary of the major limitations and gaps in the research base is important for a clear understanding of what is known about farmworker housing in the eastern US.

The Housing Assistance Council, in collaboration with Farmworker Health Services, Inc., completed a regional study of migrant farmworker housing in the eastern US (Holden 2000). Data were collected from December 1997 through October 1998 by Farmworker Health Services, Inc., outreach staff as part of their outreach activities. Participants were migrant farmworkers residing in 1,566 housing units in Connecticut, Florida, Kentucky, Massachusetts, Maryland, North Carolina, New Jersey, New York, South Carolina, and Virginia. The largest number of units, 605, was in Florida. The survey included farmworkers living in employer-owned and private market units. Data were collected with survey interviews and observational evaluation of housing quality, and included structure type, location, exterior quality, interior quality, number of rooms, and appliances.

The analysis completed by Early et al. (2006) used data from four surveys of farmworker communities conducted from 2001 to 2003 to document aspects of housing quality that could affect farmworker family health. Three housing domains were considered: dwelling characteristics, household characteristics, and household behaviors. Two of these studies were conducted in five counties of northwest North Carolina (Alleghany, Ashe, Avery, Mitchell, and Watauga), with some participants recruited from three counties of southwest Virginia (Smyth, Grayson, and Carroll). Two of the studies were conducted in eastern North Carolina, with participants recruited from Duplin, Harnett, Johnston, Sampson, Wake, and Wayne counties.

Data for the first northwest North Carolina study were collected in 2001. Forty-one households participated. Eligible households included at least one adult employed as a farmworker within the last 12 months and at least one child between 12 and 84 months of age. Assessments included in-depth interviews, survey interviews, and limited observation of housing quality. Wipe samples to assess environmental pesticide exposure were also collected (Quandt et al. 2004; see Sect. 8.2.4). Data for the second northwest North Carolina study were collected in 2003, and included the dwellings of 117 farmworker households. An eligible household had to include at least one farmworker and at least one child aged 13 years or younger. All participants were involved in a lay health advisor intervention, and housing data were collected as part of a baseline survey that measured characteristics of the participating households and their dwellings.

Data for the first eastern North Carolina study were collected in 2002. In-depth and survey interviews were conducted with 25 farmworker households that included at least one farmworker and at least one child. Included in the interviews were fixed response interview items and observations about living conditions such as number of years in residence, type of structure, and house cleaning. Data for the second eastern North Carolina study were collected in 2003 as part of an effort to document lead exposure in farmworker dwellings (see Sect. 8.2.4). Eligible households had to have at least one adult who had done farm work within 12 months and at least one child under the age of 6 present. Data, including survey interviews, interviewer observations about housing quality, and lead wipe samples, were collected from 51 households.

The study by Gentry et al. (2007) was completed from July through August, 2004. Its primary objective was to evaluate the quality of housing among farmworker families. Participants included 186 farmworker households in Duplin, Harnett, Johnston, Sampson, Wake, and Wayne counties in eastern North Carolina. Eligible households included at least one adult who had been employed in farm work during the previous year and at least one child under the age of 18 years. Survey interview data included dwelling type, proximity to farm fields, number of rooms, excluding kitchen and bathroom, number of bedrooms, number of bathrooms, structural conditions, condition of windows, condition of doors, condition of paint, type of heating system, lack of appliances and fixtures, and presence of vermin or rodent infestation.

Data for the study completed by Arcury et al. (unpublished data) were collected from May through October, 2005. The primary purpose of this study was to evaluate the prevalence and risk factors for skin disease among farmworkers (Arcury et al. 2007). The sample included 304 Latino farmworkers (300 men, 4 women) from 45 camps in a nine-county area of eastern North Carolina that included Edgecombe, Greene, Harnett, Johnston, Lenoir, Sampson, Nash, Pitt, and Wilson counties. Data collection was based on an interviewer-administered questionnaire. Housing measures included two laundry items (number of working washing machines in camp and number of working clothes dryers in camp) and three crowding items (people per showerhead, number of people sharing sleeping room, and number of people living in the camp).

Each of these four studies provides insight into the quality of farmworker housing in the eastern US. However, these studies also have several important limitations that constrain knowledge about the condition of farmworker housing. First, only four studies of farmworker housing have been published. No comprehensive study of housing across the region has been completed. Other than North Carolina, no studies of farmworker housing have been completed in specific states. Second, the sample design for each study limits generalization of results. Data collection for the Housing Assistance Council's regional study was completed by Farmworker Health Services, Inc., outreach workers. Therefore, areas not served by Farmworker Health Services, Inc., could not be included in the study. The North Carolina studies reported by Early and Gentry were limited to farmworker households that included a child; many, but not all, of these families were seasonal farmworkers. Also excluded are the majority of migrant farmworkers who are unaccompanied men. The North Carolina study by Arcury and colleagues was limited to migrant farmworkers living in farmworker camps; therefore, seasonal farmworkers and those living in other housing could not be included. Third, the data collected by each study were largely limited to interviews and observation. No measurement or formal inspection of housing quality was conducted. Finally, none of the studies include measures that would allow evaluating associations of housing quality and health.

3.4   Farmworker Housing Conditions in the Eastern United States

3.4.1   Tenure

Although sources differ in the information describing farmworker housing tenure, it is clear that farmworkers seldom control the housing in which they live. About 75% of the rural US population, and 69% of the general US population, own the homes in which they live (US Census Bureau 2006). Farmworkers are less likely than the average US resident to own their homes. The 2004 National Agricultural Worker Survey found that only 23% of farmworkers in the eastern US own their home, while 45% rent their housing (Gabbard 2006). Studies completed in North Carolina report as few as no farmworkers and as many as a quarter of farmworker families own their homes (Early et al. 2006; Gentry et al. 2007). The Housing Assistance Council survey found that more than half of farmworkers lived in dwellings owned by their employer, with between 75 and 96% of farmworkers in most states living in employer-owned dwellings (Table 3.1) (Holden 2000). Florida (22%) and Kentucky (33%) were the only states in which less than three fourths of surveyed dwellings were employer-owned. Nearly two thirds of employer-owned housing units were provided free of charge; Florida (1.5%) and Connecticut (28%) are the only states with less than 60% of employer-owned housing being provided at no cost to workers.

Employer-provided housing is rare in some states, particularly those that are the home states for many farmworkers or those in which year-round labor is needed for the state's major crops. In contrast, employer-provided housing is common in North Carolina, New York, and Pennsylvania (HAC 1996). The Housing Assistance Council (1996) estimated that one fifth to one third of farmworkers in the US live in employer-provided housing.

Even in states such as New York where employer-provided housing is common, the number of beds available is often insufficient to meet the housing needs of all

Table 3.1 Variability between states in the eastern United States of housing tenure and quality measures: Results from Housing Assistance Council's 1997–1998 survey (Holden 2000)

State	Mean length of stay in state (months)	Median monthly net income ($)	Percent of units with crowding[a]	Percent of units with housing cost burden[b]	Percent of units employer-owned	Percent of employer-owned units severely inadequate[c]	Percent of private market units severely inadequate[c]
Connecticut	3.0	1,000	65	0	96	2	0
Florida	6.7	750	89	31	22	43	48
Kentucky	5.6	950	83	2	33	55	39
Massachusetts	5.5	1,010	100	0	89	50	0
Maryland	4.7	813	82	8	94	22	25
North Carolina	5.0	638	77	0	92	28	46
New Jersey	5.3	890	86	11	77	18	46
New York	2.5	900	66	4	83	25	20
South Carolina	6.7	960	75	0	77	31	25
Virginia	3.1	1,000	90	0	90	50	44
Total Sample	*5.3*	*850*	*85*	*14*	*55*	*32*	*45*

[a]Crowding is defined as a mean of more than 1 person per room, excluding kitchens and bathrooms
[b]Households that pay more than 30% of their income on housing costs, including utilities, have housing cost burden
[c]A dwelling is considered severely inadequate if it has serious plumbing problems such as a lack of indoor plumbing or broken sinks, toilets, or showers, broken heating elements, damaged electrical systems, and both interior and exterior structural damage

migrant farmworkers during the peak of the agricultural season (Rural Opportunities, Inc. 2000). For example, in Suffolk County 600 beds were available in 40 on-farm labor camps, but employers in the county reported hiring 2,601 seasonal and migrant farmworkers (Rural Opportunities, Inc. 2000).

Studies differ as to whether employer-provided or rental housing is more likely to meet housing standards. The Housing Assistance Council survey showed that private market units were more likely to be severely inadequate than employer-provided units (45% vs. 32%) (Holden 2000). This may be because temporary labor camp standards require preoccupancy inspections for employment-related housing, whereas housing codes in rural areas may not be very strict and probably do not require inspection before renters move in. In contrast, the study by Gentry et al. (2007) on family housing in North Carolina found that farmworkers who own or rent their home had better housing conditions than those who lived in employer-provided housing.

Migrant farmworkers may live in several housing units in different states during a given year. The mean length of stay in the housing occupied when workers were surveyed for the HAC survey ranged from 2.5 months in New York to 6.7 months in Florida and South Carolina (Holden 2000). In North Carolina, 46.8% of farmworker families had moved at least once during the previous year, and one third moved at least once to follow crops (Gentry et al. 2007). The quality and type of housing in each new location is likely to differ.

Migration to follow the crops is associated with poorer housing conditions (Gentry et al. 2007). Migrants must either depend on housing provided free of charge by an employer or find a temporary home in the private housing market. When housing is provided free of charge, many workers do not feel entitled to complain about substandard conditions. The temporary nature of the housing is also a disincentive to making complaints.

3.4.2   Types of Farmworker Housing

Mobile homes (32%) and dormitories or barracks (30%) are the most common types of farmworker housing in the eastern US (Holden 2000) (Figs. 3.1a, b and 3.2a–c). The dominant housing type varies by state. In Florida, which is the main home base state in the eastern US, the most common housing type is the mobile home (56%); duplex (16%) is the second most common, and single-family home ranks third (15%) (Figs. 3.3a, b and 3.4). Mobile homes (85.2%) are a common type of dwelling for North Carolina farmworker families with children (Gentry et al. 2007). Farmworker families in North Carolina and Virginia were more likely to live in mobile homes (54% and 71%, respectively), than farmworkers nationally (15%), rural US residents (15%), or US residents (7%) (Early et al. 2006; Holden 2000, 2001).

Some housing types are more likely to have substandard conditions than are others. For example, the Housing Assistance Council surveys found that mobile homes were more likely than other types of dwellings to be substandard or crowded,

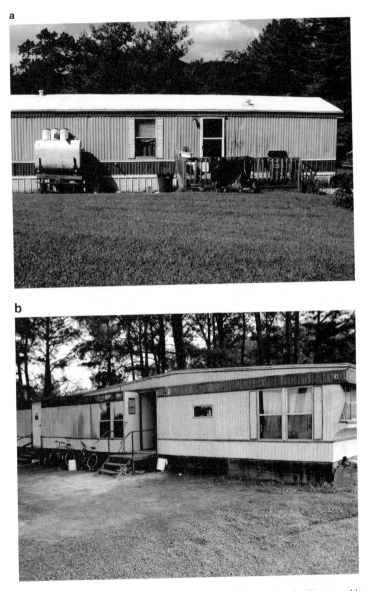

Fig. 3.1 Mobile homes occupied year-round by a seasonal farmworker family (**a**) and by migrant workers (**b**), North Carolina. Copyright, Thomas A. Arcury

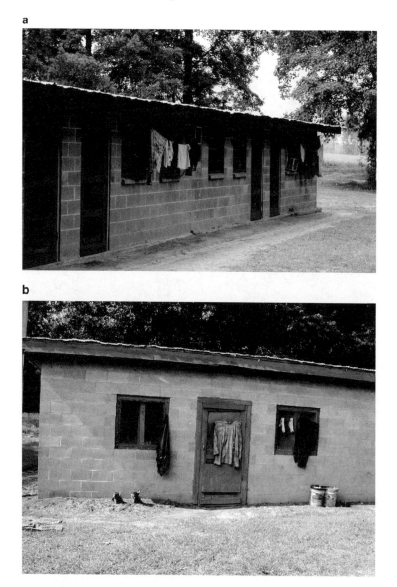

Fig. 3.2 (a–c) Three examples of barracks housing occupied by migrant workers, North Carolina. Copyright, Thomas A. Arcury

c

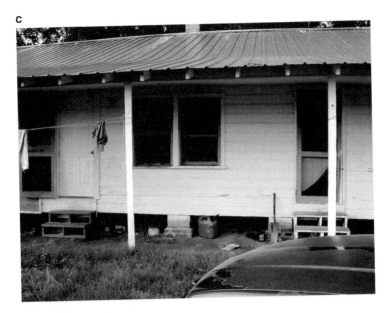

Fig. 3.2 (continued)

a

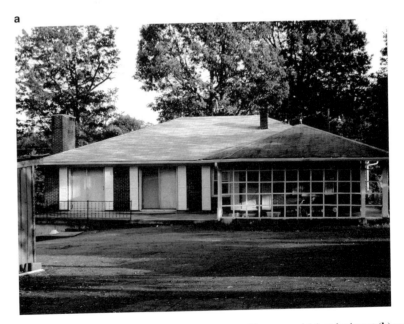

Fig. 3.3 Two examples showing the variety of houses used by seasonal (**a**) and migrant (**b**) workers, North Carolina. Copyright, Thomas A. Arcury

b

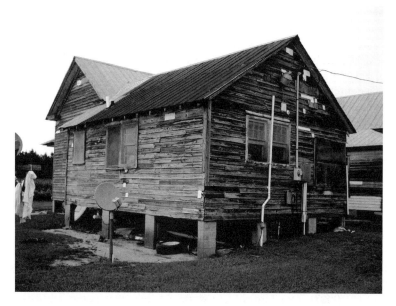

Fig. 3.3 (continued)

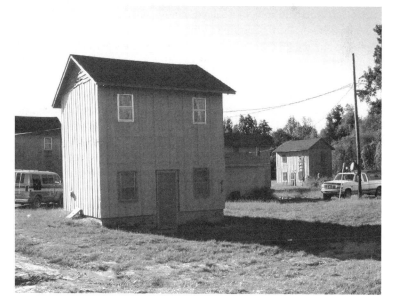

Fig. 3.4 Tobacco curing barn converted to migrant housing in North Carolina. Copyright, Thomas A. Arcury

with nearly half having water damage, 43% having peeling paint, more than one third having holes in the walls, more than one fifth having exposed wiring, and 15% having holes in the floor large enough to be deemed tripping hazards (Holden 2000, 2001). Mobile homes were more likely than other dwelling types to have four or more exterior problems (Holden 2000). They were also the most likely dwelling type to have three or more interior problems and to meet the American Housing Survey's definition of severely inadequate; more than half of mobile homes in the eastern US were severely inadequate.

3.4.3 Crowding

Most (85%) farmworker housing in the eastern US is crowded (more than one person per room, excluding kitchen and bathrooms) (Holden 2000). Crowding rates vary substantially between states, from 21% in Connecticut to 100% in Massachusetts (Holden 2000). North Carolina studies confirm that overcrowding is a serious problem. More than two thirds of North Carolina farmworker families live in crowded conditions, with nearly half having more than two people per bedroom (Gentry et al. 2007). Two thirds of farmworkers living in temporary labor camps in North Carolina share a sleeping room with three or more farmworkers, with almost one quarter sharing a bathroom with six or more persons; 11% of workers reported sharing a showerhead with more than ten people (Arcury et al. unpublished data). The level of crowding in temporary labor camps changes across the agricultural season; while 48% of North Carolina farmworkers reported three or more persons per sleeping room and 12% reported six or more persons per showerhead in May, 67% reported three or more persons per sleeping room and 42% reported six or more persons per showerhead in August and September.

Crowding is often associated with higher housing costs. In states or areas where rents are high, workers attempt to lower their housing costs by increasing the number of residents (Holden 2002). Owing to the discrepancy between the number of beds available in employment-related housing and the number of workers temporarily employed, most farmworkers rely on private housing markets, the majority of which are unable to meet the high demand for inexpensive short-term housing that occurs during the peak agricultural season (HAC 1996; Rural Opportunities, Inc. 2000). Farmworkers in the Eastern US who pay for housing experience high rates of housing cost burden (spending more than 30% of household income on housing) (Holden 2000). The prevalence of farmworker households with housing cost burden varies considerably from state to state. Connecticut, Massachusetts, North Carolina, South Carolina, and Virginia had no units in the Housing Assistance Council survey with housing cost burden, whereas Florida had 31%, New Jersey 11%, and Maryland 8% of units with housing cost burden.

Crowding is especially prevalent in housing that is considered substandard. Using the American Housing Survey physical quality measures, 38% of farmworker housing units in the eastern US were severely inadequate (Holden 2000). To be considered severely inadequate, a dwelling must have serious plumbing problems such as a lack of indoor plumbing or broken sinks, toilets, or showers; broken heating elements; damaged electrical systems; and both interior and exterior structural damage. Crowding was present in 90% of these substandard units, and children were living in 42% of them (Holden 2000).

The estimated prevalence of crowding among farmworker households (36–85%) is much higher than the prevalence of crowding among the population of the rural US (4%) (Early et al. 2006; Holden 2000, 2001), and, based on calculations from data collected in the 2005 American Housing Survey, the general US population (2.4%) (US Census Bureau 2006). Crowding among farmworker households in the eastern US is also much more prevalent than it is among Latino/Hispanic house-holds in the US (13%) (Bradman et al. 2005).

3.4.4 Broken or Missing Appliances and Facilities

It is common for farmworker households in the eastern US to lack access to impor-tant appliances and facilities. The stove, refrigerator, bathtub/shower, or toilet was broken in almost one fifth of dwellings in the Housing Assistance Council survey (Holden 2000). These dwellings commonly lacked appliances necessary for safe storage and preparation of food; more than one quarter of households lacked a working oven, 12% lacked a working stove, and 8% lacked a working refrigerator. Toilets were missing or broken in 15% of housing units, and nearly 7% of units lacked bathing facilities. An indoor toilet was not present in 5% of farmworker family dwellings in North Carolina; 28% did not have adequate facilities for food preparation and refuse disposal; two thirds did not have adequate space and lacked lockable doors and windows; and 58% lacked equipment for safe and adequate heating (Gentry et al. 2007).

Farmworker housing commonly lacks laundry equipment. The lack of washing machines is especially important to farmworker families because not having easy access to laundry facilities makes it more difficult to launder clothes to remove pesticide residues (Grieshop et al. 1994). The North Carolina studies reported that one third or more of farmworker family households did not have washing machines (Early et al. 2006; Gentry et al. 2007). The percentage of farmworker households that lacked access to washing machines is nearly twice as high as the percentage of households in the US (18%) (US Census Bureau 2006).

Many farmworker residences, especially those that are employer-provided, lack telephone service. Only 41% of dwellings in the Housing Assistance Council's survey of eastern farmworker housing had access to a telephone (Holden 2000), while a mere 3% of households in the US lacked a telephone in 2005 (US Census Bureau 2006).

According to calculations from the 2005 American Housing Survey data, only 2% of households in the US lacked complete kitchen facilities, including sink, refrigerator, and oven or burners (US Census Bureau 2006). Less than 1% of households in the US lacked a stove, oven, or refrigerator. The majority of American households have complete plumbing facilities. Very few households lacked a complete bathroom in the 2005 American Housing Survey; 0.1% lacked a tub and shower, 0.1% lacked a flush toilet, and 0.2% did not have hot piped water. Very few households in the US (less than 1%) lack central heating equipment. An awareness of the dramatic difference between the prevalence of such substandard conditions among farmworkers and that among the general population leads one to question why American society is willing to accept such an unequal burden of exposure to potentially health-damaging conditions among farmworkers.

3.4.5 Structural Problems

Over one quarter of farmworker housing in the eastern US had evidence of serious structural problems such as sagging roof, frame, or porches (Holden 2000). More than three fourths of dwellings had at least one exterior problem; 29% of dwellings had four or more problems; and 13% had six or more problems. Common exterior problems included peeling paint (50%), damaged windows (43%), trash in the yard (36%), problems with gutters or downspouts (34%), problems with the roof (16%), and foundation damage (14%). The damaged roof, gutters, and downspouts can lead to moisture problems in the dwellings. In contrast to farmworker housing, only 18% of housing units surveyed in the 2005 American Housing Survey had structural damage, only 8% had roof problems, and 2% had foundation problems (US Census Bureau 2006).

Two thirds of farmworker dwellings in the eastern US had at least one interior problem; 29% had three or more interior problems (Holden 2000). Common interior problems included peeling paint (36%), broken plaster (36%), and evidence of water leakage (35%). Of the homes with peeling paint, 35% had children present. Over half of the housing units that included children had peeling exterior or interior paint, which may expose children to lead.

The majority of farmworker dwellings had multiple interior and exterior structural problems. At least one interior and one exterior problem were identified in almost two thirds of dwellings in the eastern US (Holden 2000). That one fifth of dwellings had four or more exterior and three or more interior problems is even more alarming.

Among family dwellings in North Carolina, a third had damaged structural features such as roof, interior and exterior walls, and floors (Gentry et al. 2007). Peeling paint was also common in farmworker family housing; it was present on the exterior of over a third, and on the interior and on window frames in nearly a quarter of dwellings surveyed.

Farmworker housing is also more likely than US housing in general to have interior quality problems. Only 2% of homes in the US in general had interior problems (US Census Bureau 2006). Farmworkers were 16 times more likely than other rural residents to live in severely inadequate housing, 38% of farmworker dwellings compared to 2% of rural homeowners and 2% of rural renters (Holden 2000).

3.4.6   Infestations

Dampness and insufficient refuse disposal and food storage facilities, which have been documented in farmworker housing, can lead to infestation problems. Housing that has structural damage such as holes and cracks in the foundation, floors, and exterior and interior walls is vulnerable to infestations. Moisture and water damage, peeling paint, and crowding also increase the risk of infestations (Bradman et al. 2005). A study in an agricultural community in California reported that rodent infestations were more than twice as likely in homes with peeling paint, two and a half times as likely in homes with water damage, and twice as likely in homes with mold. Cockroach infestations were almost four times as likely in homes with peeling paint, more than twice as likely in homes with water damage or a leak under the sink, 1.7 times as likely in homes with mold, and nearly three times as likely in crowded homes (Bradman et al. 2005).

Given the prevalence of these conditions in farmworker housing, it is not surprising that a large portion of farmworker homes in the eastern US have problems with insect and rodent infestations. One North Carolina study on farmworker family homes showed that nearly three fourths had rodent or vermin infestations (Gentry et al. 2007). The Housing Assistance Council survey recorded unsanitary conditions, including signs of insect and rodent infestations, in more than one third of housing units (Holden 2000).

Signs of infestation are also more common in farmworker housing units than in the households in the US in general. Only 7% of homes in the US (US Census Bureau 2006) had signs of rats, mice, or other rodents, compared with one third of farmworker housing (Holden 2000).

3.4.7   Proximity to Agricultural Fields

Residents of homes that are adjacent to agricultural fields are at increased risk of exposure from pesticides drifting into the homes when they are applied to nearby fields (Bradman et al. 1997; Curl et al. 2002; Fenske et al. 2002; McCauley et al. 2001; Quandt et al. 2004). The Housing Assistance Council found that 39% of farmworker households in the eastern US were located adjacent to fields (Holden 2000). Adding to the concern about housing located near fields is the fact that 4% of such units had a missing or broken bath or shower and 72% had a missing or broken washing machine. Convenient access to bathing and clothes laundering facilities is essential for farmworkers to be able to reduce their own and their families' exposure to pesticides by washing pesticide residues off their bodies and clothes as quickly as possible.

3.4.8   Variability in Farmworker Housing

Rates of crowding, substandard conditions, and housing cost burden varied across states in the Housing Assistance Councils' survey of farmworker housing in the eastern US (Table 3.1) (Holden 2000). Rates of substandard housing varied from 3% in Connecticut to 56% in Florida. Much of this variation may be attributable to the differences in the types of housing available in different states. In Florida, the majority of farmworkers must rent or purchase housing on the private market; and there is very little housing in the state that is provided by employers. Private market housing is not regulated at the federal level but, rather, by local housing codes. In contrast, housing that is provided by agricultural employers or is employment-related is regulated by the OSHA's temporary labor camp standards and must be inspected before it is occupied each year. The majority of housing in Connecticut is provided by employers and is subject to annual preoccupancy inspections. This variability may be evidence that, when housing is subject to inspection, it is likely to be of higher quality.

3.5   Farmworker Housing Conditions: Eastern US and National Data Compared

The substandard housing conditions common in the eastern US are common in other parts of the country. Farmworkers across the US face similarly abysmal housing conditions and often have no choice but to live in crowded, dilapidated housing units. Although many farmworkers have shared experiences, there are also marked differences between the overall housing conditions, housing availability, the types of housing that are common, and the housing assistance resources that are available in the East, Midwest, and West. Table 3.2 outlines the housing conditions that have been documented among farmworkers in the eastern US and in the US as a whole.

The Housing Assistance Council conducted surveys to characterize regional farmworkers' housing conditions (Holden 2000, 2001). The results show that substandard housing conditions are more common in the eastern US than they are in farmworker dwellings in the US as a whole. The eastern US had a higher prevalence of severely substandard units (20–38% in the East, compared to 17% in the US) and of moderately substandard units (23% in East, compared to 16% in the US). Farmworker housing units in the East are also more likely to be crowded, to lack a living room, and to lack a working toilet.

More than three fourths of farmworker dwellings in the eastern US lacked a washing machine, compared to just over half in the nation as a whole. Dwellings in the eastern US were also more likely to be located near agricultural fields (39%) than were dwelling in the US as a whole (26%). Both of these conditions may lead to greater levels of exposure to pesticides. Eastern dwellings were less likely to have telephone access, and interior and exterior structural problems were slightly more prevalent in the eastern US.

Table 3.2 Housing conditions documented among eastern US farmworkers, all US farmworkers, and the general US population

Housing condition	Eastern US farmworkers	All US farmworkers[a]	General US population[b]
Structure type (%)			
Mobile home	32[c]	15	6[d]
Barracks	30[c]	4	–
Single family	16[c]	42	64 (detached) 6 (attached)[d]
Apartments	17[a]	21	24 (2–50 units per structure)[d]
Tenure (%)			
Private market/renter occupied	45[c]	75	31[d]
Owner occupied	0.3[a]	3	69[d]
Employer owned	55[c] 43[a]	25	–
Free of charge	63[c]	57	–
Mean length of stay (months)	5.3[c]	7.6	–
State with longest	Florida: 6.7[c]	Washington: 10.7	–
State with shortest	New York: 2.5[c]	Michigan, Missouri: 3.2	–
Housing cost burden (%)	14–22 (excluding those provided free of charge)[c]	29–34 (excluding those provided free of charge)	34[d]
Children present (%)	66[c] 66[c]–79[a]	86	–
Crowding (>1 person per room excluding bathrooms and kitchens) (%)	72[a]–85 (excluding dorms and barracks)[c]	52 (excluding dorms and barracks)	2 (all US households)[a,d]; 3 (nonmetropolitan households)[a]
Crowded units with children[e] (%)	40[a]–50[c]	74	–
Missing or broken appliance or fixture (%)	18[c]–25[a]	22	2 (lack complete kitchen facilities)[d]
No working stove	12[c]	10	1[a]
No working refrigerator	8[c]	6	0.2[d]
No working bath/shower	7[c]	8	0.1[d]
No working toilet	15[c]	9	0.1 (no flush toilet)[d]; 2 (no working toilet some time past 3 months)[d]
Detached bathroom (%)	29[c]	9	–
No bathroom (%)	3[c]	2	0.5 (no complete bathrooms)[d]
No living room (%)	41[c]	17	–
No working laundry machine (%)	77[c]	52	18[d]
No working telephone (%)	60[c]	43	3[d]
Adjacent to agricultural fields (%)	39[c]	26	–

(continued)

Table 3.2 (continued)

Housing condition	Eastern US farmworkers	All US farmworkers[a]	General US population[b]
Children present (%)	27[c]	60	–
Exterior problems (at least one) (%)	80[c]	–	18[d]
Serious structural problems (sagging roof, house frame, porch)	27[c]	22	3 (sagging roof or sloping outside walls)[d]
Holes or shingles missing in roof	16[c]	15	6[d]
Foundation damage	14[c]	10	2[d]
Windows with broken glass or screens	43[c]	36	4 (broken windows)[d]
Exterior peeling paint	49[c]	41	–
Gutters or downspouts missing or damaged	34[c]	26	–
Interior problems (%)	–	–	–
Peeling paint or broken plaster	36[c]	29	2[d]
Evidence of water leakage	35[c]	29	19 (water leakage last 12 months)[d]
Holes in walls	30[c]	22	5[d]
Unsanitary conditions (signs of rodent or insect infestation)	33[c]	19	7[d]
Electrical hazard (e.g., frayed wiring)	11[c]	9	0.6[d]
Substandard housing (%)	43[a]	33	–
Private market	45[c]	33	–
Employer owned	32[c]	32	–
Mobile homes	53[c]	26	–
Children present	42[c]	65	–
Crowded	-	63	–
Severely substandard (lack indoor plumbing and have number of interior and exterior problems)	20[a]–38[c]	17	2[a]
Moderately substandard (number of interior and exterior problems)	23[a]	16	5[a]

[a]HAC 2001
[b]US Census Bureau 2006
[c]Holden 2000
[d]Author's calculations from American Housing Survey for the United States: 2005 data (US Census Bureau 2006)
[e]Percentage of crowded housing units in the survey that had children present in the home

Eastern farmworkers fared better than farmworkers nationwide in a few housing measures. They have lower rates of housing cost burden. This can be attributed, in part, to the prevalence of employer-provided housing, which tends to be provided free of charge (Holden 2000). Farmworker households that have substandard conditions are less likely in the East than in the nation as a whole to have children present.

In general, farmworkers in the eastern US tend to have worse housing conditions than their counterparts in other areas of the country. This may be because the western and midwestern parts of the country have a long history of addressing the needs of Latino/Hispanic agricultural workers, whereas eastern states have experienced the growth of the Latino/Hispanic farmworker population during the past two decades. There is a great need for efforts to address housing conditions in the eastern US. It may be useful to look to efforts that have been made in the West and Midwest for ideas of effective approaches toward improving farmworker housing conditions.

3.6   Health Effects of Substandard Housing

Although the prevalence of substandard housing conditions among farmworker housing units is well documented, very little research has explored the association between substandard housing conditions and health among farmworkers. One study found that migrant farmworkers who indicated that they lived in poor housing conditions had significantly higher levels of anxiety symptoms than did those who did not experience poor housing conditions (Magaña and Hovey 2003). An association between inadequate sanitation and water facilities or lack of laundry facilities with the exposure of farmworkers' family members to pesticides has also been identified (Meister 1991). This is presumably because inadequate water facilities and the absence of laundry facilities make it more difficult for workers to bathe and wash work clothes (Villarejo and Schenker 2006).

Although evidence of the association between housing conditions and health in farmworkers is limited, a number of studies in other populations have identified associations between substandard housing conditions and a number of health outcomes, including stress, depression, asthma and other respiratory problems, infectious diseases, and injury. One can expect that being exposed to the same substandard housing conditions would lead to similar health outcomes among farmworkers.

Crowded living conditions have been associated with a doubling of the prevalence of psychological distress, including anxiety, nervousness, and depression (Guite et al. 2006). Crowding has been linked to social withdrawal and is also related to measures of physiological stress such as elevation in blood pressure and deteriorated interpersonal relationships in adults (Evans et al. 1998; Evans and Lepore 1993; Lepore et al. 1991). Crowded living conditions are also associated with the spread of infectious diseases such as tuberculosis and respiratory infections, influenza, and parasitic infections (Krieger and Higgins 2002; Holden 2002; MacIntyre et al. 1997; Villarejo and Schenker 2006).

Housing conditions that lead to infestations also produce unsanitary conditions, and these housing conditions contribute to the spread of infectious diseases (Krieger and Higgins 2002; Mood 1993; Howard 1993). Insects and rodents can transmit infectious diseases such as West Nile Virus, eastern equine encephalitis, St. Louis encephalitis, plague, typhus, leptospirosis, rickettsialpox, and rat-bite fever (CDC and HUD 2006; Howard 1993).

In addition to the risk of respiratory problems and infectious diseases, infestations are problematic because they lead residents to apply pesticides to their homes in order to eliminate the pests (Bradman et al. 2005; Whyatt et al. 2002; Chew et al. 2006). Infestations, combined with occupational contamination and close proximity to agricultural fields, can lead to the presence of pesticides at home. Several studies have documented high levels of both agricultural and residential pesticides in farmworker homes (Fenske et al. 2000; McCauley et al. 2001; Quandt et al. 2002, 2004; see Chap. 4).

Poor ventilation and lack of safe equipment for heating or cooling a dwelling can lead to temperature extremes in a home. Extreme heat could increase a resident's likelihood of experiencing heat exhaustion, heat stress, or heat stroke. Extreme cold temperatures could lead to cold stress or hypothermia (CDC and HUD 2006). Exposure to temperature extremes is also associated with mental health consequences (Collins 1993).

The presence of structural damage such as holes in walls and floors and of electrical hazards such as exposed wires increases residents' risk of injury from falls and electric shock (Bradman et al. 2005). Broken glass in windows and doors can result in cuts (Holden 2002). The absence of functional locks on doors and windows makes it easier for criminals to gain access to farmworker residences.

The presence of peeling paint in housing constructed before 1978 can potentially pose a lead exposure hazard (see Sect. 8.2.4). Lead exposure is especially dangerous to children because lead affects neurological development (Berney 1996; Bellinger 2004; Holden 2000; Millstone 1997; Shen et al. 2001).

Not having access to a telephone can pose a very serious hazard in case of medical emergencies. Workers who spend long hours laboring in the sun in crops that may have been treated with pesticides during seasons with high average temperatures should have access to telephones in case a worker displays symptoms of heat stress or pesticide poisoning. The inability to call for emergency medical service could increase the likelihood that a person would die before receiving needed medical care. Lack of telephone access has also been linked to poor mental health (Grzywacz et al. 2006; see Sect. 7.5.4).

3.7   Housing Quality Standards

The quality of temporary labor camps, which are defined as farm housing directly related to the seasonal or temporary employment of farmworkers, is regulated by OSHA's Occupational Safety and Health Standards for temporary labor camps. These standards are, in many ways, similar to housing quality standards that have been established by the US Department of Housing and Urban Development (HUD) to regulate dwellings that house people who participate in the Section 8 housing voucher program. Although the regulations are similar, there are important areas in which the temporary labor camp standards allow much poorer conditions than are permitted by HUD. Many of these areas are far worse than those seen in typical housing units in the US. Although the Section 8 housing quality standards are not applied to farmworker housing, they can be used to describe the minimum components that the US government has determined to be necessary for a healthy home. Table 3.3 contrasts these with federal temporary labor camp standards to highlight the disparities that exist between the two sets of housing regulations.

3.7.1 Adequate Space

One requirement indicating a willingness to accept poorer conditions for farmworkers than for the general public is the required amount of space per resident. The temporary labor camp standards state that all sleeping rooms should contain at least 50 sq ft of floor space per occupant and have at least a 7-foot ceiling; if a room is used for cooking, living, and sleeping, it should provide at least 100 sq ft per person (OSHA 2005). In contrast, HUD Housing Quality Standards (2008a) require that a dwelling contain at least one bedroom or living/sleeping room per every 2 residents and specify that no more than 12 residents may share a dwelling. Many employer-owned farmworker housing units are barracks style and lack indoor common areas, apart from a kitchen and dining room. Employment-related mobile homes and houses that are used to house farmworkers are often crowded and common areas such as living rooms frequently double as sleeping rooms for some of the residents.

Calculations using data from the US Census Bureau's 2005 American Housing Survey (2006) show that a mere 2% of households in the US have less than 200 sq ft per person. In a dwelling in which the bedroom is the primary location where residents can spend time, 50–100 sq ft per person is well below the amount of space that 98% of residents of American households enjoy.

3.7.2 Plumbing, Water Supply, and Toilet Facilities

Temporary labor camp standards do not require that dwellings have flush toilets. The regulations state that an adequate (35 gallons per person per day) and convenient water supply approved by the local health authority must be provided in each camp; if water is not piped to shelters, water outlets should be within 100 ft of each shelter (OSHA 2005). The standards also specify that toilet facilities should be

Table 3.3 Comparison of OSHA temporary labor camp standards with HUD Section 8 housing quality standards

Requirement category	Temporary labor camp standards[a]	HUD Section 8 standards[b]
Shelter	Provide protection against the elements.	Not specified.
Windows	Living quarters should have windows that cover 1/10 of floor area; can be opened for ventilation.	Each bedroom or living/sleeping room should have at least one window. Free of signs of severe deterioration.
Paint	Not specified.	In pre-1978 housing with resident under age 7: all interior and exterior paint stable and free of cracking, scaling, chipping, peeling or loose paint.
Exterior openings	Must be screened. Screen doors should be self-closing if present.	Should be lockable and be in good repair to provide protection against the elements.
Exterior structure	Not specified.	Sound and free from hazards (includes walls, chimney, foundation, stairs, porches, railings, roofs, gutters, and downspouts).
Water supply	35 gallons per person per day; if not piped to shelter, water outlet should be within 100 ft of each shelter; approved by local health authority.	Approved by local health authority; adequate supply of heated and unheated water, under pressure.
Plumbing	Not specified.	Free of leaks, corrosion, and sewer backup.
Electricity	At least one ceiling light fixture and one outlet in each habitable room (where electric service is available).	All rooms should be free of electrical hazards; at least 2 working electrical outlets or 1 outlet and 1 working permanently installed light fixture.
Heating equipment	If dwelling inhabited during cold weather, adequate heating equipment shall be provided.	Capable of providing adequate heat to all rooms used for living.
Living room	Not specified.	At least 1 room per unit intended for living, sleeping, cooking, or eating purposes.
Living space	At least 50 sq ft of floor space per occupant; 100 ft per occupant if room used for sleeping, living, and cooking; 7-foot ceilings.	One living or sleeping room per every 2 residents.
Beds	Include beds, cots, or bunks; elevated 12 in. from floor, spaced 36 in. apart (48 in. if double bunk); triple bunks not allowed.	Not specified.

Kitchen/meal preparation area	If room used for cooking, living, and sleeping, it should provide at least 100 sq ft of floor space per occupant. Should include the following: 1. An adequate and convenient supply of water for cooking purposes, approved by appropriate health authority 2. One stove burner per 10 persons in a closed and screened space; should meet local and state regulations 3. If present, oven should meet state and local regulations 4. Sanitary facilities for storing and preparing food	At least 1 present per unit. Should include the following: 1. A sink with hot and cold water under pressure and connected to approved sewer/septic system 2. Stove with all burners working 3. Oven in working condition 4. Space for food storage and preparation 5. At least 1 working refrigerator with some freezing capability
Bathroom	Shared facilities acceptable.	For exclusive use of unit occupants.
Toilet	Privy is acceptable toilet facility; located within 200 ft of each sleeping room; toilet fixtures, water closets, chemical toilets or urinals should not be located in room used for other purposes.	Toilet in working condition and connected to approved sewer/septic system and water supply.
Sink/washbasin	1 per family shelter or per 6 persons in shared shelters.	Required in bathroom, connected to hot and cold water under pressure and connected to approved sewer/septic system and water supply.
Tub or shower	Floors, walls, and partitions smooth and impervious to moisture up to height of splash; floors should have a drain; hot and cold running water required; one showerhead per 10 persons.	Hot and cold water under pressure, connected to approved sewer/septic system and water supply.
Vent or window	Working vent or openable window required.	Working vent or openable window required.
Alternate fire exit	Not specified.	Required.
Infestation	Effective rodent and infestation control measures should be taken.	Free of severe infestation by rats, mice, or vermin.
Indoor air pollution	Not specified.	Free of abnormally high levels.
Garbage and debris	At least 1 approved fly-tight, rodent-tight container for refuse disposal per shelter; located within 100 ft of shelter on wood, metal, or concrete stand; emptied when full and kept clean.	Free of heavy accumulation inside and outside.

(continued)

Table 3.3 (continued)

Requirement category	Temporary labor camp standards[a]	HUD Section 8 standards[b]
Special requirements for shared housing		
Adequate space	At least 50 sq ft of floor space per occupant in sleeping rooms; 7-foot ceilings.	At least one bedroom per family; one bedroom for every 2 persons in a family; common space for shared use by all residents; 12 residents maximum.
Toilet facilities	Separate facilities for both the sexes; one toilet per 15 persons; adequate supply of toilet paper; sanitary condition, cleaned at least daily.	Not specified.
Special requirements for congregate housing		
Central kitchen	Should meet requirements of OSHA Food Service Sanitation Ordinance and Code; adequate in size; separate from sleeping quarters.	Large enough to accommodate all residents; refrigerator adequate size for all residents; sanitary food storage; sanitary disposal of food waste and refuse.

[a]OSHA 2005
[b]HUD 2008a

accessible without any individual passing through a sleeping room and should be located within 200 ft of each sleeping room (OSHA 2005). Privies or outhouses and chemical toilets are acceptable toilet facilities according to the standards.

HUD Housing Quality Standards (2008a) require that a dwelling contain a bathroom for the exclusive use of the occupants. The bathroom should have a working toilet, washbasin, and tub or shower, all of which are in good working order and connected to an approved/approvable private or public water supply and sewer system. Sinks and bathing facilities should have an adequate supply of heated and unheated water that is under pressure. Water heaters should be installed and located in a safe manner. All plumbing should be free of major leaks or corrosion and free from sewer or septic system backup (HUD 2008a).

Failing to require flush toilets is another example of OSHA accepting living standards that are far poorer than those that are typical in the US. Less than 0.1% of households in the 2005 American Housing Survey lacked a flush toilet (US Census Bureau 2006). It is disturbing that the US government is willing to accept a lack of such important facilities for farmworkers when such conditions are extremely rare in American housing.

3.7.3 Lighting and Electricity

The standards for lighting and electricity in migrant housing are prefaced by the stipulation "where electric service is available" but require that each habitable room be provided with at least one ceiling light fixture and one outlet. The HUD housing quality standards are similar but do not allow for a dwelling to lack electricity and include a requirement that dwellings be free of electrical hazards. The temporary labor camp standards include no requirement that dwellings be free of electrical hazards.

3.7.4 Food Preparation Facilities

The temporary labor camp standards require that food handling facilities in camps with central dining operations meet requirements of the Food Service Sanitation Ordinance and Code (OSHA 2005) and should be adequate in size and separate from sleeping quarters. Congregate housing in the Section 8 program should include a central kitchen and a central dining facility that is large enough to accommodate all residents and containing a refrigerator of adequate size for all residents. The central kitchen should also include adequate facilities and services for sanitary storage and disposal of food waste and refuse (HUD 2008a).

Migrant farmworkers' dwellings that do not have central dining operations are allowed to have a single room that is used for cooking, sleeping, and living, as long as the room provides at least 100 sq ft per person. HUD housing standards state that all units must have a kitchen or kitchen area for meal preparation that contains a sink with hot and cold running water that is in good working order and is connected to an approved sewer system, a working refrigerator with some capability of freezing food, a working oven, a stove with all burners working, and some space available to store and prepare food. Federal temporary labor camp standards do not require a refrigerator, sink, or oven in housing that does not have central dining operations. They do, however, require a stove with one working burner per ten residents and sanitary facilities for storing and preparing food.

3.7.5   Safety and Structural Quality

HUD standards require that the exterior of a dwelling, including walls, chimney, foundation, stairs, porches, railings, roof, gutters, and downspouts, be sound and free from hazards (HUD 2008a). In all dwellings that were built before 1978 in which a child under age 7 will live, all interior and exterior paint should be stable and free of cracking, scaling, chipping, peeling, or loose paint (HUD 2008a). For health and safety reasons, a housing unit should have an acceptable alternate fire exit; be free of severe infestation by rats, mice, or vermin; be free of abnormally high levels of indoor air pollution; and be free of heavy accumulation of garbage or debris inside and outside (HUD 2008a). Doors and windows accessible from outside should be lockable and free of signs of severe deterioration that would impede their ability to provide reasonable protection from the weather.

Temporary labor camp standards do not specify requirements that dwellings be free of structural damage or peeling paint. Nor do they require that windows and doors be lockable or that an alternate exit be provided for fire safety. Temporary labor camp standards do not mention indoor air pollution but do require that dwellings and sites be free of garbage and debris. Temporary labor camp standards also require that effective infestation controls be used.

3.8   Enforcement and Effectiveness of Migrant Housing Regulations

Although federal regulations established by OSHA apply to all employment-related housing for temporary agricultural laborers, regardless of who provides the housing, the quality of temporary housing for farmworkers varies significantly from state to state and, within states, from camp to camp. The agencies charged with enforcing temporary labor camp standards are different in each state and include OSHA, state departments of labor, state and local health departments, and state departments of agriculture. Each state must establish and enforce its own set of housing regulations, which must be at least as stringent as the federal standards. Some states have adopted regulations that are more stringent than those set forth by OSHA, but many simply follow the federal standards.

In North Carolina, the state Department of Labor conducts preoccupancy housing inspections of employer-owned housing. In New York, the responsibility for inspecting farmworker housing is shared by the US Department of Labor and the New York State Department of Health. The US Department of Labor is responsible for preoccupancy inspections of housing that has four or fewer occupants and housing provided to foreign workers with an H2A visa. (An H2A visa allows an individual to enter the US to work in agriculture for a specified period of time for a particular farmer, who is obligated to provide an average of 35 h of work per week, a specific hourly wage, and to meet all safety requirements. Employers who hire H2A workers are required to provide housing to the workers.) Preoccupancy inspections of housing that has five or more occupants are conducted by the New York State Department of Health (Rural Opportunities, Inc. 2000). Off-farm housing in New York does not receive inspections, and employers and contractors in the state are not required to report year-round housing (Rural Opportunities, Inc. 2000). In Florida, the Florida Department of Health is the sole organization responsible for enforcing farmworker housing standards. All migrant labor camps and migrant residential housing must be issued a permit of operation. State regulations state that all migrant labor camps and migrant residential housing be inspected at least twice quarterly during periods of occupancy. Inspections are conducted and permits issued by the Environmental Health office of county health departments (State of Florida 2008). Despite the requirement that housing be inspected twice quarterly, those who are interested in farmworker housing in the state believe that there is a need to improve enforcement of health and housing regulations (Flock and Burns 2006).

Regardless of how stringent migrant housing regulations are in a given state, they have limited effectiveness for ensuring the quality of farmworker housing because some employers fail to register housing in which their workers are housed with the agencies responsible for enforcing regulations. In New York, it has been reported that some employers house groups of migrant workers for only a few months in housing that is registered as year-round and, therefore, does not require inspection (Rural Opportunities, Inc. 2000). Other employers have avoided registering housing by placing employees in dwellings that are owned by relatives who charge rent and by placing workers in units of four or fewer occupants (Rural Opportunities, Inc. 2000). Most agencies responsible for enforcing farmworker housing regulations have limited staff and lack the resources needed to seek out unregistered camps (HAC 1996; Rural Opportunities, Inc. 2000). A limited number of inspectors also makes it difficult for agencies to inspect all of the housing that is registered in a given state. The North Carolina Department of Labor is not able to inspect all registered housing before it is inhabited and very rarely is it able to conduct inspections of housing that had violations at the preoccupancy inspection to ensure the quality of the housing once it is inhabited (Buhler et al. 2007).

Farmworkers face many barriers to reporting poor housing conditions in rental housing. Migrant workers new to an area are unlikely to be familiar with the local housing codes. Nor are they likely to know where to inquire about such codes. If they do not read or speak English or have limited literacy skills, they may not be able to read housing codes if they were available to them. If poor housing conditions exist and other housing options in the area are limited, the fear of losing one's housing may make a resident hesitant to report poor housing. Undocumented workers may fail to report poor housing conditions because of a fear of government officials in general or a fear that their landlord will retaliate against them by reporting them to immigration officials (Ortiz 2002). Therefore, a system that relies upon farmworkers to address poor housing conditions by reporting them to government officials is insufficient.

3.9 Housing Assistance Programs

There have been attempts nationwide to create programs to assist farmworkers with obtaining safe and affordable housing. These include federal programs that fund the construction and rehabilitation of housing for farmworkers, as well as a number of nonprofit, development, and farmworker advocacy organizations that have undertaken programs to improve farmworker housing in their service areas. However, only a small portion of farmworkers in the eastern US benefit from the housing assistance programs available for farmworkers.

The US Department of Agriculture's 514/516 Rural Development – Farm Labor Housing Loan and Grant Program provides loans and grants to finance the purchase, construction, improvement, or repair of housing for farm laborers. This program has limited reach because of strict eligibility standards that exclude workers who are in the country on an H2A agricultural guest worker visa and those who are undocumented (HAC 2006). In addition, the program is not funded at a level sufficient to meet the demand. In 2005, the Farm Labor Housing Program had $58 million in funding and received applications for two to three times that amount (HAC 2006; NFA 2005). This shows that many agricultural employers are interested in improving the housing they provide to their workers but need financial assistance to do so. Only a small portion of those who seek funding to construct or improve housing can receive the assistance they need. Furthermore, the Housing Assistance Council conducted an analysis of the 514/516 program and found that the majority of the housing units that have been funded through the program are now at least 15 years old and are beginning to show signs of deterioration (HAC 2006).

Some communities, including Orange County and Ulster County, New York, have been able to use HUD Community Development Block Grant funds to provide matching grants to employers for rehabilitating their on-farm housing (Rural Opportunities, Inc. 2000). Although the block grant program is not targeted at farmworker housing, some projects that address the quality of farmworker housing may qualify for this program.

Two other programs that target rural housing needs and may include farmworkers are the US Department of Agriculture Rural Housing Service Self-Help Housing Technical Assistance Program (Section 523) and the HUD Rural Housing and Economic Development Program (National Farmworker Alliance 2005). The purpose of the Self-Help Housing program is to "sponsor groups which will locate and work with families who will build their own homes under the self-help method. Families earn 'sweat equity,' providing many their only homeownership opportunity. Most are very low-income, minority families and nearly all obtain Section 502 Direct loans (ExpectMore.gov 2007)." In 2007, the program provided funding to build 1,277 homes; the number of those homes built by farmworkers is unspecified. The Rural Housing and Economic Development Program "provides for capacity building at the state and local level for rural housing and economic development and to support innovative housing and economic development activities in rural areas" (US Department of Housing and Urban Development (HUD) 2008b). In 2005, the program's $23.68 million budget was used to fund 103 grants, an unspecified number of which were used to provide housing assistance to farmworkers (HUD 2008b).

These programs are a valuable resource and provide much needed assistance to a small portion of farmworkers. Although these programs are beneficial to those farmworkers who are able to access them, they do not come close to meeting the vast need for improvements to farmworker housing that exists in the eastern US.

3.10   Discussion

Although regulations are in effect to ensure the quality of housing provided to farmworkers and there are a number of programs aimed at constructing high-quality farmworker housing or improving the quality of existing housing, farmworkers in the eastern US are exposed to substandard housing conditions at much higher rates than are the general US population. Studies conducted with nonfarmworker populations show that exposure to substandard conditions such as crowding, structural damage, lack of facilities and appliances, and infestations is related to a number of health problems, including stress, anxiety, respiratory problems, and infectious diseases.

OSHA's temporary labor camp standards are not successfully ensuring that farmworkers have access to safe, healthy, affordable housing. Areas in which the temporary labor camp standards are less stringent than HUD standards should be strengthened. Privies should not be considered acceptable toilet facilities. The allowance for dwellings to not have electricity should be removed. Kitchen facilities that include a sink with hot and cold running water, a refrigerator, and an oven should be required. The minimum amount of space per resident should be increased. Given the importance of bathing to remove pesticide residues, the requirement of one showerhead for every ten persons is inadequate and should be decreased to one showerhead per five persons. Because farmworkers tend to work very long hours, it is difficult for them to wash their clothes by hand. Many lack the transportation to go to laundromats on their own. Therefore, a requirement that washing machines be provided and maintained would also help to decrease workers' exposure to pesticides. For the safety of workers, locks on all doors and windows and an alternate fire exit should be required.

It is important to strengthen the temporary labor camp standards and to ensure that the standards are better enforced. Agencies should require inspectors to focus on locating unregistered housing. In addition, the consequences for failing to register housing should be more severe; it is currently a fine that is often forgiven if efforts to get housing up to standard are made. These consequences are not severe enough to make employers hesitate to take the risk that they will be discovered if they fail to follow the law.

Another avenue to improve the quality of employment-related housing would be to focus on postoccupancy inspection of farmworker housing. In many states, current enforcement of housing standards involves conducting inspections of dwellings that will be used to house farmworkers prior to their arrival. Often, if a violation is found, the employer must send a letter certifying that repairs were made before he can receive a certificate of occupancy. Owing to limited staff, the certificate of occupancy is often issued without an inspector confirming in person that the repairs were actually made. Although most employers are honest and are likely to make needed repairs whether or not their property will be reinspected, this system makes it easier for employers to be dishonest. In addition to not making needed repairs, it would be easy for an employer to house more workers in a dwelling than the number for which it is certified. Another problem with conducting only preoccupancy inspections is that it fails to ensure that housing conditions do not deteriorate during the agricultural season. With the heavy use of facilities and appliances that is common in group housing, it is expected that some things will break and need to be repaired. The current system does little to provide incentives to employers to make such repairs or to impose consequences on them for failing to do so.

An example of an incentive program to encourage agricultural employers to provide housing that meets standards is a tax credit program in which employers could claim a tax credit for all money invested in building or improving housing for their employers. This would make it easier for employers to finance high-quality housing without having to go through the application process for programs such as the US Department of Agriculture's 514/516 Rural Development program. Another possibility would be to provide employers with tax incentives for hiring a housing manager who lives in or near the camp and is responsible for ensuring that cleaning and maintenance tasks are completed regularly. The presence of a housing manager was found in a Colorado survey of farmworker housing to be associated with lower prevalence of substandard conditions (Vela-Acosta et al. 2002).

Even if the temporary labor camp standards were completely successful in eliminating substandard housing conditions for migrant farmworkers who live in employment-related housing, they would still be insufficient to guarantee quality housing for all farmworkers. While there remain a number of farmworkers who migrate along the eastern US to follow the availability of work in agriculture, these workers no longer represent the majority of farmworkers in this region of the country. The number of agricultural employers who are providing housing to their temporary laborers is decreasing. More needs to be done to guarantee the quality of housing available to those workers who must rent their housing in the private market. Creative housing solutions are needed that address the need of all farmworkers for safe, healthy, and affordable housing. Strong, well-funded programs that address rural housing quality and supply would likely be successful in improving farmworkers' access to safe housing.

Any program that attempts to ensure quality housing for all farmworkers needs to address the problem of undocumented workers, who do not qualify for federally funded programs. Federal immigration reform is needed that will allow people from foreign countries who are willing to work in US agriculture to obtain documentation status to fill agricultural jobs that cannot be filled from within the country. The current system with its demand for inexpensive labor that is not available in the US creates many problems. Undocumented workers are easy to exploit and have limited access to services that are needed to keep them healthy. Undocumented workers are susceptible to intimidation and are unlikely to report housing violations and other conditions that may be hazardous to their health.

Research is needed to determine whether farmworkers' exposure to substandard housing conditions is associated with health problems. Positive evidence will serve to strengthen the argument that farmworkers' exposure to substandard housing conditions needs to be addressed. Because any programs or changes in housing quality standards are likely to be costly, additional justification for improvement will increase the likelihood that new programs will be created. Such research would also help identify specific areas in which housing quality has the greatest effect on health so that programs can target those areas.

References

Arcury TA, Feldman SR, Schulz MR et al. (2007) Diagnosed skin diseases among migrant farmworkers in North Carolina: prevalence and risk factors. J Agric Saf Health 13:407–418

Bellinger DC (2004) Lead. Pediatrics 113(4 suppl):1016–1022

Berney B (1996) Epidemiology of childhood lead poisoning. In: Pueschel SM, Linakis J, Anderson AC (eds) Lead poisoning in childhood. Brookes, Baltimore

Bradman MA, Harnly ME, Draper W et al. (1997) Pesticide exposures to children from California's Central Valley: results of a pilot study. J Expo Anal Environ Epidemiol 7:217–234

Bradman A, Chevrier J, Tager I et al. (2005) Association of housing disrepair indicators with cockroach and rodent infestations in a cohort of pregnant Latina women and their children. Environ Health Perspect 113:1795–1801

Buhler WG, Langley RL, Luginbuhl RC et al. (2007) Violations of pesticide use and worker safety regulations in North Carolina. J Agric Saf Health 13(2):189–203

Centers for Disease Control and Prevention and US Department of Housing and Urban Development (2006) Healthy housing reference manual. US Department of Health and Human Services, Atlanta

Chew GL, Carlton EJ, Kass D et al. (2006) Determinants of cockroach and mouse exposure and associations with asthma in families and elderly individuals living in New York City public housing. Ann Allergy Asthma Immunol 97(4):502–513

Collins KJ (1993) Cold- and heat-related illnesses in the indoor environment. In: Burridge R, Ormandy D (eds) Unhealthy housing: research, remedies and reform. Spon, New York

Curl CL, Fenske RA, Kissel JC et al. (2002) Evaluation of take-home organophosphorus pesticide exposure among agricultural workers and their children. Environ Health Perspect 110:A787–A792

Early J, Davis SW, Quandt SA et al. (2006) Housing characteristics of farmworker families in North Carolina. J Immigr Minor Health 8(2):173–184

Evans GW, Lepore SJ (1993) Household crowding and social support: a quasiexperimental analysis. J Pers Soc Psychol 65:308–316

Evans GW, Lepore SJ, Shejwal BR et al. (1998) Chronic residential crowding and children's well-being: an ecological perspective. Child Dev 69(6):1514–1523

ExpectMore.gov. Detailed information on the mutual self-help housing – technical assistance grants assessment. http://www.whitehouse.gov/omb/expectmore/detail/10002038.2004.html. Cited 1 May 2008

Fenske RA, Lu C, Simcox NJ et al. (2000) Strategies for assessing children's organophosphorus pesticide exposures in agricultural communities. J Expo Anal Environ Epidemiol 10(6 Pt 2):662–671

Fenske RA, Lu C, Barr D et al. (2002) Children's exposure to chlorpyrifos and parathion in an agricultural community in central Washington State. Environ Health Perspect 110:549–553

Flocks JD, Burns AF (2006) Stakeholder analysis of Florida farmworker housing. J Agromed 11:59–67

Gabbard S (2006) Emerging trends in farmworker demographics: Results from the National Agricultural Workers' Survey. Presentation at the NACHC National Farmworker Health Conference (May), San Antonio, TX

Gentry AL, Grzywacz JG, Quandt SA et al. (2007) Housing quality among North Carolina farmworker families. J Agric Saf Health 13(3):323–337

Grieshop JI, Villanueva NE, Stiles MC (1994) Wash day blues: secondhand exposure to agricultural chemicals. J Rural Health 10:247–257

Grzywacz JG, Quandt SA, Early J et al. (2006) Leaving family for work: ambivalence and mental health among Mexican migrant farmworker men. J Immigr Minor Health 8:85–97

Guite HF, Clark C, Ackrill G (2006) The impact of the physical and urban environment on mental well-being. Public Health 120(12):1117–1126

Holden C (2000) Abundant fields, meager shelter: findings from a survey of farmworker housing in the eastern migrant stream. Housing Assistance Council, Washington, DC. http://www.ruralhome.org/pubs/farmworker/ecoast/execsummary.htm. Cited 23 Jul 2008

Holden C (2001) Migrant health issues: housing. In: Migrant health issues monograph series. National Center for Farmworker Health, Buda, TX

Holden C (2002) Bitter harvest: housing conditions of migrant and seasonal farmworkers. In: Thompson CD, Jr., Wiggins MF (eds) The human cost of food: farmworkers' lives, labor, and advocacy. University of Texas Press, Austin

Housing Assistance Council (1996) Fitting the pieces together: an examination of sources related to farmworker housing. Housing Assistance Council, Washington, DC. http://www.ruralhome.org/pubs/farmworker/pieces/fittingbody.htm. Cited 7 Feb 2008

Housing Assistance Council (2001) No refuge from the fields: findings from a survey of farmworker housing conditions in the United States. Housing Assistance Council, Washington, DC

Housing Assistance Council (2006) USDA section 514/516 farmworker housing: existing stock and changing needs. Housing Assistance Council, Washington, DC

Howard M (1993) The effects on human health of pest infestations in houses. In: Burridge R, Ormandy D (eds) Unhealthy housing: research, remedies and reform. Spon, New York

Krieger J, Higgins DL (2002) Housing and health: time again for public health action. Am J Public Health 92:758–768

Lepore SJ, Evans GW, Schneider ML (1991) Dynamic role of social support in the link between chronic stress and psychological distress. J Pers Soc Psychol 61:899–909

MacIntyre CR, Kendig N, Kummer L et al. (1997) Impact of tuberculosis control measures and crowding on the incidence of tuberculosis infection in Maryland prisons. Clin Infect Dis 24:1060–1067

Magaña CG, Hovey JD (2003) Psychosocial stressors associated with Mexican migrant farmworkers in the midwest United States. J Immigr Health 5:75–86

McCauley LA, Lasarev MR, Higgins G et al. (2001) Work characteristics and pesticide exposures among migrant agricultural families: a community-based research approach. Environ Health Perspect 109:533–538

Meister JS (1991) The health of migrant farm workers. Occup Med 6:503–518

Millstone E (1997) Lead and public health: the dangers for children. Earthscan, London

Mood EW (1993) Fundamentals of healthful housing: their application in the 21st century. In: Burridge R, Ormandy D (eds) Unhealthy housing: research, remedies and reform. Spon, New York

National Farmworker Alliance (NFA) (2005) Fairness for farmworkers agenda: a migrant and seasonal farmworker initiative. Washington, DC. http://www.foodandfarmworkers.org/fairness.htm. Cited 23 Jul 2008

Office of the High Commissioner for Human Rights. Fact sheet no. 21, the human right to adequate housing. United Nations, Geneva. http://www.unhchr.ch/html/menu6/2/fs21.htm. Cited 7 Feb 2008

Ortiz P (2002) From slavery to Cesar Chavez and beyond: farmworker organizing in the United States. In: Thompson CD, Wiggins MF (eds) The human cost of food: farmworkers' lives, labor, and advocacy. University of Texas Press, Austin

Quandt SA, Arcury TA, Mellen BG et al. (2002) Pesticides in wipes from farmworker residences in North Carolina. In: Levin H (ed) Proceedings of Indoor Air 2002, Vol 4. Santa Cruz, CA

Quandt SA, Arcury TA, Rao P et al. (2004) Agricultural and residential pesticides in wipe samples from farmworker family residences in North Carolina and Virginia. Environ Health Perspect 112:382–387

Shen X, Wu S, Yan C (2001) Impacts of low-level lead exposure on development of children: recent studies in China. Clin Chim Acta 313(1/2):217–220

State of Florida (2008) Migrant farmworker housing. Retrieved 25 Jul 2008 from http://www.doh.state.fl.us/Environment/community/migrant-labor/index.html

US Census Bureau (2006) Current housing reports, Series H-150, American housing survey for the United States: 2005. US Government Printing Office, Washington, DC

US Department of Housing and Urban Development (HUD) (2008a) Housing quality standards. HUD, Washington, DC. http://www.hud.gov/local/shared/working/r10/ph/hqs.cfm?STATE=wa. Cited 23 Jul 2008

US Department of Housing and Urban Development (HUD) (2008b) Rural housing and economic development. HUD, Washington, DC. http://www.hud.gov/offices/cpd/economicdevelopment/programs/rhed/. Cited 23 Jul 2008

US Occupational Safety and Health Administration (OSHA), US Department of Labor (2005) Regulations (Standards – 29 CFR) Temporary labor camps. 1910.142. http://www.osha.gov/pls/oshaweb/owadisp.show_document?p_table=STANDARDS&p_id=9790. Cited 23 Jul 2008

Vela-Acosta MS, Bigelow P, Buchan R (2002) Assessment of occupational health and safety risks of farmworkers in Colorado. Am J Ind Med Suppl 2:19–27

Villarejo D, Schenker M (2006) Environmental health policy and California's farm labor housing. John Muir Institute on the Environment, Davis, CA

Whyatt RM, Camann DE, Kinney PL et al. (2002) Residential pesticide use during pregnancy among a cohort of urban minority women. Environ Health Perspect 110:507–514

Chapter 4
Occupational Injury and Illness in Farmworkers in the Eastern United States

John J. May

Abstract Farmworkers experience high rates of occupational injury and illness in an industry with fatality rates seven times higher than the national average. This chapter addresses key occupational health challenges encountered by farmworkers in the eastern United States. Some are common problems likely to be encountered by those working any commodity, while others are unique to the particular mix of crops produced in this region. This chapter reviews common occupational health problems of farmworkers, including heat stress, musculoskeletal injuries, skin disease, hearing loss, eye injury, and transportation-related injuries. Because some knowledge of geographic, commodity-specific, and other patterns of illness and injury occurrence can be of considerable assistance to the clinician, examples of prominent occupational challenges associated with selected commodities are also presented. These include orchard work, tobacco production, dairy farming, and vegetable and berry production. Recommendations for more effective protections for farmworkers and for further research are presented.

4.1 Introduction

Few populations of workers in the United States (US) are so readily acknowledged to be socially and economically disadvantaged as the nation's migrant and seasonal farmworkers. Agriculture as a whole is a dangerous industry, with rates of occupational fatality and injury that are seven times the national average (Bureau of Labor Statistics 2007a). Migrant and seasonal farmworkers often face the worst working conditions within this dangerous industry.

Data on the degree to which the migrant and seasonal farmworker population experiences occupational injuries and illnesses are quite limited and generally inadequate. The traditional sources of such data simply do not provide reliable information for this population of workers. Injury logs used for reporting to the Occupational Safety and Health Administration (OSHA) and Workers' Compensation statistics are at best suspect with this group of workers. The problem of underreporting is substantial and leads to very limited information being available to assess the issue of occupational illness and injury affecting workers in the eastern US (Azaroff et al. 2002).

T.A. Arcury and S.A. Quandt (eds.), *Latino Farmworkers in Eastern United States*,
DOI: 10.1007/978-0-387-88347-2_4, © Springer Science+Business Media, LLC 2009

Migrant and seasonal farmworkers are hired on a temporary basis, most without benefits or the protections other workers enjoy. Manual crop work often requires prolonged repetitive motions, lifting heavy weights, holding awkward postures for extended periods, exposure to toxic chemicals, and use of sharp tools. These workers may be paid piece-rate, which under the pressure of the short harvest period, discourages adequate breaks and rest. Basic hydration and hygiene facilities are often not readily available at the work site. Workers' cultural and linguistic isolation and their uncertain legal status add to their extreme dependency upon the employer. This marked imbalance of power serves to enhance their susceptibility to occupational safety risks (Wilk 1988; Mobed et al. 1992). Given the organizational structure of these jobs, it is unlikely that OSHA reporting mechanisms will ever accurately reflect illness and injury rates.

Agricultural work exposes the worker to myriad occupational health challenges. The problem of pesticide exposure has been the focus of most occupational health concerns in farmworkers for decades (Chap. 5). Recent data indicate a number of other significant occupational threats for these workers. Some of these are issues familiar to the occupational health practitioner: people being forced to fit the job, rather than vice versa; employers focused entirely upon short-term issues of production and costs; unhealthy rates of work; and unhealthy work conditions. Other occupational problems for migrant farmworkers in the eastern US may be less familiar to occupational health professionals: chemical intoxications, heat stress, unusual working conditions, limited access to care, and linguistic and cultural differences. These are complex issues that would challenge most occupational health experts. Currently, they are routinely presented to primary care practitioners who often feel ill-equipped to address them effectively. The unavailability of appropriate support for these workers and health professionals reflects the lack of respect our society affords these essential workers.

This chapter provides an overview of some of the more significant occupational health problems experienced by migrant and seasonal farmworkers as they grow and harvest large proportions of eastern states' overall agricultural production. Examined first are some of the problems that may occur commonly in a number of locations and with many commodities. Subsequent discussion of selected specific commodities illustrates how each can present unique challenges that require the health professional to have some understanding of the specific work process. Throughout the chapter limited comments on treatment and prevention are provided. Recommendations on steps to improve the understanding and prevention of occupational health problems in farmworkers in the eastern US are provided at the end of this chapter. Clearly, a full appreciation of the health problems for this population of workers can only be gained by carefully reviewing information on pesticides, mental health, infectious diseases, and other challenges discussed in subsequent chapters.

4.1.1   The Role of Culture in Farmworker Occupational Injury

Farmers have their own culture (see Sect. 2.4.2), as do farmworkers (see Sect. 2.6). The farmer–farmworker interaction represents the intersection of these two distinct cultures – neither readily understood by the health professional or outside observer.

Farmers have a remarkably high tolerance for risk, believing that most things will work out in the end (Sorensen et al. 2008). While acknowledging the dangers inherent in farming, farmers often adopt an optimistic bias with regard to hazard (Weinstein 1988). Farmers generally place greater priority on efficient production than on safety, and they see most safety measures as contributing little to their efficiency and productivity. At the same time, farmers express considerable concern regarding the safety of spouses, children, and employees. This attitude is reflected in decisions to personally undertake the most risky tasks and in the resultant elevated rates of injuries to farmers, compared to employees on small family farms (Pratt et al. 1992).

The farmer's high tolerance of risk, denial of susceptibility, and skepticism regarding safety measures may contribute significantly to the woes encountered by some of the farmworker employees. The exposure of these workers to hazards, such as heat, chemicals, and falls, often reflects the farmers' personal approach to risk and prevention. Farmworkers' beliefs and values may exacerbate the potential for occupational injury. Their beliefs about the role of fate and supernatural factors in their health and safety, their recognition of limited power relative to their employers, their expectation that work will be physically demanding, and their financial need to keep their jobs and maximize income often lead them to continue working in the face of imminent pain, injury, and illness.

4.1.2 Data on Migrant Occupational Illness and Injury

Throughout the remaining discussion, apologies regarding the paucity of data will be ubiquitous. In part, this reflects the overall situation in agriculture. However, in the case of farmworkers, this problem is compounded. Papers in the literature are few, particularly when one focuses upon the experience of workers in the eastern US. Published rates are virtually nonexistent; for most of this work there are significant questions regarding both numerators and denominators.

4.1.2.1 Numerator Problems

Many farmworkers are not particularly interested in being studied (Earle-Richardson et al. 1998). When they are injured, they have limited access to health care, and for financial, social, and legal reasons, may avoid interactions with the medical establishment. Both the cost of care and the time lost from work are important financial considerations. Many workers may not completely accept medicine as practiced in the US and are likely to use home remedies or seek treatment from healers within their community. Certainly those who are undocumented will have a powerful disincentive to seek medical care or to participate in any research projects. This population can be hard to access and much of the literature relies upon sampling that is little better than convenience sampling, with all of its attendant biases. In recent years several methodologies have been developed that represent an improvement

(Arcury et al. 2003b; Earle-Richardson et al. 2008), but these continue to have limitations. The camp sampling methods used in North Carolina can suffer if some camps are not identified or are not sampled for reasons that might inject unrecognized biases. The selection of those within the camp to sample can result in data that are not fully representative. The review of medical charts from migrant clinics and emergency rooms presumes that those seeking care at these sites are representative of all farmworkers in the region. Problems can arise with accurate recognition, diagnosis, and sufficient documentation in the notes to enable identification of an occupationally related injury or illness in subsequent chart reviews. All of these issues lead to some uncertainty regarding the number of adverse health events actually being experienced by migrant farmworkers in the eastern US.

Further complicating matters is the migratory nature of some of this work force. Does a musculoskeletal injury in a Pennsylvania orchard worker relate to orchard work? Might this injury actually relate to cucumber work done previously in North Carolina? In some unknown number of cases an identified health problem relates more directly to activities done further downstream in the recent or remote past. In other cases an injury may have occurred in one work setting, but then have been further exacerbated by different work in a different location.

4.1.2.2 Denominator Problems

Although figures are quoted repeatedly throughout the literature and throughout this book, in fact there is no clear understanding of how many farmworkers are employed in the eastern US or elsewhere in the country. The literature often refers to estimates produced by the Health Resources and Services Administration (HRSA) in the late 1980s (HRSA 1990). Alternate estimates are based upon the Larson's minimum labor demand methodology (Larsen and Plascencia 1993; Larson 2000). Using figures relating the number of hours of worker time required to produce a given amount of a commodity product, Larson was able to estimate the total number of workers required in each state to account for its reported agricultural production of a series of different labor-intensive commodities.

Each state currently makes various estimates of the number of migrant farmworkers employed. In New York estimates are now made by both the Department of Agriculture and Markets and the Department of Labor. The traditional estimates made by the Department of Labor rely upon mandatory reporting by any farm employing more than five workers or any contractor employing any number of workers. Comparison of these figures with those derived using Larson's methodology shows considerable divergence, with the minimum labor demand calculations estimating nearly twice as many workers (Earle-Richardson et al. 2005a). Efforts based upon accumulating counts from various farmworker advocacy and support organizations have proven equally difficult (Borjan et al. 2008). These examples of the underlying uncertainty regarding the number of workers illustrate the significant challenges in any efforts aimed at establishing rates of specific injuries or illnesses in farmworkers.

The general absence of reliable numerator and denominator figures represents a substantial challenge to establishing priorities for intervention. Subsequently, this problem will also complicate the assessment of effect of any interventions that are implemented. Assessment of long-term outcomes of either exposures or of interventions is substantially challenged by the migratory nature of this workforce.

4.2 Access to Optimal Health Care

Access of farmworkers and their families to appropriate health care is a matter of social justice. These workers are as entitled as any other workers in America to health care that is suitable to address their occupational exposures (American College of Occupational and Environmental Medicine 1993). Often this is not the case. In some cases these workers may receive excellent primary care services through various migrant health programs or other sources. However, as will be noted in this and subsequent chapters, farmworkers are at risk for a number of specific health problems related to their work and living situations. Most clinicians caring for these workers and families, despite expertise in primary care, may have limited comfort in the areas of occupational health (Institute of Medicine 1988), toxicology, complex infectious diseases, and cultural and psychological issues affecting Latino/Hispanic workers. Recent data from farmworkers in New York and Maine indicate that roughly 60% of workers obtain care from either a local emergency department or, more commonly, from a nearby migrant health facility (Earle-Richardson et al. 2008). Surveys of clinicians working in migrant clinics have documented quite limited training in occupational health and some level of discomfort in diagnosing and treating these problems (Liebman and Harper 2001). Yet reviews of migrant clinic charts in New York and Pennsylvania demonstrated that more than 10% (and in some clinics considerably more) of all visits related to occupational problems (Earle-Richardson et al. 2004).

A similar situation exists regarding the diagnosis and treatment of pesticide exposures. *The National Strategies for Health Care Providers: Pesticides Initiative* is a partnership of the Environmental Protection Agency, the US Departments of Health and Human Resources, Labor and Agriculture, and the National Environmental Education and Training Foundation begun in 1998 to address concerns that clinicians are poorly prepared to deal with occupational and environmental exposures to pesticides (Institute of Medicine 1993). Publications from this group have included a publication on recognition and treatment of poisonings (Reigart and Roberts 1999) and more recent practice guidelines for physicians and nurses (The National Environmental Education and Training Foundation 2003).

Addressing the many social inequities relating to health-care access will require improved availability for all farmworkers to culturally sensitive, affordable primary care services. These must be enhanced by provision of appropriate skills and support to clinicians caring for farmworkers and their families to assure that the important problems linked to this population's work exposures and life style can be adequately addressed.

4.3   Common Occupational Health Problems

Although many of the occupational hazards encountered by migrant farmworkers are universal issues affecting workers across commodities and across the eastern US, others are quite specific issues encountered only in a specific commodity. The following discussion addresses the problems that tend to be generalized first. This is followed by examples of selected commodities known to have unique occupational health challenges.

4.3.1   Heat Stress

4.3.1.1   Heat Hazards for Farmworkers

Farmworkers acquire heat from the environment and from solar radiation, but mainly from heat generation arising from strenuous muscular activity. Hyperthermia occurs with the failure of various regulatory mechanisms that might normally compensate for this heat loading. Definitive data on the incidence of heat stress and heat stroke are unknown for farmworkers. Migrant health programs in the US reported more than 1,000 visits for dehydration or heat–cold exposures in 2006, and it is likely that this is an underestimate (HRSA 2007). During 1992–2006, 68 crop workers died from heat stress; these deaths occurred at a rate 20 times greater than for the entire US civilian work force (Luginbuhl et al. 2008). On the basis of factors known to increase risk, this is a population of concern, with particular risk encountered by those working in the southern half of the eastern US.

The farmworker's primary defense against overheating is evaporative heat losses from the skin surface. Peak sweating rates may be as high as 2 L h^{-1} (Bouchama and Knochel 2002). The efficiency of evaporation has an important effect upon heat loss. Determinants affecting this include clothing, hydration, and the ambient relative humidity. As humidity increases, evaporation slows and cooling is impaired.

Important factors determining a farmworker's risk for hyperthermia include ambient temperature and humidity; the effect of solar radiation as moderated by both cloud cover and clothing; the intensity of muscular work; the impact of clothing choices on heat loss via radiation, convection and evaporation; and adequate fluid volume for both redistribution of blood flow to the skin and maximal sweat production. Another important consideration is acclimatization. Over the course of several weeks of thermal stimulation, the worker's fluid intake increases, kidney mechanisms shift toward fluid preservation, blood volume increases, maximal sweat production goes up, and clothing and heat avoidance behaviors become refined. Once acclimatized, the worker is less susceptible to the risk of hyperthermia (Bouchama and Knochel 2002).

4.3.1.2   Diagnosis and Treatment of Heat Stress

Farmworkers developing problems related to heat initially manifest dehydration related to excessive losses and inadequate fluid intake. Declining urine output and rising urine concentration serve as useful indicators of inadequate hydration. The appearance of heat cramps, particularly affecting calves and abdomen, is the first obvious symptom that might warn the farmworker of impending heat-related problems. Heat exhaustion is present when body temperature exceeds 37°C and headache, muscle pain, and lightheadedness appear. The onset of confusion, nausea, and vomiting at this stage is particularly onerous because it removes the potential for oral rehydration. Heat stroke is associated with hot, dry skin and confusion, convulsions, or coma (Bouchama and Knochel 2002). This is a potentially disastrous occurrence that can lead to damage of multiple organs and even death.

Treatment focuses upon cooling and support of organ-system function. Cooling efforts should involve removal of clothing and application of cooling packs to armpits, groin and neck. Use of a fan or other source of moving air will enhance convective heat losses, and spraying the skin with water will enhance evaporative losses. Aggressive rehydration with intravenous fluids is of great importance, although the total volume depletion may be less than would be expected in many of these patients (Seraj et al. 1991). The risk of serious complications in these workers is considerable and prompt medical evaluation is needed.

4.3.1.3   Prevention of Heat Injury

Farmworkers must have ready access to ample potable water. One half to one quart of water per hour may be needed as the temperature increases from 80 to 90°F. During periods of high risk, farmworkers should hydrate to the point that they are urinating frequently with light-colored, dilute urine. One potentially unanticipated problem with provision of water to workers is the belief among some groups that hot–cold imbalance leads to illness (Flores 2000). This may cause workers to hesitate to drink sufficient volumes of water (which is considered metaphorically "cold") while working in hot weather.

Those supervising the work must be aware of the effects of temperature and humidity. Short work breaks and use of shade are encouraged. Employers, contractors, and workers must recognize the heightened sensitivity of those who have not undergone the 2–3 weeks of acclimatization. It is important to assure use of hats and appropriate clothing to limit heat acquisition from the sun while not greatly impairing heat losses. In general, lightweight, loose-fitting, light-colored, breathable clothes are favored. Recognition of early warning signs such as cramping, muscle pain, weakness, and lightheadedness should prompt immediate cessation of physical exertion, aggressive oral hydration, and removal to a cooler environment.

4.3.2 Musculoskeletal Injuries and Illness

4.3.2.1 Musculoskeletal Injuries Affecting Farmworkers

Work-related musculoskeletal disorders are among the most common problems affecting farmworkers. The National Institute for Occupational Safety and Health (NIOSH) defines these as "injuries or disorders of the muscles, nerves, tendons, joints, cartilage, and spinal discs." Among these are "sprains, strains, tears; back pain, … carpal tunnel syndrome" and other problems occurring in response to "bending, climbing, crawling, reaching, twisting, overexertion, or repetitive motion" (NIOSH 2004). These disorders include a broad spectrum of problems that can be placed into three groups: (1) peripheral neuropathies arising from carpal and cubital tunnel syndromes; (2) tendonitis and epicondylitis; and (3) other musculoskeletal disorders, including strains and muscle pain, rotator cuff injuries, bursitis, and others (Morse et al. 2005). Major factors are excessive load, rapidly repeating motions, and sustained awkward postures, which are all common experiences for the farmworker.

Musculoskeletal disorders account for nearly half of all agricultural occupational illnesses and injuries (Bureau of Labor Statistics 2007c). In most cases, these musculoskeletal disorders represent an accumulation of microtrauma in a setting of insufficient opportunity to recover. Any activity requiring moderate or greater force, work cycles of 30 s or less, or consistently less recovery time than work time in a cycle places the worker at considerable risk of musculoskeletal disorders (Latko et al. 1999; Stock 1991).

In the case of farmworkers in the eastern US, the neck, shoulders, upper extremities, and back are affected by the repetitive, work-related overloading of selected muscle groups. More than 200 physicians caring for migrant workers in Georgia rated musculoskeletal problems as the fourth most common problem seen (Tedders et al. 1998). In the Northeast, Earle-Richardson et al. (2003) used a methodology based upon systematic review of medical visits to migrant health facilities and emergency rooms in Pennsylvania and New York to identify occupational injury/illness cases over a 2-year period (1997–1999). Of 516 cases identified, 162 (31%) related to muscle or joint injuries. Three quarters of these affected the trunk and shoulders, with the remainder involving the extremities. Subsequent work using systematic interviews of all workers in randomly selected New York camps has validated the clinic record surveillance methodology and suggests a somewhat higher proportion (45%) of musculoskeletal disorders (Earle-Richardson et al. 2008). As per clinic notes, the vast majority of these injuries related to overwork, overuse, or awkward posture; and many of these injuries seen in the Northeast related to work in apple orchards. Given the extent of orchard work done by farmworkers from Maine to Florida, it seems reasonable to assume that large numbers of farmworkers in the eastern US are at risk of musculoskeletal disorders.

Other commodities have been associated with different types of musculoskeletal disorders. Data from blueberry rakers in Maine have suggested that the tendonitis and epichondylitis pattern is common here. Harvesting of some vegetables involves combined motions of spinal flexion and extension, partial rotation of the trunk, and throwing of the produce back over the shoulder. All of this is repeated several times a minute for long days with very limited recovery time. Mushroom work often requires sustained difficult postures. Harvesting mushrooms exposes workers to highly repetitive movements at high rates of speed. Tobacco harvesting, particularly the lowest leaves, involves continuous forward bending of the spine.

4.3.2.2 Diagnosis and Treatment of Musculoskeletal Disorders

Diagnosis of musculoskeletal disorders is seldom challenging for the health professional who has even limited insight into the nature of the work being performed. Usually a few extra moments learning from the patient about the motions and forces associated with any repetitive tasks can readily explain the etiology of most musculoskeletal complaints. The intensity of the worker's symptoms generally correlates well with the intensity of the work. For some of these disorders the role of underlying medical conditions such as diabetes, hypothyroidism, obesity, and arthritis must be considered.

Musculoskeletal disorders are caused by overuse and are ideally treated with rest, anti-inflammatory agents, and when appropriate, splinting, physical therapy, and gradual rehabilitation. Unfortunately, farmworkers are subject to considerable pressure, both internal and external, to continue to work at highly productive rates. Advice that they rest more and slow down is not helpful. Ready access to joint injections, splinting, physical therapy modalities, and rehabilitation is possible for some workers in America, but not the farmworker population. Many farmworkers currently rely upon home remedies and over–the-counter anti-inflammatory agents while they continue injurious repetitive work activities.

4.3.2.3 Musculoskeletal Disorder Solutions

Clearly, one solution to physically demanding, highly repetitive agricultural work is increased mechanization. In commodities in which this approach has been taken, the small number of remaining workers may be exposed to a new set of mechanical hazards, while the majority of workers no longer have a job. Other commodities continue to rely upon manual labor based upon considerations of capital expenditures, terrain, availability of reliable workers, and various social and economic considerations. The challenge is to address those aspects of the work that are most demanding and most likely to induce musculoskeletal disorders.

Interventions ranging from administrative changes to altered work procedures to redesign of commonly used tools can reduce the hazard from physically demanding repetitive tasks (Baron et al. 2001). Job redesign efforts in California reduced awkward postures, forceful thumb-finger pinches, and repetitive bending and twisting (Janowitz et al. 1998). Introduction of hourly 5-min rest breaks significantly decreased musculoskeletal disorders symptoms in California farmworkers (Faucett et al. 2007). Adoption of different tools and processes led to less musculoskeletal disorder hazards with equal or improved production among midwestern vegetable producers (Chapman et al. 2004). Community-based approaches can effectively combine the expertise of ergonomists and researchers with the expertise of the workers, farm owners, and cooperative extension personnel (Scharf et al. 1998; Hawkes et al. 2007). Process and tool redesign approaches can be considered and interventions can be systematically tested. With key contributions from northeastern farmworkers and their employers, this approach has led to successful redesign of the picking bucket used in orchard work (Earle-Richardson et al. 2005b) and the rake used for harvesting blueberries (May et al. 2008).

4.3.3   Skin Disease

4.3.3.1   Skin Disorders Affecting Farmworkers

Occupational dermatitis occurs much more commonly in production agriculture than in the general population of American workers (Bureau of Labor Statistics 2007b). Rates are particularly high for the "crop production" category, especially greenhouse, nursery, floriculture, and fruit farming. Among farmworkers in the eastern US, this has been best studied in North Carolina, where more than half of the farmworkers described skin problems. Sunburn and fungal infection led the list, followed by acne, "skin rash," and "itching" reported by more than 40% (Vallejos et al. 2008). It appears that these problems may evolve over the course of the growing season, rising from nearly 25% early to 37% late in the season (Arcury et al. 2003a). Dermatological examination of residents of two camps in North Carolina documented the presence of skin disease in 47 of 59 (80%) workers examined (Krejci-Manwaring et al. 2006).

Fungal infection of the skin, scalp, and nails is commonly reported. In the 47 cases noted above, fungal infections of the feet and nails accounted for 28 (nearly 60%) of the cases. These infections can be readily transmitted from person-to-person, from animals or contaminated surfaces. The housing conditions and shared shower facilities in many migrant farmworker camps (Early et al. 2006) likely play a significant role in the persistence and spread of these problems.

Six to twelve percent of skin disease noted in surveys of North Carolina farm-workers related to contact dermatitis (Krejci-Manwaring et al. 2006; Arcury et al. 2008). In 2006, the federally funded migrant health programs reported roughly 14,000 contact dermatitis cases (HRSA 2007). This could be a response to a primary irritant or to an allergic sensitizing agent. Irritant contact dermatitis (80% of all contact dermatitis) is a nonallergic reaction appearing within minutes of contact with a wide variety of irritating substances. The itchy eruptions affecting the upper extremity flexor surfaces of North Carolina tobacco workers, noted by Abraham et al. (2007), may well be examples of irritant-induced contact dermatitis. These reactions may occur to endogenous plant components or to chemicals that have been applied to the plants (Schuman and Dobson 1985).

Allergic contact dermatitis requires a period of 1–3 weeks for the initial sensitization. With subsequent contacts, dermatitis appears within hours or days. As most people do not react to the majority of sensitizers, allergic contact dermatitis is relatively uncommon. An exception to this is urushiol, the allergen found in poison ivy, oak, and sumac, to which a majority of the population reacts. This most certainly includes farmworkers who are likely to be exposed while working in orchards and other sites.

The ultraviolet waves of the sun are a significant skin hazard. Phototoxic or photoallergic reactions to a sensitizing agent (topical or systemic) can cause itching, local redness, and blistering in sun-exposed workers. Antibiotics and other drugs, as well as a number of plant-derived compounds, can be responsible for these reactions. Typically these occur on the sun-exposed surfaces of individuals with relatively limited pigment in their skin. The occurrence of premalignant and malignant skin lesions is fairly common in farmers. At public screening events in New York and Pennsylvania roughly 25% of farmers are typically referred to a dermatologist for evaluation of a lesion (Evans and May, unpublished data). The vast majority of these prove to be premalignant changes such as actinic keratoses, generally appearing upon sun-exposed surfaces of the face, ears, or upper extremities. While there is clearly a selection bias in these public screening events, the more systematic selection involved in the New York Farm Family Health and Hazard Survey yielded quite similar findings (May, unpublished data). Of the malignancies detected, two thirds were basal cell cancers and nearly all others were squamous cell cancers. It should be noted that these findings apply to a population composed largely of family farmers of northern European ancestry. There are remarkably little data regarding the rates of these problems in eastern farmworkers and this should be an area of future study.

4.3.3.2 Skin Disease Solutions

Ideally solar radiation should be avoided. The use of light, loose-fitting clothing, and appropriate hats can do much to reduce skin damage from UVA and UVB light. Topical sun-blocking agents can substantially reduce exposure, but it is not likely that most farmworkers will routinely apply sufficient amounts to make this an effective strategy. While clothing worn in the field can reduce some of the contact dermatitis problems, it also is potentially contaminated and needs to be removed promptly at the end of the workday and laundered separately from other noncontaminated clothing. Use of gloves (watching for latex allergy!) when feasible for the job may be helpful in reducing some of the mechanical and chemical trauma to the skin. Daily showering and routine use of nonirritating cleansing agents are recommended.

4.3.4 Hearing Loss

4.3.4.1 Hearing Loss Occurring in Eastern Agriculture

Hearing loss, typically noise-induced, is very common among farm populations (Marvel et al. 1991; Gomez et al. 2001). Substantial noise has been documented around agricultural equipment in New York (Dennis and May 1995). Information

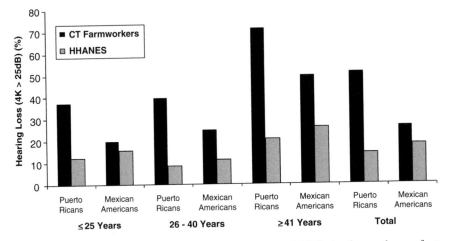

Fig. 4.1 Prevalence of hearing loss at 4,000 Hz by age category. Male Latino farmworkers perform consistently worse than Hispanic males in the Hispanic Health and Nutrition Examination Survey (HHANES) (Rabinowitz et al. 2005)

on hearing loss for farmworkers in the eastern US is limited to one report focusing upon a self-selected group of 150 predominantly Mexican men (mean age, 34 years) in Connecticut River Valley migrant camps (Rabinowitz et al. 2005). The majority of these people were tobacco workers; smaller proportions worked in nursery and fruit orchards. They were thoroughly evaluated with a survey questionnaire, tympanometry, and pure tone audiometry. Twelve percent of these workers met criteria for hearing impairment and more than half showed evidence of deficits (≥25 dB) at one or more frequencies. Subjectively, 35% complained of difficulty hearing or understanding speech. When compared with the findings of the 1982–1984 Hispanic Health and Nutrition Examination Survey (HHANES), the farmworkers demonstrated consistently worse high-frequency perception in all age groups (Fig. 4.1).

4.3.4.2 Causes of Hearing Loss in Farmworkers

The obvious cause of these findings is exposure to hazardous noise (>80 dB) in the work environment, particularly as only 14% of workers, mainly nursery, reported using appropriate hearing protection. However, currently no data regarding the level of noise encountered by these workers are available, and it might be expected that because of less exposure to farm machinery, their total noise exposures would be less than other agricultural workers. Baseline information on rates of hearing loss in their native populations would be of interest in light of the ready access to antibiotics and other agents that affect hearing in some countries of origin. The effects of recreational noise, agrichemicals, and other toxin exposures need further investigation. A better understanding of other nonagricultural occupational exposures encountered by these workers might provide important insight into their increased levels of hearing loss.

4.3.4.3 Hearing Loss Solutions

As in other prevention situations, engineering approaches to hearing loss are preferred. In agriculture, tightening a few screws to reduce metal vibration on machinery and replacing defective mufflers can do much to reduce ambient noise. However, the most apparent solution to this problem is provision of inexpensive hearing protection for workers and instruction on its proper use. Earmuffs can be easily put on and off, but are bulky and can be misplaced, and so earplugs are preferred by many workers. These should be available in any settings where background noise requires workers to raise their voices to be heard. Attention must be given to proper insertion techniques and to cleanliness of the earplugs after repeated use. Care must be taken to avoid contamination with agrichemicals prior to insertion in the ear. Further audiometric assessment of other migrant populations would be of considerable interest as would systematic area or personal noise sampling of the various work environments commonly encountered.

4.3.5 Eye Injury

4.3.5.1 Eye Injuries Affecting Eastern Farmworkers

Eye injuries have been reported in agriculture for many decades (Smith 1940). These certainly can affect farmworkers. Penetrating ocular injuries or other acute trauma can result from contact with plants, particularly in orchard work, or tasks such as the sharpening of a hoe. Chronic eye problems, such as irritation, pterygium, and cataract, can arise from the combination of wind, dust, and UV light that is nearly ubiquitous in most commodities. The US Department of Labor has documented nearly 37,000 eye injuries affecting American workers in 2004 (Harris 2006). Of these, 700 involved reports from agricultural operations. However, capture of these injuries by BLS is suspect. It is estimated to be less than a quarter of the actual number of events (Lacey et al. 2007). The data on eye injuries affecting migrant farmworkers in the eastern US are few.

Exposure to agrichemicals poses some specific risks for workers. Data from pesticide applicators in North Carolina and Iowa suggest that several types of fungicide are related to retinal degeneration in both applicators and their wives (Kirrane et al. 2005). The most common specific agents were three dithiocarbamate compounds: maneb, mancozeb, and ziram. The Japanese literature describes a series of disorders ("Saku Disease") related to organophosphate agents, which can be readily absorbed into the chambers of the eye following topical application, eventually reaching the cells of the retina (Boyes et al. 1994). Manifestations of these exposures range from problems at the level of the lens to pathologic changes in the retina (Dementi 1994).

4.3.5.2   Chronic Irritation of the Eyes

Most commonly farmworkers experience problems with chronic conjunctivitis affecting the tissue covering the eye, or blepharitis, an inflammation affecting the margin of the lid. When North Carolina farmworkers from randomly selected housing sites were interviewed over the course of a growing season, they noted the presence of a number of eye symptoms. This predominantly Mexican group of 197 tobacco and cucumber workers experienced eye pain (40%), redness (43%), itching (25%), and blurred vision (13%). More than 98% of these workers wore no sunglasses while in the fields. Half stated that sunglasses interfered with their work and their ability to differentiate ripe from green leaves (Quandt et al. 2001b). Vegetable workers (and farm owners) in New York complain that the fine black soil of the region produces eye irritation. A cohort of 99 of these workers described proportions of eye symptoms similar to those found in North Carolina: eye pain (44%), redness (35%), itching (35%), and blurred vision (34%). Following early season trainings, the use of sunglasses or protective eyewear ("sometimes" or "always") was in the range of 90% (May, unpublished data).

4.3.5.3   Cataract and Pterygium

Although there are no reports on cataract rates in eastern farmworkers, their extensive exposure to solar ultraviolet radiation would be expected to result in elevated risk for the opacities of the lens. Another effect of solar radiation, combined with other sources of chronic irritation (wind, dust), is the development of pterygium. This wedge-shaped fleshy growth of conjunctival tissue extends across the surface of the eye, typically extending from the inner corner of the eye toward the pupil. These may grow to be large enough to actually obscure vision, though this is rare. More commonly pterygia cause ongoing irritation and redness by interfering with the normal lubricating mechanism of the eye. In the only relevant study of this problem, digital photographs of 304 North Carolina farmworkers documented a 23% prevalence (10% bilateral) of this problem (Taylor et al. 2006). Treatment of these lesions may require surgery if it becomes so extensive as to obscure vision, though more often lubricating eye drops, possibly topical steroid drops, and sunglasses or protective UV-blocking glasses are recommended.

4.3.5.4   Eyesight and Eye Care

Good vision is important for safety in hazardous occupations such as farm work. Only a single study has documented the general eyesight of farmworkers in the eastern US and the eye care they have received. Using interviews conducted with

79 farmworkers recruited at clinics in North Carolina, Quandt et al. (2008) found that 21.3% of these farmworkers reported fair or poor eyesight. More than 11% reported difficulty in recognizing a friend across the street, and 19.5% reported difficulty in reading. About 20% of these farmworkers reported each of several eye symptoms. At the same time, only 4 of the 79 farmworkers reported wearing glasses or contact lenses, and 38% reported never having visited any eye care professional. It is apparent that farmworkers in the eastern US have a high level of unmet need for both routine preventive eye care and treatment or correction of vision problems.

4.3.5.5 Eye Injury Solutions

Relying entirely upon protective equipment is not viewed as desirable in occupational health, but in this case use of carefully selected protective glasses is the most realistic solution. Such eyewear should provide protection from both UVA and UVB rays, thus reducing risk of problems such as cataract and pterygium. These high-impact glasses have side shields to limit the risk of foreign bodies and trauma from plants and also to reduce exposure of the conjunctiva and cornea to the effects of dust and wind. North Carolina workers have avoided use of glasses (Quandt et al. 2001b), for many of the same concerns about appearance, discomfort, perspiration and fogging, slowing work processes, and interference with vision voiced by workers in the Midwest (Forst et al. 2006).

The experience with workers in New York parallels that of Midwestern farmworkers who adopted use of safety glasses after distribution of eyewear and training by community health workers (Forst et al. 2004). Initially, New York vegetable workers experienced fogging and discomfort with some designs and problems seeing spoilage on lettuce leaves with dark lenses. But after some trial and error, they settled upon a design that was comfortable and socially acceptable. They were able to identify lens colors (yellow) that did not interfere with their work efficiency. As the wearing of protective glasses became a social norm, general acceptance increased substantially. The use of small plastic vials of sterile saline solution for immediate eye irrigation and moisturizing further reduced irritative symptoms (May, unpublished data). The use of camp health aides to model behavior and provide peer-to-peer education stimulated increased positive perception of protective eyewear among Florida citrus workers (Luque et al. 2007) (Fig. 4.2). A recent review from the Midwest notes the situations in which redesign of aspects of the tasks or selection of alternate tools may reduce the risk of eye injury (Lacey et al. 2007).

4.3.6 Transportation

4.3.6.1 Transportation Injuries Affecting Farmworkers

There is remarkably little in the literature regarding transportation deaths in migrant farmworkers, particularly in the eastern US. This is surprising as motor vehicle incidents are the leading contributor to overall occupational fatality and appear to

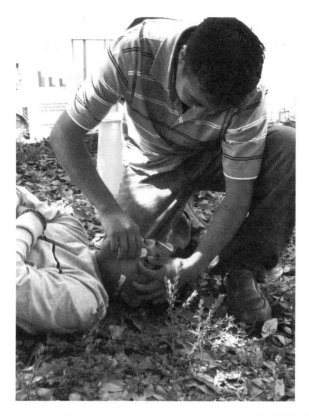

Fig. 4.2 Camp health aide demonstrates emergency use of eye wash in the fields (Photograph by Jason Lind)

be a significant source of fatality among migrant farmworkers (NIOSH 2003). In a 2001 report of farmworker deaths across 24 states, farmworkers from the Northeast and Southeast accounted for nearly 60% of the total. Of the injury-related deaths in the group, 53% were due to motor vehicles (Colt et al. 2001). The agriculture, forestry, and fishing sector consistently has rates of highway fatalities that are second only to the transportation industry itself (MMWR 2004). Considerable confusion surrounds the interpretation of "transportation fatalities," and the distinction of "vehicle" vs. "machinery" in some of the published literature. Unfortunately, the Bureau of Labor Statistics has further confounded the situation by distributing tractor-related fatalities among the vehicle, machinery, and several other categories in the Census of Fatal Occupational Injuries (CFOI) statistics (Murphy and Yoder 1998). To compound the problems, the determination of when a highway collision is "occupational" is also arbitrary. The CFOI database excludes incidents that occur during the commute to or from work, unless traveling from a camp.

While substantial numbers of tractor-motor vehicle crashes have been documented in North Carolina, it is unlikely that many of these involve migrant farmworkers, who typically do not operate farm machinery (Luginbuhl et al. 2003). What does appear to be certain is that farmworkers, particularly those born outside the US and whose English language skills are limited, are at risk on rural highways when they are going to and from work or traveling between fields. A study on farmworkers in California's Central Valley assessed driving behaviors by using both questionnaires and unobtrusive systematic observations of 126 vehicles being driven in Central Valley labor camps. This work documented an increased incidence of adverse outcomes (including revoked licenses, citations and crashes) and unsafe driving behaviors among those licensed in Mexico and those driving without licenses. Among all drivers, 79% were licensed. Only 58% learned to drive in the US and those who learned to drive in Mexico learned at an early age (20% between ages 8 and 14 years.) Observed use of seat belts was 37%, and compliance with belting of passengers, children, and use of child seats was low (Stiles and Grieshop 1999). In Steinhorst's study on Hispanic farmworkers admitted to a North Carolina trauma center, 51% of injuries were related to motor vehicle crashes, though the vast majority of these were not work-related. Significant factors in the incidence and severity of these injuries included the low rates of seat belt and airbag usage (40%) and the high rates of positive blood alcohol levels (66%) (Steinhorst et al. 2006).

It is likely that the factors traditionally associated with fatal crashes (running off the road or failing to stay in the proper lane, driving over the speed limit or too fast for conditions, driver inattention, and driver drowsiness [MMWR 2004]) are involved in these farmworker crashes as well. Compounding the problem are factors relating to social justice: poverty, education, and social problems. These workers often have little recourse other than the use of old and poorly maintained vehicles that are often overcrowded. Poor understanding of traffic laws, unavailability of seatbelts or lack of seatbelt use and, in some cases, the use of alcohol certainly contribute to the hazard. When incidents do occur, payment of medical costs, lost work, and even repatriation of remains often fall upon the farmworker and family.

4.3.6.2 Transportation Solutions

In situations where farmworkers are being transported by the employer or by a contractor, strict enforcement of licensing requirements for drivers, of inspection and safety requirements for vehicles, and of occupancy and seatbelt laws for passengers by local and state police is needed. Substantial fines from local traffic enforcement and from OSHA are entirely appropriate. Similar enforcement is appropriate for farmworkers driving personal vehicles, but educational interventions might also be used in an effort to reduce both crashes and problems with law enforcement. Undocumented farmworkers' inability to obtain drivers licenses may not restrict their driving, but certainly restricts opportunities to train and regulate their driving. In response to the problem of inadequate driving skills among some migrant farmworkers, the

University of California, Davis, has produced the *La Loteria del Manejo Seguro* driver safety program for use in community education programs.

4.4 Commodity-specific Occupational Illness and Injury

With the obvious exception of pesticide exposures (Chap. 5), the occupational health challenges described above are those that might generally be expected to affect farmworkers in nearly any work setting. In addition to these universal problems, there are a number of exposures and health problems that are specific for a given commodity. These relate both to the individual characteristics of the plants involved and to the nature of the work required for harvesting of produce. Although virtually every commodity has its own specific hazards, the following represent work that is quite common in the eastern US or present unique and interesting occupational health challenges.

4.4.1 Orchard Work

Orchard fruits are major production commodities in much of the eastern US. Citrus production, which is largely limited to Florida, accounts for nearly 70% of the nation's total acreage of citrus orchards. Other significant orchard fruits include peaches (Georgia, South Carolina, Pennsylvania, New York), pears (Pennsylvania, New York), and apples (Pennsylvania, New York).

4.4.1.1 The Nature of Orchard Work

The vast majority of the manual labor associated with orchard production relates to the harvesting of the fruit. Some ergonomic exposures are associated with off-season pruning and some potential exposures are related to application of pesticides and plant hormones prior to harvest. However, the number of workers exposed is far less than the number associated with harvest.

Orchard work is quite similar across commodities, with the main variation in the work relating to the size of the trees and the nature of the fruit. Some fruits are increasingly grown on dwarf trees, which reduce the ladder work, but may increase the amount of stoop work. The durability of the fruit also dictates some of the specific practices. Because apples bruise after any impact, they are harvested in buckets smaller than those for citrus. At about 45 lb, a full apple bucket weighs considerably less than a full citrus bag. The citrus worker can stand upright while dumping the bag of fruit, while the apple harvester must fully flex forward with a loaded bucket to gently release the apples from the bottom of the bucket into the apple bin.

Detailed ergonomic data are available on the harvesting process. A standardized time sampling technique demonstrated that New York apple harvesters spend 63% of their time with one or both arms extended above the head reaching for apples. Often this is with a nearly filled bucket on the shoulder. Buckets are at least partially loaded nearly 80% of the time. Nearly 10% of the time is spent with the spine acutely forward flexed over the edge of bin as the buckets are emptied (Earle-Richardson et al. 2004).

Unless dwarf trees are being harvested, the ladder is a major component of the job. Motivated in part by the piece-work pay strategy, workers try to minimize the number of times the ladder is repositioned. Harvesters will place one foot off to the side of the ladder upon a convenient branch to extend their picking range without having to move the ladder. Often this involves repeated shifts of the bag or bucket from one hip to the other. Conditions in the orchard for the first half of each day tend to be wet from dew in the grass and trees, so that footing on ladders and branches can be insecure. The demand for reaching highly placed fruit and for extending reach means that workers routinely use the top two steps of the ladder, thus reducing its stability and increasing their chances of falling (Salazar et al. 2005).

4.4.1.2 Occupational Health Problems Associated with Orchard Work

On the basis of review of charts from migrant health programs and from nearby emergency departments, a cohort of 303 work-related injuries affecting apple workers has been analyzed. Sixty percent of these related to musculoskeletal strain, 11% to contact with an irritant material, and 8% to falls. The most common medical diagnoses are shown in Fig. 4.3. These include musculoskeletal disorders from the repetitive motions, load bearing, acute flexion, and overhead work noted above. Eight percent of injuries relate to falls, probably a common occurrence that often does not result in a medical visit, but can result in sprains, contusions, and broken bones. These falls may relate to inadequate maintenance of ladders, to wet and slippery footwear, to overreaching, and to inadequate attention to the proper placement of the ladder. A smaller number of eye injuries may follow trauma from vegetation in the trees and from rebounding branches. This risk is present early in the season when a small number of workers are pruning and at harvest when a large number of workers are on the trees.

4.4.1.3 Orchard Work Injury Solutions

In the orchard, as in other work sites, respect for the worker and sensitivity to the safety challenges of the work might substantially reduce the risk of injury (Salazar et al. 2005). Some of the solutions here could relate to reengineering of the job or the equipment. Others might be addressed by administrative changes in the pay structure of the job. Reliance upon protective equipment is perhaps the most direct approach to the issue of eye injury. The use of polycarbonate lenses with side guards will greatly reduce the risk of eye trauma related to tree branches.

Falls from ladders are more complex, being related to the condition of both the ladder and the worker's footwear. Behaviors such as the setting of the ladder, the

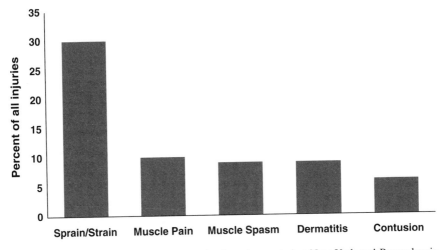

Fig. 4.3 Distribution of 303 injuries to orchard workers noted at New York and Pennsylvania migrant health program chart audits (From: A Migrant Farmworker Occupational Health Reference Manual. The New York Center for Agricultural Medicine and Health. Accessed at http://www.nycamh.com/resources/manualindex.htm)

height ascended, the extent of reach beyond the ladder and behaviors such as stepping onto adjacent branches and shifting of a loaded bucket also are key determinants of risk. To reduce falls, each of these issues must be optimized. Unsafe ladders need to be retired. The positioning and use of ladders cannot be hurried. The use of piece-rate pay strategies encourages inappropriate haste and shortcuts and may well heighten injury risk. More data on the unrecognized costs of piece-rate strategies would be of interest in discussing this practice with farmers.

Redesign efforts aimed at addressing some of the ergonomic challenges of orchard picking may well result in decreased frequency of musculoskeletal disorders. Redesign of the apple-picking bucket to permit partial support by attaching and detaching from a hip belt has been shown to effectively reduce the forces required of the shoulder and back muscles (Earle-Richardson et al. 2005b). Modification of the collecting bins, even of the trees, such as shifting toward dwarf trees, may effectively reduce exposures to musculoskeletal disorders.

4.4.2 Tobacco Production

The termination of the USDA tobacco program has caused substantial changes in tobacco production. Despite a 27% decline in US production, ~640 million pounds of tobacco is still produced annually. Although some states in the Northeast are involved in production, burley in Pennsylvania and "shade tobacco" used for wrapping cigars in the Connecticut River Valley, the majority of the nation's production occurs in the Southeast (Capehart 2006).

4.4.2.1 The Nature of Tobacco Production Work

The process of tobacco production extends from setting the plants and early cultivation to curing and baling the harvested leaves toward the end of the season (Arcury and Quandt 2007). Over the middle third of the season, workers remove flowers ("topping" the plants) to direct the growth to the leaves, cultivate and begin to harvest the earlier maturing leaves. Harvesting varies with the type of tobacco. Burley is harvested by the entire stalk, while flue-cured tobacco is harvested by the leaf ("primed"). This begins with the larger lower leaves that contain less nicotine. Typically about three leaves are taken with each cycle of picking. As each is picked, it is placed with others in a stack held under the worker's arm. Toward the end of the season, the smaller "tip" leaves containing the highest concentrations of nicotine are taken. "Curing" the leaves begins as it is picked. For burley tobacco several entire tobacco plants are attached to long wooden poles and lifted up four or five levels above the ground for air curing into the rafters of the barn. For flue-cured tobacco, curing involves packing the tobacco into "bulk barns" in which the heat and humidity are automatically controlled. Cured leaves are then retrieved from the different barns: for burley tobacco the leaves are manually stripped from the stalks and the leaves are baled; for flue-cured tobacco the leaves are removed from the barns and baled.

4.4.2.2 Occupational Health Problems Associated with Tobacco Production

For a review of occupational health problems, see Arcury and Quandt (2006). Areas of potential hazard in this process include repetitive motion and sustained awkward postures, as ergonomic challenges are associated with planting in the initial weeks of the season. A variety of potentially toxic chemicals are applied to tobacco over the course of the growing season, including insecticides and growth regulators. Heat and humidity are significant problems for workers throughout the most active portions of the season. Harvest work is associated with repetitive motion and repeated ergonomically challenging work postures, throughout the burley tobacco harvest and early in the harvest of flue-cured tobacco when lower leaves are harvested. For burley tobacco, potential hazards include lacerations from the "knives" used to cut the tobacco stalks and "spear points" put on the sticks that allow impaling the stalks. Harvest is also associated with considerable dermal contact with the tobacco leaves. Recent work used digital photography of face, hands, arms, and feet to look specifically for skin rash in 304 systematically selected workers followed at 3-week intervals through the season. More than 40% of participants reported symptoms of itch or skin rash (the two were highly correlated). A dermatologist reviewed the photographs and noted traumatic skin lesions in 16.8% of workers and contact dermatitis in 12.2% (Arcury et al. 2008). For burley tobacco, the curing process requires considerable climbing on barn rafters while holding poles with the attached leaves. Although there are no data available on fall rates associated with the suspending of leaves from barn rafters, there is clearly risk here.

Green tobacco sickness is a common occupational illness that results from tobacco work. It results from the effects of increased levels of nicotine related to absorption through the skin from plant leaves and nicotine-containing dew or rain water saturating the workers' clothes (Gehlbach et al. 1975). Over the course of the season, roughly one quarter of tobacco workers are likely to experience at least some of the symptoms of nicotine intoxication. These include nausea, vomiting, abdominal pain, diarrhea, dizziness, palpitations, and headache. Most commonly noted are headache, dizziness, and nausea occurring in the evening or night following a day of working with tobacco (Arcury et al. 2001). Levels of the nicotine breakdown product cotinine in workers' saliva and the incidence of green tobacco sickness symptoms have been found to increase across the course of the season, likely related to the progressively more intense dermal contact associated with the common methods of harvest (Quandt et al. 2001a). Work conditions associated with increased occurrence of symptoms and levels of salivary cotinine include specific tasks, late season, and wet leaves (Arcury et al. 2003). Wearing water-repellent garments that block dermal contact with the nicotine source reduces exposure (Arcury et al. 2002). Other worker characteristics that have been associated with increased risk of green tobacco sickness include age, experience, nonoccupational exposure to nicotine, and type of tobacco work (Quandt et al. 2001a). Older, more experienced workers have fewer symptoms, likely reflecting both learned avoidance behaviors and some "healthy worker" effect. The 40% of Hispanic farmworkers who smoke (Spangler et al. 2003) or use chewing tobacco have notably lower rates of green tobacco sickness symptoms (Arcury et al. 2001). The presence of self-reported skin rash significantly increased the odds of green tobacco sickness (OR, 3.30; 95% CI 2.17, 5.02) (Arcury et al. 2008). Possibly because shade tobacco leaves are generally not harvested wet and, once picked, are handled minimally by workers, neither symptoms nor measurable increases in salivary cotinine levels have been documented (Trape-Cardoso et al. 2005).

Dizziness or headache and nausea or vomiting in the setting of recent tobacco work are adequate for diagnosis if other potential causes have been eliminated. The illness is self-limited once continuous dermal absorption of nicotine is interrupted. Removal of saturated garments, showering, and symptomatic treatment are generally all that is required.

4.4.2.3 Occupational Health Solutions in Tobacco Production

Use of water-repellent clothing can reduce the incidence of symptoms, but this presents a potential hyperthermia problem. Use of gloves and changes in how the leaves are held after picking (i.e., not under the arm) can reduce skin injury and nicotine absorption. Changing out of wet clothing during the day or most certainly at the end of the day and showering immediately after work should reduce nicotine exposure as well.

4.4.3 Dairy Farming

The number of milk cows in the Northeast is roughly three times that in the Southeast. Pennsylvania and New York are among the nation's leading milk-producing states, with considerable production in Vermont and Maryland. Dairy is a significant commodity in Florida, Virginia, and Kentucky as well. A problem of increasing severity for dairy producers in the past few decades has been the scarcity of reliable labor to assist an aging farm owner population. The recent influx of Latino/Hispanic workers has done much to address this issue. In the Northeast these workers are predominantly males in their late twenties with considerably less dairy experience than their American counterparts. These Spanish-speaking workers work an average of 50–60 h per week. When tracked with quarterly phone calls over a 2-year period, those on large farms consistently worked 14 hours per week more than the non-Hispanic group (Stack et al. 2006). In Pennsylvania, New York, and Vermont, there is a clear trend toward increasing employment of Spanish-speaking workers, and by 2010 more than half of those employed on large northeastern dairy farms will be Latino/Hispanic (Jenkins et al. 2009).

4.4.3.1 The Nature of Dairy Work

Dairy work on most operations combines animal husbandry with the fieldwork required to produce feed required for the animals. Thus throughout the year, diary operations devote considerable effort to feeding, milking, and a variety of animal care and in-barn housekeeping tasks. These tasks are assigned to Latino/Hispanic workers much more commonly than the more machinery-intensive and seasonal fieldwork. Milking, feeding, and bedding practices vary with the design of the barn. In "stanchion" barns each animal is individually tethered in its own stall. A milker will kneel, squat, or stoop an average of five times for each of the cows milked (which occurs 2–3 times daily). The weight of the milking head and repeated over-head reaches to attach it to the milking pipeline represent other ergonomic challenges. In a "free stall" barn, the animals roam at will and then are herded toward a milking parlor twice daily for milking. Here milkers usually stand about 4 ft below the level of the cows and have access to the udders of multiple cows without having to stoop. In a parlor arrangement, one worker can be milking several cows simultaneously in a standing position. This work involves highly repetitive tasks often requiring one or both arms to be elevated. Fieldwork involves use of tractor-drawn implements to prepare the soil, distribute seed, cultivate the plants, and eventually harvest them. At present, Latino/Hispanic workers on northeastern farms are seldom involved in fieldwork tasks (Stack et al. 2006).

4.4.3.2 Occupational Health Problems Associated with Dairy Work

Dairy farmers are at risk of injury from animals and from machinery. They are exposed to substantial amounts of organic dust associated with silos and baled feed, with resultant asthma and chronic bronchitis. Silage can generate dangerous levels of noxious fumes, most notably nitrogen dioxide. Stored manure can generate dangerous levels of hydrogen sulfide, methane, and carbon monoxide. Rates of hearing loss and arthritis, particularly of the knee and shoulder, are elevated in dairy farmers (NY FFHHS – report to NIOSH 1998). There are very limited data on the extent to which Latino/Hispanic workers are affected by these hazards. Several of these are chronic problems that would not yet be seen in a population that has begun to appear on farms only over the past one to two decades. Other health problems result from trauma associated with animals or machinery. As Latino/Hispanic workers have much greater contact with animals than with machinery, most of their hazard exposure occurs in the course of interacting with the animals. Crush injuries, contusions, musculoskeletal injuries, and lacerations are the most common types of injuries in this setting (Boyle et al. 1997). Reliable data on the rates of these injuries in Latino/Hispanic dairy workers are not currently available.

4.4.4 Vegetables

Tomatoes, melons, beans, cucumbers, peppers, and cabbage are among the leading vegetable commodities in the eastern US (USDA 2007). Each of these requires substantial input of farmworker labor. There can be no single description for vegetable work, but many commodities do share some similar tasks that can be associated with occupational health problems. Planting of vegetables may involve seeding but often involves the planting of seedlings while riding on the back of a slowly moving tractor. This work involves the ergonomic challenges of rapid, continually repeated movements, often in the setting of an awkward sustained posture. Depending upon the use of plastic mulch, more or less cultivating and thinning may be required. In some situations this can be done mechanically, but more often it is done either manually or chemically, both of which can represent potential occupational problems for farmworkers. Harvest work usually involves the use of blades with associated risk of lacerations. Issues of posture and repetitive motions are likely to be prominent in harvest work as well. Farmworkers are at risk of skin and eye injury related to sun, and heat problems throughout most vegetable work.

4.4.5 Berries

4.4.5.1 The Work of Harvesting Blueberries

Blueberry production in other states centers upon bush fruit, while Maine blueberries are "wild", growing on scrubby plants no higher than 6–8 in. off the ground. The terrain is sometimes rocky and quite irregular. The berries are harvested in midsummer by "raking" with comb-like metal rakes with an attached collecting box. These

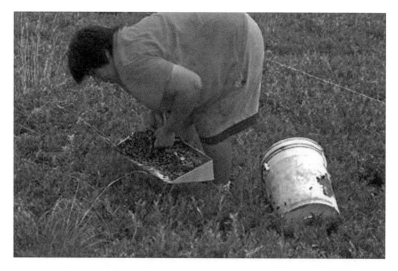

Fig. 4.4 The traditional center-handled rake used in harvesting of wild blueberries

rakes come in varying widths, and usually weigh 3.5–10 lb. The traditional rake has a single, short, horizontally oriented central handle (Fig. 4.4) that requires repeated forceful motions of the wrist to engage the foliage with the rake and then to pull directly up. Bending at the waist and working at a rate often exceeding 30 cycles per minute, the raker might pause only intermittently to empty the rake's collecting box. Considerable force is required to pull the rake up through the foliage.

4.4.5.2 Occupational Injury Associated with Berry Work

Evidence from a variety of sources shows that the traditional approach to blueberry raking is associated with ergonomic challenges and related worker injuries (Tanaka et al. 1994; Estill and Tanaka 1998). Ergonomic problems affecting the elbows, shoulders, and particularly in the back and wrist have been previously noted in association with blueberry raking (Millard et al. 1996). Chart review data from the Maine Migrant Health Program showed 86 clinic visits for complaints identified as related to blueberry raking. Sixty-five of these (76%) were musculoskeletal problems. Of these 38% related to back problems, 32% to shoulder, wrist, and hand problems, and 18% related to knee problems (Hawkes et al. 2007). Twelve percent related to skin problems.

4.4.5.3 Solutions for Injuries in Berry Work

In recent years, a work team composed of farmworkers and farm owners worked to systematically examine various alternative designs of the rake. A long-handled design (Fig. 4.5) was found to enhance productivity and was preferred by the workers,

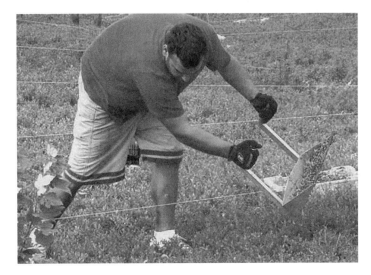

Fig. 4.5 A blueberry rake with 12-in. handle extensions

who noted less force required and less pain associated with harvest work. Currently, rake manufacturers are offering long-handle models and are selling inexpensive handle conversion kits for traditional rakes (May et al. 2008).

4.5 Conclusions

As agriculture evolves, shifts in commodities and modification of production methods will change some of the hazards experienced by migrant farmworkers. Work in tobacco may decline, while work in dairy and other commodities is quite likely to increase. Severe acute injury and fatality may become more significant threats as farmworkers experience increased exposure to large animals and machinery. The more traditional highly repetitive manual labor will certainly remain in many commodities. Occupational health threats relating to heat, musculoskeletal injury, and injury to eyes, ears, and skin will continue to be challenges for this population of workers and for those providing support for them.

That people who work this hard and provide such a vital service to our society remain at the very bottom of America's economic and social order is a curious and unfortunate phenomenon. The social and economic inequities imposed on these workers certainly compound the occupational hazards inherent in their work. To some degree the problems experienced by farmworkers relate directly to the behaviors of some of their employers. However, on a larger scale, farmworkers and farmers alike are victims of both economic policies and evolving market forces. The phenomenon of vertical integration (for example, a firm marketing chicken meat owns the chicks, provides the feed and bedding, and controls the entire process, simply renting the farmer's space and labor) and the impact of competition from subsidized foreign producers are just two recent and powerful factors that threaten the existence of many farms. While some operations thrive, many chronically operate on very thin margins. It is easy and sometimes appropriate to view the farm owner as the cause of the farmworkers' problems, but this approach can be both incorrect and counterproductive. In many ways the producer shares the same concerns as the farmworker. They both want the farm to stay in business and provide employment. They want the workers to be productive and to avoid injuries. Most farm owners want their workers to stay through the season and return for the next. Many employers can be effective partners in seeking ways to keep their employees safe. The combined wisdom and experience of farmworkers and farm owners can be invaluable in devising solutions to the daunting problems described above. The challenge for the farmworker advocate is to seek just treatment for workers without squandering the possibilities for effective collaboration with farm owners.

4.6   Recommendations

A variety of initiatives would likely enhance our understanding of the causes and remedies for some of the occupational health challenges discussed above. These include the following:

- Increased access to occupational health support and expertise for migrant clinicians.
- Increased health and safety training for farmworkers.
- Enhanced access to the workers' compensation system for farmworkers.
- Improved surveillance of occupational illness and injury in farmworkers.
- Data on the true costs and benefits of various work strategies (for example, piece-rate pay strategies) in terms of injuries, medical expenses, retention of work force, and overall productivity.
- Efforts to define the most effective ways to promote farmworkers' use of appropriate protective equipment.
- Community-based approaches that involve farmworkers and growers in defining problems and seeking solutions. The labor-management safety committee is an accepted approach to enhancing worker safety in many industries.
- Policy changes to assure adequate resources to federal and state agencies for development of interventions demonstrated to effectively reduce occupational injury and illness in farmworkers.

References

Abraham NF, Feldman SR, Vallejos QM et al. (2007) Contact dermatitis in tobacco farmworkers. Contact Dermat 57:40–43
American College of Occupational and Environmental Medicine Board of Directors (1993) ACOEM Code of Ethical Conduct. http://www.acoem.org/codeofconduct.aspx. Cited 26 May 2008

Arcury TA, Quandt SA (2007) Health and social impacts of tobacco production. J Agromed 11:71–81

Arcury TA, Quandt SA, Preisser JS et al. (2001) The incidence of green tobacco sickness among Latino farmworkers. J Occup Environ Med 43(7):601–609

Arcury TA, Quandt SA, Garcia DI et al. (2002) A clinic based, case–control comparison of green tobacco sickness among minority farmworkers: clues for prevention. South Med J 95(9):1008–1011

Arcury TA, Quandt SA, Mellen BG (2003a) An exploratory analysis of occupational skin disease among Latino migrant and seasonal farmworkers in North Carolina. J Agric Saf Health 9(3):221–232

Arcury TA, Quandt SA, Preisser JS et al. (2003b) High levels of transdermal nicotine exposure produce green tobacco sickness in Latino farmworkers. Nicotine Tob Res 5(3):315–321

Arcury TA, Vallejos QM, Schulz MR et al. (2008) Green tobacco sickness and skin integrity among migrant Latino farmworkers. Am J Indust Med 51:195–203

Azaroff LS, Levenstein C, Wegman DH (2002) Occupational injury and illness surveillance: conceptual filters explain underreporting. Am J Public Health 92:1421–1429

Baron S, Estill CF, Steege A et al. (eds) (2001) Simple Solutions: ergonomics for Farmworkers. National Institute for Occupational Safety and Health, Washington, DC

Borjan M, Constantino P, Robson MG (2008) New Jersey migrant and seasonal farm workers: enumeration and access to healthcare study. New Solut 18(1):77–86

Bouchama A, Knochel JP (2002) Heat Stroke. N Engl J Med 346(25):1978–1988

Boyes WK, Tandon P, Barone S, Jr et al. (1994) Effects of organophosphates on the visual system of rats. J Appl Toxicol 14:135–143

Boyle D, Gerberich SG, Gibson RW et al. (1997) Injury from diary cattle activities. Epidemiology 8(1):37–41

Bureau of Labor Statistics (2007a) Fatal occupational injuries, employment, and rates of fatal occupational injuries by selected worker characteristics, occupations, and industries, 2006. http://www.bls.gov/iif/oshwc/cfoi/CFOI_Rates_2006.pdf. Cited 30 Mar 2006

Bureau of Labor Statistics (2007b) Illness rates by type of illness – detailed industry, 2006. http://www.bls.gov/iif/oshwc/osh/os/ostb1760.txt. Cited 30 Mar 2008

Bureau of Labor Statistics (2007c) OSHA work-related injuries and illness involving days away from work, 2006. Table R1: Number of nonfatal occupational injuries and illnesses involving days away from work. http://stats.bls.gov/iif/oshwc/osh/case/ostb1793.txt. Cited 27 Mar 2008

Capehart T (2006) US tobacco sector regroups. Amber Waves, United States Department of Agriculture, Economic Research Service. http://www.ers.usda.gov/AmberWaves/February06/Findings/findings_mt1.htm. Cited 13 Mar 2008

Chapman LJ, Newenhouse AC, Meyer RH et al. (2004) Evaluation of an intervention to reduce musculoskeletal hazards among fresh market vegetable growers. Appl Ergon 35(1):57–66

Colt J, Stallones L, Cameron LL et al. (2001) Proportionate mortality among US migrant and seasonal farmworkers in twenty-four states. Am J Indust Med 40:604–611

Dementi B (1994) Ocular effects of organophosphates: a historical perspective of Saku disease. J Appl Toxicol 14:119–129

Dennis JW, May JJ (1995) Occupational noise exposure in dairy farming. In: McDuffie HH et al. (eds) Agricultural Health and Safety: Workplace, Environment, Sustainability. Lewis, Boca Raton

Earle-Richardson G, May JJ, Ivory JF (1998) Planning study of migrant and seasonal farmworkers in New York State: understanding the occupational safety environment using focus groups. J Agric Saf Health, Special Issue (1):111–119

Earle-Richardson G, Jenkins PL, Slingerland DT et al. (2003) Occupational injury and illness among migrant and seasonal farmworkers in New York State and Pennsylvania, 1997–1999: pilot study of a new surveillance method. Am J Indust Med 44:37–45

Earle-Richardson G, Fulmer S, Jenkins P et al. (2004) Ergonomic analysis of New York apple harvest work using a Posture-Activities-Tools-Handling (PATH) work sampling approach. J Agric Saf Health 10:163–176

Earle-Richardson G, Jenkins PL, Stack S et al. (2005a) Estimating farmworker population size in New York State using a minimum labor demand method. J Agric Saf Health 11(3):335–345

Earle-Richardson G, Jenkins P, Fulmer S et al. (2005b) An ergonomic intervention to reduce back strain among apple harvest workers in New York State. Appl Ergon 36:327–334

Earle-Richardson GB, Brower MA, Jones AM et al. (2008) Estimating the occupational morbidity for migrant and seasonal farmworkers in New York State: a comparison of two methods. Ann Epidemiol 18(1):1–7

Early J, Davis SW, Quandt SA et al. (2006) Housing characteristics of farmworker families in North Carolina. J Immigr Minor Health 8(2):173–184

Estill CF, Tanaka S (1998) Ergonomic considerations of manually harvesting Maine wild blueberries. J Agric Saf Health 4(1):43–57

Faucett J, Meyers J, Miles J et al. (2007) Rest break interventions in stoop labor tasks. Appl Ergon 38(2):219–226

Flores G (2000) Culture and the patient–physician relationship: achieving cultural competency in health care. J Pediatr 136:14–23

Forst L, Lacey S, Chen HY et al. (2004) Effectiveness of community health workers for promoting use of safety eyewear by Latino farm workers. Am J Indust Med 46:607–613

Forst L, Noth IM, Lacey S et al. (2006) Barriers and benefits of protective eyewear use by Latino farm workers. J Agromed 11:11–17

Gehlbach S, Williams W, Perry L et al. (1975) Nicotine absorption by workers harvesting green tobacco. Lancet 305:478–480

Gomez MI, Hwang SA, Sobotova L et al. (2001) A comparison of self-reported hearing loss and audiometry in a cohort of New York farmers. J Speech Lang Hear Res 44:1201–1208

Harris PM (2006) Nonfatal occupational injuries involving the eyes, 2004. http://www.bls.gov/opub/cwc/sh20060823ar01p1.htm. Cited 22 Mar 2008

Hawkes L, May J, Earle-Richardson G et al. (2007) Identifying the occupational health needs of migrant workers. J Comm Pract 15(3):57–76

Health Resources Services Administration (1990) An Atlas of State Profiles which Estimates the Number of Migrant and Seasonal Workers and Members of Their Families. Health Resources Services Administration, Washington, DC

Health Resources Services Administration (2007) Uniform data system. Table 6: Selected diagnoses and services rendered. http://ftp.hrsa.gov/bphc/pdf/uds/2006Migrantuds.pdf. Cited 10 Apr 2008

Institute of Medicine (1988) Role of the Primary Care Physician in Occupational and Environmental Medicine (IOM Publication No 88–05). National Academy Press, Washington, DC

Institute of Medicine (1993) Environmental Medicine in the Medical School Curriculum. National Academy Press, Washington, DC

Janowitz I, Meyers JM, Tejeda DG et al. (1998) Reducing risk factors for the development of work-related musculoskeletal problems in nursery work. Appl Occup Environ Hyg 13(1):9–14

Jenkins P, Stack S, Earle-Richardson G, May J (2009) Growth of the Spanish-speaking workforce in the northeast dairy industry. J Agromed 14(1) (accepted)

Kirrane EF, Hoppin JA, Kamel F et al. (2005) Retinal degeneration and other eye disorders in wives of farmer pesticide applicators enrolled in the agricultural health study. Am J Epidemiol 161:1020–1029

Krejci-Manwaring J, Schulz MR, Feldman SR et al. (2006) Skin disease among Latino farm workers in North Carolina. J Agric Saf Health 12(2):155–163

Lacey S, Forst L, Petrea R et al. (2007) Eye injury in migrant farmworkers and suggested hazard controls. J Agric Saf Health 13(3):259–274

Larsen AC, Plascencia L (1993) Migrant enumeration project. Migrant Legal Services, Office of Migrant Health, Bureau of Primary Health Care, Health Resources and Services Administration, Washington, DC

Larson AC (2000) Migrant and seasonal farmworkers enumeration profiles study. Migrant Health Program, Bureau of Primary Health Care, Health Resources and Services Administration. http://www.ncfh.org/00_ns_rc_enumeration.php. Cited 30 Mar 2008

Latko WA, Armstrong TJ, Franzblau A et al. (1999) Cross-sectional study of the relationship between repetitive work and the prevalence of upper limb musculoskeletal disorders. Am J Ind Med 36:248–259

Liebman A, Harper S (2001) Environmental health perceptions among clinicians and administrators caring for migrants. MCN Streamline 7(2):1–4

Luginbuhl RC, Jones VC, Langley RL (2003) Farmers' perceptions and concerns: the risks of driving farm vehicles on rural roadways in North Carolina. J Agric Saf Health 9(4):327–348

Luginbuhl RC, Jackson LL, Castillo DN et al. (2008) Heat-related deaths among crop workers – United States, 1992–2006. MMWR 57(24):649–653

Luque JS, Monaghan P, Contreras RB et al. (2007) Implementation evaluation of a culturally competent eye injury prevention program for citrus workers in a Florida migrant community. Prog Community Health Partnerships 1(4):359–369

Marvel ME, Pratt DS, Marvel LH et al. (1991) Occupational hearing loss in New York dairy farmers. Am J Indust Med 20(4):517–531

May J, Hawkes L, Jones A et al. (2008) Evaluation of a community-based effort to reduce blueberry harvesting injury. Am J Indust Med 51(4):307–315

Millard PS, Shannon SC, Carvette B et al. (1996) Maine students' musculoskeletal injuries attributed to harvesting blueberries. Am J Public Health 86(12):1821–1822

MMWR (2004) Work-related roadway crashes – United States, 1992–2002. Morbidity and Mortality Weekly Report 53(12):260–264

Mobed K, Gold EB, Schenker MB (1992) Occupational health problems among migrant and seasonal farm workers. West J Med 157(3):367–373

Morse T, Dillon C, Kenta-Bibi E et al. (2005) Trends in work-related musculoskeletal disorder reports by year, type and industrial sector: a capture–recapture analysis. Am J Ind Med 48(1):40–49

Murphy D-J, Yoder AM (1998) Census of fatal occupational injury in the agriculture, forestry and fishing industry. J Agric Saf Health 1:55–66

National Environmental Education and Training Foundation (2003) National pesticide practice skills guidelines for medical and nursing practice. National Environmental Education and Training Foundation, Washington, DC

National Institute for Occupational Safety and Health (2003) Work-related roadway crashes – Challenges and opportunities for prevention, NIOSH Publication No. 2003–119. National Institute for Occupational Safety and Health, Cincinnati, OH

National Institute for Occupational Safety and Health (2004) Worker Health Chartbook. National Institute for Occupational Safety and Health, Cincinnati, OH. NIOSH Publication No. 2004–146

Pratt DS, Marvel LH, Darrow D et al. (1992) The dangers of dairy farming: the injury experience of 600 workers followed for two years. Am J Indust Med 21:637–650

Quandt SA, Arcury TA, Preisser JS et al. (2001a) Environmental and behavioral predictors of salivary cotinine in Latino tobacco workers. J Occup Environ Med 43(10):844–852

Quandt SA, Elmore RC, Arcury TA et al. (2001b) Eye symptoms and use of eye protection among seasonal and migrant farmworkers. South Med J 94:603–607

Quandt SA, Feldman SR, Vallejos QM et al. (2008) Vision problems, eye care history, and ocular protective behaviors of migrant farmworkers. Arch Environ Occup Health 63:13–16

Rabinowitz PM, Sircar KD, Tarabar S et al. (2005) Hearing loss in migrant agricultural workers. J Agromed 10(4):9–17

Reigart JR, Roberts JR (1999) Recognition and Management of Pesticide Poisonings, 5th edn. EPA No. 735-R-98–003. US Environmental Protection Agency, Washington, DC. http://www.epa.gov/oppfead1/safety/healthcare/handbook/handbook.htm. Cited 17 Jul 2008

Salazar MK, Keifer M, Negrete M et al. (2005) Occupational risk among orchard workers: a descriptive study. Fam Community Health 28(3):239–252

Scharf T, Kidd P, Cole H et al. (1998) Intervention tools for farmers – safe and productive work practices in a safer work environment. J Agric Saf Health, Special Issue (1):193–203

Schuman SH, Dobson RL (1985) An outbreak of contact dermatitis in farm workers. J Am Acad Dermatol 13:220–223

Seraj MA, Channa AB, al Harthi SS et al. (1991) Are heat stroke patients fluid depleted? Importance of monitoring central venous pressure as a simple guideline for fluid therapy. Resuscitation 21(1):33–39

Smith FPE (1940) Eye injuries in agriculture. Trans Opthalmol Soc UK 60:252–257

Sorensen JA, May J, Purschwitz M et al. (2008) Encouraging farmers to retrofit tractors: a qualitative analysis of risk perceptions among a group of high-risk farmers in New York. J Agric Saf Health 14(1):105–117

Spangler JG, Arcury TA, Quandt SA et al. (2003) Tobacco use among Mexican farmworkers working in tobacco: implications for agromedicine. J Agromed 9(1):83–91

Stack SG, Jenkins PL, Earle-Richardson G et al. (2006) Spanish-speaking dairy workers in New York, Pennsylvania and Vermont: results from a survey of farm owners. J Agromed 11(2):37–44

Steinhorst B, Dolezal JM, Jenkins N et al. (2006) Trauma in Hispanic farm workers in eastern North Carolina: 10-year experience at a level I trauma center. J Agromed 11:5–14

Stiles M, Grieshop J (1999) Impacts of culture on driver knowledge and safety device usage among Hispanic farm workers. Accid Anal Prev 31:235–241

Stock SR (1991) Workplace ergonomic factors and the development of musculoskeletal disorders of the neck and upper limbs: a meta-analysis. Am J Indust Med 19(1):87–107

Tanaka S, Estill CF, Shannon SC (1994) Blueberry rakers' tendinitis. N Engl J Med 331(8):552

Taylor SL, Coates ML, Vallejos Q et al. (2006) Pterygium among Latino migrant farmworkers in North Carolina. Arch Environ Occup Health 61(1):27–32

Tedders SH, Schafer E, Eveland AP et al. (1998) Some physician perceptions of migrant and seasonal farm worker health in 45 rural Georgia counties. J Agromed 5(3):61–77

Trape-Cardoso M, Bracker A, Dauser D et al. (2005) Cotinine levels and green tobacco sickness among shade tobacco workers. J Agromed 10(2):27–37

United States Department of Agriculture (2007) Quick Stats. http://www.nass.usda.gov/Data_and_Statistics/Quick_Stats. Cited 17 Jun 2008

Vallejos QM, Schulz MR, Quandt SA et al. (2008) Self report of skin problems among farmworkers in North Carolina. Am J Indust Med 51:204–212

Weinstein ND (1988) The precaution adoption process. Health Psychol 7(4):355–386

Wilk VA (1988) The occupational health of migrant seasonal farmworkers in the U.S.: progress report. Farmworker Justice Fund, Washington, DC

Chapter 5
Pesticide Exposure Among Farmworkers and Their Families in the Eastern United States: Matters of Social and Environmental Justice

Thomas A. Arcury and Sara A. Quandt

Abstract Pesticides are found in the workplaces and living quarters of farmworkers and their families. Despite federal regulations designed to reduce pesticide exposure among farmworkers, research conducted in farmworker communities in the eastern US shows that such regulations are only partially enforced. Farmworker knowledge and beliefs about pesticides are often contrary to safety behaviors encouraged in this population. While studies documenting exposure of farmworkers to pesticides and the dose received are limited, they indicate that most farmworker housing is contaminated with a broad range of pesticides, exposing workers as well as family members to pesticides. Most workers and family members have absorbed measurable doses of pesticides. The health implications of different levels of pesticide exposure and dose are not known, but epidemiological studies indicate that lifetime exposure is associated with significant health effects. Because social and environmental factors place farmworkers at a disproportionate risk of pesticide exposure, this hazard of farmwork is both a social and environmental injustice for which solutions are needed.

5.1   Introduction

Pesticides are poisonous substances to which farmworkers in the eastern United States and the members of their families are exposed. Farmworkers have little knowledge of their pesticide exposure and, thus, little control over when and whether they are exposed. Pesticides, as toxins, have the potential to affect the health of all members of the farmworker community, including farmworkers themselves, spouses and partners not employed in farm work, and children. In contrast to many other low-wage workers, farmworkers must work and their families must live in environments contaminated by pesticides in order to make a living. The exposure of all members of the farmworker community to pesticides and the potential adverse health effects in a context of having limited control over the circumstances of exposure make farmworker pesticide exposure a matter of social and environmental justice.

The goals of this chapter are to document current pesticide exposure among farmworkers in the eastern United States and to present recommendations for needed policy and research to reduce pesticide exposure and the health affects of this exposure in this population. General information about pesticides – why pesticides matter and why farmworker pesticide exposure is a matter of social and environmental justice – is presented first. Current knowledge about farmworkers' exposure pathways and a description and critique of the safety regulations that have been implemented to protect workers are reviewed. Research on the remote and immediate predictors of pesticide exposure (beliefs about pesticides and behaviors that result in exposure) is reviewed, as well as the limited studies that have actually measured exposure and documented health outcomes.

5.1.1 Pesticides Defined

Pesticides are pervasive in the environment, and most people experience pesticide exposure on a daily basis. While people generally recognize insecticides when discussion turns to pesticides, pesticides include a large number of substances with diverse targets. The United States Environmental Protection Agency (US-EPA) defines pesticides as "any substance or mixture of substances intended for preventing, destroying, repelling, or mitigating any pest." Pests can be insects, mice and other animals, unwanted plants (weeds), fungi, or microorganisms like bacteria and viruses. Though often misunderstood to refer only to *insecticides*, the term pesticide also applies to herbicides, fungicides, and various other substances used to control pests. Under United States law, "a pesticide is also any substance or mixture of substances intended for use as a plant regulator, defoliant, or desiccant" (http://www.epa.gov/pesticides/about/#what_pesticide accessed February 17, 2008). Therefore, many common household products such as chlorine bleach and disinfectants are pesticides, as well as insect repellents, insect traps, and spray cans. Within agriculture, pesticides that are widely used include insecticides, herbicides, fungicides, fumigants, nematicides, rodenticides, and plant growth regulators. Pesticide use in agriculture includes application to crops in the fields, to livestock, and to product storage.

Most pesticides to which workers are exposed are "nonpersistent" pesticides. In contrast to older "persistent" pesticides like DDT, which remain in the human body and in the environment for a long time, nonpersistent pesticides are metabolized in the body within days (up to three days for organophosphorus pesticides). Those in the environment degrade when exposed to sun and water. Pesticides can enter the body through ingestion and inhalation, but the primary route of entry is usually absorption through the skin. Pesticides vary in their toxicity; in the US, labels carry warnings of *caution* (slightly toxic), *warning* (moderately toxic), and *danger* (highly toxic).

Pesticides are political. Pesticides and their use have been politically charged since the publication of Rachel Carson's *Silent Spring* in 1962. It is often difficult to discuss the use of pesticides in agriculture without raising an emotional response from farmers who feel that pesticides are required for the efficient production of food and fiber. Most farmers believe that they are knowledgeable about pesticides and their application. They perceive that the removal of a specific pesticide or threats to remove all pesticides will cripple their ability to make a living. Farm organizations have become involved in the regulatory and political process surrounding pesticide use. Environmentalists may also respond emotionally when discussing pesticides. They document the misuse of pesticides, their presence in food, and their effects on human health, as well as their effects on wild species. However, statements that all pesticides should be banned immediately indicate a lack of knowledge of the variety of substances that are pesticides and the variety of circumstances for which these substances are used.

Farmworkers and the members of their families are exposed to pesticides at home as well as at work. Everyone who works on a nonorganic farm in the United States is exposed to pesticides, and farmworkers are no exception. The level of exposure to pesticides and the dose that is absorbed vary by the levels of safety and hygiene employed on a particular farm. Farmworkers are also exposed to pesticides in their homes. Housing available to farmworkers is often in disrepair (Holden 2000; Early et al. 2006; Gentry et al. 2007; see Chap. 3). Much of this housing is old and contains the accumulation of pesticides brought into the dwelling in the past through drift during nearby agricultural application; deposition from pesticide-contaminated boots, clothing, and containers; and residential pesticide application. Many pesticides, including those considered nonpersistent, can remain viable in houses for years because they are not exposed to elements (e.g., ultraviolet light) which lead to decomposition. Further, because the housing is dilapidated and located in rural areas, it is subject to infestations by insects and rodents, for which farmworkers or landlords often apply pesticides.

While pesticide exposure is generally recognized to be a threat to the health of farmworkers and their families, research on farmworker pesticide exposure has been conducted in only three southern states in the eastern United States: North Carolina (e.g., Arcury et al. 2006; Quandt et al. 2004a), South Carolina (Halacre-Hitchcock et al. 2006), and Florida (e.g., Flocks et al. 2007; Kamel et al. 2003). This research has examined a broad set of issues related to farmworker pesticide exposure, but with little depth. Topics addressed are farmworker beliefs and perceptions of their occupational and residential pesticide exposure, farmer beliefs about farmworker pesticide exposure, enforcement of pesticides regulation for farmworkers, environmental and biological measures of pesticide exposure for farmworkers and their families, potential health outcomes for farmworkers due to pesticide exposure, and educational programs on pesticide safety for farmworkers.

5.1.2 Pesticide Exposure Matters

Pesticide exposure has the potential to affect the immediate and long-term health of farmworkers and the members of their families. In this respect, farmworkers are no different from farmers and other people. "Pesticide exposure" is generally used to refer to two distinct concepts: pesticide exposure and pesticide dose. Exposure is the amount of pesticides with which farmworkers come into contact, as in the amount in their workplace, the amount in their homes, and the amount on their clothes. Dose refers to the amount of pesticide that actually enters the body. Dose can be kept low in the face of high exposure when proper safety and hygiene procedures are implemented. However, high pesticide exposure generally results in a high pesticide dose. Exposure is an environmental measure, and dose is a biological measure, often measured as a biomarker such as a pesticide or its breakdown product in the urine.

Pesticides are known to have immediate and delayed health effects (Reigart and Roberts 1999; Sanborn et al. 2004). The severity of the immediate and delayed health effects of pesticides is a function of the strength and number of pesticide doses an individual experiences. Immediate health effects of exposure to a large dose of pesticides can be quite severe, and include loss of consciousness, coma, and death. The immediate health effects of smaller doses of pesticides can include rash, dizziness, nausea and vomiting, and muscle weakness. Immediate pesticide health effects also include negative birth outcomes, such as spontaneous abortion and deformities. Several long-term health effects of large and small doses of pesticides, particularly when these doses are repeated, are also documented. Some of these long-term health effects are readily diagnosed and include increased risk of several cancers, sterility, and neurological decline in adults. Other long-term health effects are subclinical and may not be recognized. These include retarded neurobehavioral development of children and memory loss in adults.

The effects of pesticide exposure on the health of farmworkers and the members of their families remain understudied (McCauley et al. 2006). Numerous health effects are associated with pesticide exposure. These health effects differ by age, with children being at great risk (Eskenazi et al. 1999) due to large surface to volume ratio, fast metabolism, and ongoing development. The Agricultural Health Study (Alavanja et al. 1996) has been particularly important in examining possible associations of pesticide exposure with a large variety of health outcomes. The Agricultural Health Study includes over 80,000 licensed pesticide applicators and their family members from Iowa and North Carolina. This large sample has allowed examination of the association of pesticide exposure with health outcomes that are infrequent as well as those that are common. It has shown the association of self-reported pesticide exposure to increased risk for several forms of cancer (Alavanja et al. 1994, 2004; Bonner et al. 2005, 2007; Lee et al. 2007; Mahajan et al. 2006; Purdue et al. 2007), respiratory disease (Hoppin et al. 2006b, 2007a, b, 2008; Valcin et al. 2007), vision problems (Kirrane et al. 2005), neurologic symptoms (Kamel et al. 2005, 2007), reproduction problems (Farr et al. 2004, 2006; Saldana et al. 2007), and depression (Beseler et al. 2006).

5.1.3 Farmworker Pesticide Exposure: An Issue of Justice

Environmental justice is the fair treatment and meaningful involvement of all people regardless of race, color, national origin, or income with respect to the development, implementation, and enforcement of environmental laws, regulations, and policies. EPA has this goal for all communities and persons across this Nation. It will be achieved when everyone enjoys the same degree of protection from environmental and health hazards and equal access to the decision-making process to have a healthy environment in which to live, learn, and work [http://www.epa.gov/oecaerth/environmentaljustice/index.html accessed 19 July 2008].

Like many environmental and occupational health concerns faced by communities that have little political or financial power, pesticide exposure experienced by farmworkers and their families is a matter of justice. Pesticide exposure results in ill health, and people should not have to get sick in order to make a living. Nor should people be required to live in housing that makes them and their children sick.

Pesticides do not affect the health of farmworkers more than they affect the health of other people. Farmworkers may not be more exposed to pesticides than are others who work in agriculture or who live on farms. However, it is very likely that farmworkers and the members of their families receive a greater dose of the pesticides to which they are exposed. Farmworkers and the members of their families have very limited knowledge about the pesticides to which they are exposed (Quandt et al. 1998; Arcury et al. 2002; Rao et al. 2007). They have very little control over their pesticide exposure, either at work or in their home. The grower decides what pesticides should be applied, as well as where and when they should be applied, and seldom informs the workers of these decisions. Farmworkers often live in grower-provided or rental housing and are not told about pesticides that the owner decides to apply to these dwellings. Farmworkers have very little knowledge of the potential health effects of their pesticide exposure. Regulations are not enforced; in fact, regulators often appear to identify with growers. While regulations are in place requiring that farmworkers receive pesticide safety training (the US-EPA Worker Protection Standard), this training is minimal and is often not provided (see Sect. 5.3.3). No regulations require that adults living with farmworkers (e.g., spouses) receive any information about pesticide exposure. Other regulations for pesticide safety and field sanitation, such as central posting of pesticide application information in a language that workers can understand and posting the restricted entry intervals for fields on which pesticides have been applied, are often not enforced in farmworker work settings.

Farmworkers receive small financial compensation for the jeopardy of pesticide exposure that they experience. Farmworker income seldom exceeds the poverty level (Carroll et al. 2005). Many of those who employ farmworkers do not believe that pesticides pose a danger to the health of farmworkers (Quandt et al. 1998; Rao et al. 2004). Growers believe that the danger of pesticide exposure is exaggerated by the media and the public. They feel that workers are at little risk of exposure because workers have received training and protective equipment as required by law, and because they are not in direct contact with chemicals. Growers seldom speak the same language as the workers, and they often do not recognize that linguistic, cultural, and power differences may be barriers to pesticide safety for farmworkers.

Employers often are not willing to ensure the pesticide safety of farmworkers beyond the minimum required when it increases their costs. For example, a North Carolina grower was asked during an in-depth interview if he and other growers would be willing to provide rental uniforms to their farmworkers to ensure that their clothing was adequate for reducing pesticide exposure and that work clothing soiled with pesticides would not be taken into the farmworkers' living areas. The grower responded that would create too great a cost and farmers could not afford it. During the interview, this grower was wearing a rental work uniform which he provided for his own use (Arcury unpublished data).

The residential pesticide exposure of farmworker families may be greater than that experienced by others. Farmworkers are likely to increase their exposure at home through the "paraoccupational" pathway; they unintentionally bring pesticides into their homes from work. Farmworker housing is substandard and often located in rural areas, and both of these factors increase the likelihood of infestation, which leads to the use of structural pesticides. Few farmworkers own their homes, and many live in housing provided by their employer. They have no control of the pesticides that may be applied to their homes. Finally, farmworkers are not provided with information about residential pesticide exposure and its health consequences for themselves or their families.

While an acknowledged threat to the health of farmworkers, their spouses, and their children exists, very little research has investigated pesticide exposure or its health outcomes among farmworkers. No Agricultural Health Study has been implemented that addresses the exposure and health effects of pesticides for farmworkers. Several investigators have documented the problems inherent in studying farmworker pesticide exposure, and they have published discussions of methodologies, particularly life history calendar methods (Zahm et al. 2001), to document the long-term exposure of farmworkers to pesticides and the health effects of this exposure. However, no such longitudinal study has been implemented. In North Carolina, data collection for a large scale, cross-sectional study of farmworker pesticide exposure has been completed. This study, Community Participatory Approach to Measuring Farmworker Pesticide Exposure: PACE3 (funded by the National Institute of Environmental Health Sciences; R01 ES08739), recruited 287 farmworkers and collected data to measure pesticide exposure and dose four times at monthly intervals in 2007. The analysis of the data collected by this study continues and results will be reported in the coming years.

5.2   Pathways of Pesticide Exposure

Farmworkers and their families may be exposed to pesticides through several pathways, including occupational exposure, paraoccupational exposure, environmental exposure, and residential application. The most obvious of these pathways is occupational. While at work, farmworkers are involved in loading, mixing, and applying pesticides. They work in areas in which pesticides are stored and work in fields to which pesticides have been applied. Pesticides have a restricted entry interval, the period after a pesticide is applied on a field during which no one should enter the field without wearing personal protective equipment. However, after the restricted entry interval has passed, pesticides are still present in the field, although at low levels. The paraoccupational pathway refers to exposures to occupational pesticides among those not employed in agriculture. Such exposure results when workers bring home pesticides on their skin, clothes, boots, or other objects. Individuals who are not farmworkers become exposed to pesticide through direct contact with these contaminated surfaces. They can also become exposed through contact with pesticides that are deposited from these contaminated surfaces in vehicles or in homes.

Two major sources of environmental exposure include drift and the long-term deposition of pesticides in houses and vehicles. Drift occurs when a pesticide applied in one area is spread to adjoining areas through wind or run-off. Drift can cause exposure occupationally when farmworkers working in one area are exposed to pesticides that drift while being applied to a nearby field. Drift can also affect residential exposure. The dwellings of many farmworkers are located near agricultural fields. Pesticides applied to these fields may drift into farmworker yards, outbuildings, and houses, resulting in exposure. Most pesticides remain stable and active if they are not exposed to cleaning or to ultraviolet light. Pesticides that are deposited into houses may remain for years. Therefore, farmworker dwellings often have high levels of pesticides from years of deposition. Research conducted in North Carolina shows farmworker dwellings contain large numbers of pesticides (Quandt et al. 2004), and that pesticide biomarkers collected in the urine of farmworker children in 2004 included the metabolites of pesticides banned since the 1986 (Arcury et al. 2007b).

Pesticides are often applied to the houses in which farmworkers live (Quandt et al. 2004). Farmworkers seldom own their dwellings, and many farmworkers live in camps in which housing is provided by their employer or crew leader. This housing has great potential for insect and rodent infestation (Bradman et al. 2005).

5.2.1 A Model of Predictors and Outcomes of Farmworker Pesticide Exposure

Farmworker pesticide exposure can be understood as the result of proximal, distal, and moderating forces (Fig. 5.1) (Quandt et al. 2006). The most proximal determinants are workplace and household behaviors that bring workers and their families into contact with pesticides. These behaviors are themselves the result of the corresponding environments. Thus, work environments that have regular, effective safety trainings and have an organization of work in which workers are able to exercise some degree of judgment in their work practices are more likely to have workers who exhibit good pesticide safety behaviors (e.g., regular hand-washing, not entering recently treated fields). However, beliefs (e.g., if a pesticide is not visible there is no danger) or psychosocial stressors (e.g., pressure to work as many hours as possible to send money home) may reduce the effects of a supportive environment on actual behaviors. Community factors may affect the work and home environments, as well. If pesticides are ubiquitous (e.g., crops nearby receive aerial spraying), the work and home environments may have levels of pesticides that are beyond the control of workers and other residents.

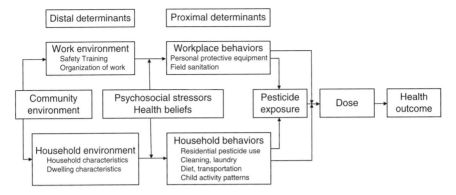

Fig. 5.1 Conceptual model of the relationship between the predictors of pesticide exposure among farmworkers and their relationship to health outcome. Reprinted with permission, Environmental Health Perspectives (Quandt et al. 2006)

5.3 Pesticide Safety Regulations

Two major sets of federal regulations are in place that are intended to reduce pesticide exposure among farmworkers. The Worker Protection Standard (WPS) specifically addresses agricultural pesticide safety (US-EPA 1992). The US Environmental Protection Agency instituted the current WPS in 1994, and a process to revise these regulations has been ongoing for several years. Housing and field sanitation regulations that affect pesticide safety have been instituted by the Occupational Safety and Health Administration.

5.3.1 The Worker Protection Standard

The WPS includes several components that address pesticide safety for all agricultural workers as well as for the environment. The major component of the WPS that is generally discussed relative to farmworkers is the requirement that agricultural workers receive training in pesticide safety. Different levels of training are required for individuals who do only field work, who are pesticide handlers (they might load, mix, and apply pesticides under the direction of a licensed pesticide applicator), and those who are licensed pesticide applicators. Migrant and seasonal farmworkers in the eastern US are seldom licensed applicators. The training for field workers is very limited. This training for field workers must be provided before the field worker accrues five days of work in fields to which restricted use pesticides have been applied in the previous 30 days. These five work days are cumulative across the individual worker's lifetime; the training must be renewed at least every five years.

Training for field workers may be provided by the employer or by a designated trainer who has passed a very limited test on the content of the WPS and provided a training plan. The training must be in the language that the worker understands, and it must cover 13 specific points (US-EPA 1992):

- Format and meaning of information on pesticide labels and in labeling, including safety information such as precautionary statements about human health hazards
- Hazards of pesticides resulting from toxicity and exposure, including acute and chronic effects, delayed effects, and sensitization
- Routes through which pesticides can enter the body
- Signs and symptoms of common types of pesticide poisonings
- Emergency first aid for pesticide injuries or poisonings
- Instructions on how to obtain emergency first aid
- Routine and emergency decontamination procedures, including emergency eye flushing techniques
- Need for and appropriate personal protective equipment
- Prevention, recognition, and first aid treatment of heat-related illness
- Safety requirements for handling, transporting, storing, and disposing of pesticides, including general procedures for spill cleanup
- Environmental concerns such as drift, runoff, and wildlife hazards
- Warnings about taking pesticides or pesticide containers home
- Other requirements: application and entry restrictions, the design of warning signs, posting of warning signs, oral warnings, the availability of specific information about applications, and protection against retaliatory acts

The training can be in any format, including a recorded presentation. To work as a pesticide handler, an individual must have received training that includes 21 specific points, the 13 points included in the training for field workers plus 8 additional points (US-EPA 1992).

Other components of these regulations refer to the entry of workers into fields after pesticides have been applied. This restricted entry interval (REI) is listed on the container label for each pesticide and indicates the number of hours or days before an individual can enter a field after the pesticide has been applied without wearing specified personal protective equipment (PPE; e.g., Tyvec suit, respirator, gloves). Employers are required to tell workers when and where they apply pesticides, the pesticide that has been applied, and the duration of the restricted entry interval, or they are to post fields with the pesticide name and restricted entry interval when pesticides are applied (Fig. 5.2). Finally, employers are required to post information about pesticide applications in a central location to which workers have access.

Other regulations refer to the storage of pesticides and the disposal of empty pesticide containers. Farmers are required to store pesticides in a locked cabinet or store room. Pesticide containers should be thoroughly washed and then disposed of properly, and not used for any other purpose. Finally, these regulations limit the application of pesticides in the face of environmental conditions, such as strong winds.

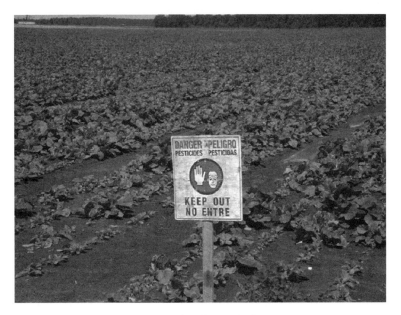

Fig. 5.2 Pesticide restricted entry interval sign. Copyright, Thomas A. Arcury

5.3.2 OSHA Field Sanitation and Housing Regulations

OSHA field sanitation and housing requirements are also very limited. The *Occupational Safety and Health Act* requires that all agricultural employers with 11 or more employees provide drinking, toilet, and washing facilities for farmworkers while they are working in a field. A supply of fresh water must be within 500 feet of the working area and must be maintained at 60°F or lower. Portable water containers are acceptable if they can be tightly closed and have a tap; water cannot be poured or dipped from the container. Toilet facilities must be located within 5-min travel time of the field. There should be separate facilities for the sexes and one toilet for each 1–20 persons of each sex. Toilet facilities should be provided with toilet paper and be kept in a sanitary condition and in working order. Hand-washing facilities should be provided and located near the toilets and within 5-min travel time of the field. Water used for hand-washing should be tested and certified to be potable. Soap and individual towels should be supplied. Housing regulations, which apply only to housing for migrant workers, are discussed in Chap. 3. These regulations address the number of bathing and laundry facilities provided for each worker.

Field sanitation and housing requirements are important to pesticide safety. Frequent hand-washing, particularly before eating and toileting, bathing immediately after finishing work, and wearing clean clothes each day all reduce the dose that results from pesticide exposure. Despite their importance, federal regulations requiring agricultural employers to provide toilets, drinking water, and hand-washing facilities to workers in the fields have only been in effect for a couple of decades. Prior to 1987, agriculture was excluded from the requirement that all employers provide such facilities (Frisvold et al. 1988, Sakala 1987). A 1985 report commissioned by the US Department of Labor, which found infectious disease levels in farmworkers equivalent to those in developing countries and attributed the rates to lack of field sanitation, led to legal action to include agriculture under the OSHA standards applied to other industries.

5.3.3 Enforcement of Pesticide-Related Regulations

While the training required for field workers, as well as other pesticide safety regulations are quite limited, research indicates that adherence to these regulations is not universal. State governments have not published evaluations of their programs to implement and monitor these regulations. Research examining implementation of the pesticide regulations in the eastern US is limited to research in North Carolina (Arcury et al. 1999, 2001, 2002), South Carolina (Halfacre-Hitchcock et al. 2006), and Florida (Flocks et al. 2001). From one-quarter to one-half of farmworkers indicate that they have not received any pesticide safety training, even when the question used to obtain this information is very broad – "Have you ever received any information or training on how to prevent or reduce your exposure to pesticides when you are working?" For example, about half of the farmworkers interviewed in 1998 and 1999 in eastern North Carolina indicated that they had received pesticide safety training (Arcury et al. 2001). In 2002–2003, three out of four women (109; 76.8%) in western North Carolina farmworker families indicated that at least one untrained worker lived in their households, including 87 households (61.3%) with no trained workers (Rao et al. 2006). In 2004, among 60 farmworkers in eastern North Carolina with children less than six years of age, 38% of mothers and 28% of fathers who do farm work had not received pesticide safety training (Arcury et al. 2007b).

Very few farmworkers can name any pesticide used where they work. Fewer than half of farmworkers interviewed indicate that they are told about pesticides that have been applied where they are working, that information on pesticides that have been applied is posted in an accessible location, or that warning signs are posted around field to which pesticides have been applied (Arcury et al. 2001).

Observations, not documented in the literature, made while visiting farms and farmworker camps support the results of the published research. Situations such as those in Fig. 5.3, in which pesticides are stored in sheds without walls, doors, or locks, have been observed on farms in all areas of North Carolina. Comments by farmers that they do not record their use of pesticides, nor do they post this information, are also commonly heard.

While research examining adherence to pesticide safety regulations in the eastern US is limited to North Carolina, South Carolina, and Florida, research in other

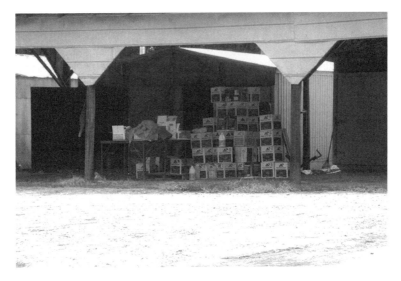

Fig. 5.3 Pesticides stored in open shed. Copyright, Thomas A. Arcury

regions has shown similar levels of compliance with training, field sanitation, and housing regulations related to farmworkers (GAO 2000). For example, only 56% of 102 mothers employed in farm work in Starr County, Texas, reported having received WPS training (Shipp et al. 2005).

Very little research has been conducted to document field sanitation conditions in the United States and evidence of conditions in the eastern US is even more limited. Arcury et al. (2001) conducted in-depth interviews and surveys with farm-workers, farmers, and Cooperative Extension agents in North Carolina. Farmworkers described frequently working in fields with inadequate field sanitation. Although most workers (90%) stated that drinking water is usually provided, fewer (66%) reported that the required disposable drinking cups are usually provided (Arcury et al. 2001). Only one third of farmworkers stated that water for washing is always or usually available, and 40% said it was seldom or never available. Furthermore, 56% of workers reported that the same water source is often provided for drinking and hand-washing (Arcury et al. 2001). This is especially problematic for those farmworkers who believe that washing themselves with cold water can cause rheu-matism, arthritis, and other illnesses because drinking water is often iced (Arcury et al. 2001). According to farmworkers' reports, toilets are often not available while workers are in the fields. Less than one third of workers said field toilets are always or usually available and over half said they are seldom or never available (Arcury et al. 2001).

Data collected during the 2007 agricultural season in North Carolina show that conditions are still worse than intended by field sanitation regulations (Arcury et al., unpublished data). Data were collected from 287 workers interviewed up to four times at monthly intervals from May until September. Water to wash hands was reportedly available on each of the three prior days for 71% of workers. However, soap and towels to dry hands were less often available (54% and 43%, respectively). Drinking water was provided in the fields in the prior three days for almost all workers (99%), but individual cups were less often (84%) available.

Farmers reported that it is difficult to move toilet and washing facilities to all of the fields where they employ workers and consider this requirement to be burdensome (Arcury et al. 2001). Some farmers reported that when they do provide sanitation facilities, such as field toilets and washing stations, workers do not use them. Cooperative Extension agents' reports were similar to those of farmers. They also mentioned that farmers provide facilities that the workers prefer not to use (Arcury et al. 2001). The lack of field toilet facilities can affect worker health. A 1981 survey in Tulare County, California found that the absence of field toilets increased gastrointestinal disorders by 60% among farmworkers (Frisvold et al. 1988).

A 1996 survey of residential sites and worksites owned by four agricultural employers in Colorado documented the continuing absence of sanitary facilities in fields and warehouses despite the federal OSHA standards (Vela-Acosta et al. 2002). Work sites were inspected by study staff and hazardous conditions were coded as no hazard, minor hazard, serious hazard, or critical hazard based on the inspector's assessment of the level of health threat posed by the conditions of the facilities. Two of the five worksites' drinking water facilities were coded as posing a critical hazard, and one was coded as a serious hazard. Two of the portable toilets were coded as minor hazards, and two were coded as serious hazards. Water for washing was coded as a serious hazard at three worksites and as a critical hazard for one site (Vela-Acosta 2002). Towels for hand-drying were coded as a serious hazard at four sites. The bathroom in the warehouse that was inspected had unhygienic conditions due to a lack of soap, towels, or running water. In addition, no drinking water was available to workers in the warehouse (Vela-Acosta 2002).

Vela-Acosta et al. (2002) also reported the farmworkers' evaluations of field sanitation conditions. According to farmworkers' reports, the provision of field sanitation facilities differed between employers. Between 18% and 81% of farmworkers at a specific work site stated that drinking water is provided at their work sites. Between 5% and 42% of farmworkers at the different work sites reported that water for washing was provided (Vela-Acosta et al. 2002). The provision of soap and towels was reported by 0–44% of workers. Just over half of workers reported that they wash their hands before using the toilet when working in the fields. Observations of workers in the fields found that 85% of workers who used the bathroom or ate during the observation washed their hands before doing so (Vela-Acosta 2002).

5.3.4 Summary of Worker Protections

Although regulations that could better protect farmworkers from pesticide exposure are limited, and analyses indicate that even these limited regulations are not followed, it is also apparent that many farmworkers do work on farms in which the work culture is geared toward a safe and responsible workplace. While as many as half of farmworkers report not receiving any training, the other half report receiving at least some training. Several agencies and organizations are dedicated to improving pesticide safety training for farmworkers. For example, the Association of Farmworker Opportunity Programs funds AmeriCorp programs specifically focused on pesticide safety training for farmworkers. Staff from US-EPA Region 4 (which includes eight southeastern states) have developed training programs for state pesticide safety inspectors that introduce these inspectors to linguistically and culturally appropriate procedures for discussing the conditions of pesticide exposure and work with farmworkers. In addition, as is discussed in Chap. 2, states in the eastern US are diverse in their regulatory and safety climates. It is not clear if the level of regulatory adherence that is documented in the literature is the same across the entire region.

5.4 Farmworker Beliefs About Pesticide Exposure

Farmworkers bring their own systems of belief and knowledge to their work. These beliefs reflect their Latino cultural background and limited formal education (see Chap. 2). The beliefs and knowledge of farmworkers surrounding pesticides apply to their actions at home (Rao et al. 2006, 2007), as well as at work (Arcury et al. 2002; Elmore and Arcury 2001; Flock et al. 2007; Halfacre-Hitchcock et al. 2006; Quandt et al. 1998), and frequently result in behaviors that are at odds with safe pesticide practices.

Farmworkers generally lack knowledge of the pesticides applied where they work: what is applied, where it is applied, and when it is applied. Even if a grower does post pesticide application information in a central location to which farmworker have access, many workers would not be able to read the information, even if it was translated into Spanish, as many are functionally illiterate and others speak a nonwritten, indigenous language. Farmers also do not always post fields with signs indicating that the restricted entry interval is in effect.

Beliefs common among farmworkers also affect their safety behaviors around pesticides. Many farmworkers state that sensory detection is necessary for there to be the potential for pesticide exposure. If pesticides are not seen, felt, or smelled, then they are not present. Smell in particular is held to be an indicator of pesticide exposure, with the strength of an odor considered an indicator of the strength and risk of pesticide exposure. Beliefs about humoral medicine are also widely held among farmworkers. Humoral medicine includes the hot–cold theory of health (Rubel 1960; Weller 1983). This presupposes that different materials have different humors, and the humors for some materials are hot while those of others are cold. Mixing hot and cold will result in illness. Hot and cold are often metaphorical rather than physical states. Because the humor for water is cold, and this could be metaphorically cold, no matter what the physical temperature, it should be avoided when the body is hot, as from work. Therefore, farmworkers often avoid washing hands during work, or showering immediately after work because they feel that they should avoid contact with water when their bodies are hot from work until they have a chance to cool (Quandt et al. 1998). In a survey of 287 farmworkers completed in North Carolina in 2008, 94.8% agreed with the statement, "One should cool the body before bathing after work" (*Debemos enfriar el cuerpo antes de bañarnos después del trabajo*), while 36.9% agreed with statement, "People should avoid washing their hands when they are at work and their bodies are hot" (*Las personas no deberían lavarse las manos cuando están trabajando y sus cuerpos están calientes*). The result can be the continued exposure to pesticides from work, and the chance of paraoccupational deposition of pesticides at home.

Health beliefs may affect pesticide safety behavior among farmworkers in other ways. For example, one quarter of farmworkers in Florida who experienced a severe incident of pesticide poisoning interpreted their symptoms in terms of the Mexican folk illness "susto" (Baer and Pensell 1993). The attribution of pesticide exposure symptoms to more familiar illnesses may limit the use of formal medical care.

Farmworkers acknowledge immediate health effects of pesticide exposure, but have little knowledge of the potential delayed and subclinical health effects of pesticides. Therefore, farmworkers generally believe that if they or coworkers have not been acutely ill, they have not been exposed to pesticides. Further, male farmworkers believe that as men they should not be concerned about injury or illness. Their strength as men will protect them from experiencing any potential ill effects of pesticide exposure; only weak men, women, and children will be harmed by pesticides. This *machismo* belief reduces some farmworkers' awareness of potential pesticide exposure hazards.

Finally, farmworkers need to work to support themselves and their families. They have little knowledge of the regulations that should protect them. If they do know the regulations, many are undocumented, and fear reporting problems to any authorities. Farmworkers often feel that they have no control of their work situations, and believe they must do what they are told to keep their jobs. This includes ignoring any pesticide exposure that they experience, and not complaining about the lack of sanitation and hygiene that could reduce this exposure. Compounding these attitudes, farmworkers often attach the value of *personalismo* in dealings with their employers; farmworkers want a personal relationship with their employer and avoid actions that would jeopardize this relationship.

Beliefs related to pesticide exposure documented for farmworkers in the eastern US are comparable to those documented among Latino agricultural workers in other regions. For example, Grieshop et al. (1996) found that farmworkers in California held that external sources of control (God and luck) were important factors in workplace safety. Salazar et al. (2004) showed that the perceptions of adolescent farmworkers in Oregon were shaped by their community context. Hunt et al. (1999) examined why farmers in Chiapas, Mexico, did not use personal protective equipment and follow occupational hygiene practices with which they were familiar, even though they understood the toxicity of pesticides and how they ought to handle these pesticides. Their analysis found that these Mexican farmers felt a lack of control in the use of pesticides due to financial pressures. These farmers also had not experienced immediate serious health effects when they had been exposed to pesticides, hence they did not believe that exposure was dangerous. Finally, they "... found that the cultural expectation that healthy males are strong and able to sustain a certain degree of hardship was a factor in the perception of personal risk. In discussing their perceptions of personal vulnerability to pesticides, several people mentioned that those who can't tolerate pesticide exposure are the very old, the very young, and pregnant women.... A man who covers up [uses PPE] to apply pesticides is a fearful man, or he is a weak man who can't tolerate a minor physical challenge" (pp. 245–246).

The knowledge and beliefs of the wives of farmworkers concerning residential pesticide exposure mirror the knowledge and beliefs of workers about occupational pesticide exposure (Rao et al. 2006, 2007). These women often do not know if their husbands or other farmworkers who live in their homes are working with or around pesticides. Unless they have done farm work themselves, generally they have not been provided with any information about the potential for paraoccupational or environmental pesticide exposure in their homes or ways that they might mitigate these sources of exposure. These women often do not think of products that they use in their homes, including consumer insecticides and rodenticides, as pesticides; pesticides are the products that their husbands use at work. Like farmworkers, these women also hold the belief that they must smell the odor of a pesticide for it to be present, and that the stronger the odor, the more powerful and dangerous the pesticide. They generally have little knowledge of the subclinical or long-term effects of pesticide exposure and only recognize immediate symptoms of exposure. Often, they have seen immediate symptoms of significant pesticide exposure in Mexican agriculture as well as in US agriculture. Therefore, they reason that, if no one in their homes has experienced the symptoms of pesticide poisoning, there is no exposure and no problem. Finally, women in farmworker households often feel they have little control over the actions of men who can introduce pesticides into their homes. These women are reluctant to tell their husbands or other adult males what they should do to reduce the potential exposure.

The beliefs of those who employ farmworkers, the farmers or growers, about farmworker pesticide exposure are also important in understanding the pesticide exposure of farmworkers (Quandt et al. 1998; Rao et al. 2004). Foremost among these beliefs is that farmers are exposed to pesticides, while farmworkers are not. Farmers reason that they generally handle, mix, and apply pesticides, and that they are therefore likely to be exposed to these pesticides. Further, farmers believe that they do not allow workers to enter fields before the restricted entry interval. Therefore, workers are not exposed to pesticides. They have been taught that pesticides are no longer a health hazard after the restricted entry interval has expired. Farmers also believe that the dangers of pesticides are exaggerated. They believe that because they adhere to all the regulations, no human health or environmental hazards result from the use of pesticides. Finally, farmers believe that they are overregulated. Many of the regulations they are forced to follow are unnecessary, and following these regulations results in a financial loss. At the same time, research consistently shows that farmers often ignore safety procedures due to constraints of time and money (e.g., Perry et al. 1999). The beliefs of farmers about farmworker pesticide exposure and the financial pressures they feel increase an unsafe work context for farmworkers.

5.5   Farmworker Behaviors that Affect Their Pesticide Exposure

Farmworker beliefs, perceptions, and knowledge about pesticide exposure, as well as those of their employers and supervisors, are important in understanding farmworker pesticide exposure. The direct correspondence of beliefs about pesticides to behaviors in the use of pesticides or safety behaviors has not been documented.

Many of the specific farmworker behaviors that might affect their pesticide exposure have not been documented. For example, studies have not documented whether farmworkers are provided with appropriate personal protective equipment (PPE) when they are working with pesticides, nor have studies documented whether farmworkers properly use PPE when it is provided. For example, the farmworkers in Fig. 5.4 are wearing appropriate PPE for their work in applying an herbicide from a back-pack sprayer. In most fieldwork situations, the appropriate pesticide PPE for farmworkers is work clothing that covers the head, body, arms, legs, and feet; that is a hat, a long-sleeve shirt that is closed around the neck, long pants, socks, and closed shoes. Research has not investigated the proportion of farmworkers who are clothed in this manner.

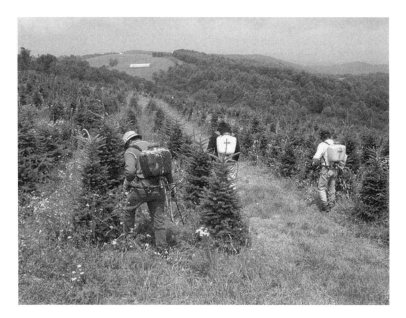

Fig. 5.4 Christmas tree workers with backpack sprayers. Copyright, Thomas A. Arcury

Research has shown that workers are often not provided with the required information that would help them avoid exposure. Fewer than half of the workers interviewed in North Carolina in 1999 indicated that they were told what pesticides had been applied where they are working, that information on pesticides that had been applied was posted in a central location accessible to workers, or that warning signs had been posted around fields to which pesticides had been applied (Arcury et al. 2001).

Bathing immediately after work is an important behavior to reduce farmworker pesticide exposure. Little information has been reported on personal hygiene behaviors among farmworkers, particularly bathing. North Carolina data from 1998 and 1999 for farmworkers living in camps indicates that almost all had access to showers where they lived (Arcury et al. 2001). Women in farmworker families interviewed in western North Carolina in 2003 and 2004 stated that almost three-quarters of farmworkers living in their homes showered within 15 minutes of arriving home.

The behaviors of women in farmworker families are safer than might be expected (Rao et al. 2006). While having limited knowledge of pesticides and of the potential of pesticide exposure for their families, the housekeeping practices of these women are such that they mitigate some potential exposures. These women also report that pesticide containers are not brought into their homes. While they have not received training that they should store and wash farm work clothes separately from other laundry, they do so simply because work clothes are so soiled. On the other hand, fewer than half report that clothes worn while doing farm work are changed outside the home, and about three-quarters of farmworkers shower within 15 minutes of arriving home. The number of women who report safe practices declines as the number of farmworkers in the house increases. Goldman et al. (2004) provide comparable results from a study of pregnant farmworkers in California. They found that among the 153 pregnant farmworkers whom they interviewed, over 40% did not store and wash clothes separately, 32% wore work shoes in the house, 45% wore work clothes more than 30 minutes before changing, and 58% bathed immediately after work.

5.6 Measurement of Actual Farmworker Pesticide Exposure

Measurement of pesticide exposure is difficult because of the short half-life of most pesticides currently in use. Because pesticides are metabolized and excreted from the body within a few days, research must be carefully timed to potential exposure. Several measurements (before and after exposure) are sometimes needed to detect exposure. These factors make exposure assessment difficult and expensive.

Given the extensive discussions of farmworker pesticide exposure, the lack of research actually measuring the levels of pesticides in the farm work environments and biomarkers of farmworker pesticides exposure is disappointing. Little such research has been conducted in any part of the US (Fenske et al. 2005; Barr et al. 2006; Hoppin et al. 2006a; Quandt et al. 2006). For farmworkers in the eastern US, this research is limited to two studies that have been reported in the literature. The first of these studies reports the numbers and levels of environmental pesticides in the houses of 41 farmworker families (Quandt et al. 2002, 2004), and pesticide urinary metabolite levels for adults and children living in nine of these houses (Arcury et al. 2005). The second study reports the pesticide urinary metabolite levels for 60 children living in farmworker households (Arcury et al. 2006, 2007). No research conducted in the eastern US has reported measures of pesticides in the environments in which farmworkers work, and no research conducted anywhere in the US has reported measures of pesticide biomarkers for a substantial sample of farmworkers.

Quandt et al.'s (2002, 2004) analysis of pesticides in the houses of 41 farmworkers in western North Carolina involved the collection of wipe sample from the floors in these houses, as well as from the toys of a focal child in each house, and from the hands of this focal child. These wipe samples were tested for 8 agricultural and 13 residential pesticides. Pesticides were found in the samples for 39 of the 41 houses, with at least one residential pesticide found in 39 houses, and at least one agricultural pesticide found in 20 houses. The pesticides included organochlorine insecticides in at least 17 of these dwellings, organophosphorus insecticides in at least 32 of these dwellings, carbamate insecticides in at least 15 of these dwellings, pyrethroid insecticides in 38 of these dwellings, and herbicides in at least 10 of these dwellings. A major concern of this study was the pathways for child pesticide exposure. As expected, the analysis showed the pathway to be from dwelling floors (39 houses, 95%), to child toys (29 houses, 71%), and then to child hands (24 houses, 55%). The detection in a house predicted detection in the toy from that house. Detection on the toy predicted detection on the hands.

Research conducted in the eastern US documenting actual exposure of farmworkers or their family members to pesticides using biomarkers is limited to two small studies in North Carolina. Arcury et al.'s (2005) study of biomarkers for family members in 9 of the 41 farmworker houses in western North Carolina was limited to the six general dialkylphosphate (DAP) metabolites of organophosporus pesticides: dimethylphosphate (DMP), dimethylthiophosphate (DMTP), dimethyldithiophosphate (DMDTP), diethylphosphate (DEP), diethylthiophosphate (DETP), and diethyldithiophosphate (DEDTP). Biomarkers for adults and children living in farmworkers' houses found that each had high levels of pesticide metabolites in their urine relative to reference data reported in the 1999–2000 National Health and Nutrition Examination Survey (Barr et al. 2004).

A study of 60 children, aged 1–6 years, living in eastern North Carolina farmworker dwellings was able to document the levels of the six general dialkylphosphate (DAP) metabolites of organophosporus pesticides, as well as those for 14 specific insecticide and herbicide metabolites (Arcury et al. 2006, 2007). The farmworker children had relatively high levels of organophosporus pesticide urinary metabolites compared to national reference data from the 1999–2000 National Health and Nutrition Examination Survey (Barr et al. 2004). For example, participating children had higher geometric means for diethylphosphate, diethylthiophosphate, and summed diethyl metabolites. Thirteen of 14 specific insecticide and herbicide metabolites were detected in these urine samples. Organophosphorus pesticide metabolites were detected in a substantial proportion of children, particularly metabolites of parathion/methyl parathion (PNP) (90.0%; geometric mean 1.00 µg/L), chlorpyrifos/chlorpyrifos methyl (TCPY) (83.3%; geometric mean 1.92 µg/L), and diazinon (IMPY) (55.0%; geometric mean 10.56 µg/L). Twenty-five of the children (41.7%) had the herbicide 2,4-D in their urine sample. The number of metabolites detected in the children's urine samples varied from 0 to 7. One child (1.7%) had no detects, 5 children (8.3%) had one detect, 1 child (1.7%) had two detects, 16 children (26.7%) had three detects, 17 children (28.3%) had four detects, 8 children (13.3%) had five detects, 9 children (15.0%) had six detects, and 3 children (5.0%) had seven detects. Also important were the number of metabolites for pesticides to which children in farmworker housing would not be expected to be exposed. The metabolite for parathion was found in urine samples from 90% of these children, yet parathion is an insecticide which is not used on crops that farmworkers cultivate or harvest. Seven of the children (11.6%) had the metabolite for coumaphos in their urine, yet this is an organophosphorus insecticide used to treat livestock. The urine of one child had the metabolite for the turf organophosphorous insecticide isazaphos; this insecticide was banned in 1998. The urine of another child had the metabolite for the herbicide 2,4,5-T; this herbicide was banned in 1986. The most plausible explanation for the number and variety of pesticides found in these farmworker children is the long-term deposition of these substances in the dwellings in which these children lived.

5.7 Health Outcomes of Pesticide Exposure Among Farmworkers and Their Families

Multiple sources suggest that pesticide exposure should affect the health of farmworkers and their families (Arcury and Quandt 1998; Eskenazi et al. 1999). However, few studies have documented the health outcomes of pesticide exposure among farmworkers or the members of their families in any part of the US (McCauley et al. 2006). Challenges in documenting any health outcomes among farmworkers have been recognized for some time (Zahm and Blair 2001). Because the most widely used insecticides, such as the organophosphorus and organochlorine pesticides, are neurotoxins, several investigators have sought to test the effects of pesticide exposure with measures of neurological development and decline. For example, recent efforts by Eskenazi and colleagues in California have begun to document developmental outcomes for children living in agricultural communities that are associated with pesticide exposure (Eskenazi et al. 2006, 2007; Fenster et al. 2007). They report that prenatal measures of the nonspecific dialkylphosphate (DAP) metabolites are inversely associated with mental development and with developmental problems at 24 months of age. They also found that prenatal exposure to the organochlorines DDT and DDE was associated with neurodevelopmental delays during early childhood; however, other analysis did not support this finding.

Research on the health outcomes of pesticide exposure for farmworkers that was conducted in the eastern US has been extremely limited. Kamel et al. (2003) completed batteries of neurobehavioral tests with adult farmworkers in Florida. While no biomarker of pesticide exposure was collected, comparisons of farmworkers with nonfarmworkers found that farmworkers had poorer performance in several of the specific tests and that longer duration of farm work was associated with worse performance. Rohlman et al. (2005) compared neurobehavioral test batteries completed by Latino children in farmworker families with Latino children from a nonagricultural community in North Carolina. They also found that the farmworker children performed more poorly on several of these tests than did children who were not from farmworker families.

Finally, an examination was conducted of birth defects for three farmworker children whose parents worked in Florida and North Carolina (Calvert et al. 2007). The three mothers worked in fields recently treated with several pesticides during the period of organogenesis. The farms on which the mothers of these babies worked have been cited for numerous pesticide safety violations. Despite the suggestion of pesticides being to blame, no causal link could be established.

5.8   Conclusions

Pesticide exposure is one of the best documented environmental and occupational health exposures for farmworkers and farmworker families in the eastern US. Multiple studies document the levels of exposure and the environment – both social and physical – that leads to exposure. The exposure of farmworkers and their families to pesticides is an injustice. Regulations exist that are designed to protect workers. However, these are either not enforced or the behaviors and environmental controls that they mandate are ineffective.

Farmworkers must be given accurate and timely information about their exposure in order to try to control it. While some researchers have described returning results of pesticide testing to farmworker families (Quandt et al. 2004), there has been little research on the best way to accomplish this. Findings published in scientific journals need to be disseminated in more accessible formats to workers. This is made difficult by the lack of firm scientific knowledge of the health effects of different doses of pesticides and of the mixtures of pesticides to which many workers are exposed.

While the research reviewed here establishes the exposure of farmworkers to pesticides and, in some cases, the dose received, few conclusions can be reached on the health effects for workers and their family members. Large samples are needed for researchers to understand the often subtle effects of pesticide exposure. For that reason, the Agricultural Health Study, active for over 15 years, is following 80,000 licensed pesticide applicators and their families. A similar study with longitudinal cohort design has not been initiated for farmworkers. The results from the Agricultural Health Study shed some light on the health risks faced by farmworkers, but they focus on different tasks and on workers with far more resources for protection (e.g., housing, health care, sanitation, control of the workplace) than farmworkers.

5.8.1 Recommendations

Based on this review of the literature on pesticides in farmworkers, we call for a variety of changes to regulations and for additional research on pesticides in farmworkers. Regulatory changes needed include revision and strengthening of the Worker Protection Standard. The current training required can be cursory. Workers typically are asked to sign a form saying they have been trained, but there is no assessment of knowledge acquired. Only field workers are trained; family members who may be affected by take-home pesticides or drift and who may be responsible for implementing some of the safety measures (e.g., washing work clothing) do not receive any training. We recommend that greater efforts be made to make all training educationally appropriate and to extend training to household members. Similarly, we recommend that the content of Worker Protection Standard training be expanded to include greater emphasis on the paraoccupational exposure pathway, pesticides being brought into the home on clothing and shoes, and on sources of environmental exposure, including drift. The Worker Protection Standard should also be expanded to include information on residential pesticide exposure pathways, including the remains of pesticides applied in homes in the past and on current residential pesticide application.

In addition to strengthening regulations for pesticides safety training mandated by the Work Protection Standard, there should be greater enforcement of regulations. A significant proportion of farmworkers in the eastern US do not receive pesticide safety education. Most enforcement is directed toward guest worker programs, leaving other farmworkers unprotected by enforcement. Other types of enforcement – e.g., proper storage of chemicals – are also needed.

Greater enforcement of field sanitation regulations is also needed. The number of workers reporting lack of field sanitation facilities continues to be substantial. Even when provision of one element, such as provision of drinking water, is improved, the accompanying elements, such as drinking cups, are not. Occupational sanitation requirements within the Worker Protection Standard and OSHA field sanitation regulations should also be expanded. Specifically, workers should be provided with facilities in which to change from work clothes and to shower. This would greatly reduce the paraoccupational pesticide exposure pathway for farmworkers and the members of their families.

States in the eastern US should follow the lead of California in establishing record keeping and reporting requirements for pesticide use. These requirements include the monthly reporting of all commercial pesticide applications including the type of pesticide applied, the amount of pesticide applied, and the location where pesticides are applied (California Department of Pesticide Regulation 2000). Such a program would make it easier to trace contamination and to investigate health effects. While growers are currently required to keep records of pesticides applied, these requirements are rarely enforced.

Policy for active monitoring of the pesticide dose experienced by farmworkers would improve health, safety, and justice. For example, Washington State has a program in which cholinesterase levels for pesticide handlers are monitored (Weyrauch et al. 2005; Hofmann et al. 2008).

Research is needed to understand better the effects of pesticides on health as such pesticides occur in practice. Most growers use multiple pesticides, but health effects studies test only one pesticide at a time. We need to know what effects the combination of multiple pesticides has on workers in both the short and long term. Research is also needed on the health effects posed by the inert ingredients in pesticides. Currently, these ingredients are proprietary information and pesticide companies need not disclose them. This makes it impossible to know if health effects seen in workers are the result of the active or inert ingredients.

We also call for research to better understand the health effects of pesticide exposure among farmworkers. This research should be a prospective cohort study, so data can be collected on exposures and dose and then compared to health effects that may occur years later. Besides data on standard risk factors, genetic data should be collected to facilitate understanding the gene–environment interactions associated with health outcomes. Because farmworkers live in housing that is frequently contaminated by take-home pesticides as well as residential pesticides, attention should be paid to residential as well as agricultural exposures.

We also call for policy changes related to use of pesticides. In the short term, improvements to pesticide labels such that they can be read and understood by all are needed. Currently, few items on the label are in Spanish, and sections that may be most necessary for individuals to protect themselves are buried amidst highly technical chemical ingredients and other information.

In the long term, efforts to reduce pesticide use in agriculture are needed. Integrated pest management holds promise as a way to reduce the contamination of the environment and to minimize human exposure. Development of pesticides that pose less threat to humans and to the environment is an alternative step.

Together these changes in regulations, research, and policy will serve to reduce the pesticide-related consequences of farm work now and in the future.

References

Alavanja MC, Akland G, Baird D et al. (1994) Cancer and noncancer risk to women in agriculture and pest control: the Agricultural Health Study. J Occup Med 36:1247–1250

Alavanja MC, Sandler DP, McMaster SB et al. (1996) The Agricultural Health Study. Environ Health Perspect 104:362–369

Alavanja MC, Dosemeci M, Samanic C et al. (2004) Pesticides and lung cancer risk in the agricultural health study cohort. Am J Epidemiol 160:876–885

Arcury TA, Quandt SA (1998) Chronic agricultural chemical exposure among migrant and seasonal farmworkers. Soc Nat Resour 11:829–843

Arcury TA, Quandt SA, Austin CK et al. (1999) Implementation of EPA's Worker Protection Standard training for agricultural laborers: an evaluation using North Carolina data. Public Health Rep 114:459–468

Arcury TA, Quandt SA, Cravey AJ et al. (2001) Farmworker reports of pesticide safety and sanitation in the work environment. Am J Ind Med 39:487–498

Arcury TA, Quandt SA, Russell GB (2002) Pesticide safety among farmworkers: perceived risk and perceived control as factors reflecting environmental justice. Environ Health Perspect 110(Suppl 2):233–240

Arcury TA, Quandt SA, Rao P et al. (2005) Organophosphate pesticide exposure in farmworker family members in western North Carolina and Virginia: case comparisons. Hum Organ 64:40–51

Arcury TA, Grzywacz JG, Davis SW et al. (2006) Organophosphorus pesticide urinary metabolite levels of children in farmworker households in eastern North Carolina. Am J Ind Med 49:751–760

Arcury TA, Grzywacz JG, Barr DB et al. (2007) Pesticide urinary metabolite levels of children in eastern North Carolina farmworker households. Environ Health Perspect 115:1254–1260

Baer RD, Penzell D (1993) Research report: susto and pesticide poisoning among Florida farmworkers. Cult Med Psychiatry 17:321–327

Barr DB, Bravo R, Weerasekera G et al. (2004) Concentrations of dialkyl phosphate metabolites of organophosphorus pesticides in the U.S. population. Environ Health Perspect 112:186–200

Barr DB, Thomas K, Curwin B et al. (2006) Biomonitoring of exposure in farmworker studies. Environ Health Perspect 114:936–942

Beseler C, Stallones L, Hoppin JA et al. (2006) Depression and pesticide exposures in female spouses of licensed pesticide applicators in the agricultural health study cohort. J Occup Environ Med 48:1005–1013

Bonner MR, Lee WJ, Sandler DP et al. (2005) Occupational exposure to carbofuran and the incidence of cancer in the Agricultural Health Study. Environ Health Perspect 113:285–289

Bonner MR, Coble J, Blair A et al. (2007) Malathion exposure and the incidence of cancer in the agricultural health study. Am J Epidemiol 166:1023–1034

Bradman A, Chevrier J, Tager I et al. (2005) Association of housing disrepair indicators with cockroach and rodent infestations in a cohort of pregnant Latina women and their children. Environ Health Perspect 113:1795–1801

California Department of Pesticide Regulation (2000) Pesticide use reporting: an overview of California's unique full reporting system. California Department of Pesticide Regulation, Sacramento

Calvert GM, Alarcon WA, Chelminski A et al. (2007) Case report: three farmworkers who gave birth to infants with birth defects closely grouped in time and place – Florida and North Carolina, 2004–2005. Environ Health Perspect 115:787–791

Carroll D, Samardick RM, Bernard S et al. (2005) Findings from the National Agricultural Workers Survey (NAWS) 2001–2002: a demographic and employment profile of United States farm workers (No. 9). US Department of Labor. http://www.doleta.gov/agworker/report9/naws_rpt9.pdf. Cited 17 Jul 2008

Carson R (1962) Silent spring. Houghton Mifflin Company, Boston

Early J, Davis SW, Quandt SA et al. (2006) Housing characteristics of farmworker families in North Carolina. J Immigr Minor Health 8:173–184

Elmore RC, Arcury TA (2001) Pesticide exposure beliefs among Latino farmworkers in North Carolina's Christmas tree industry. Am J Ind Med 40:153–160

Eskenazi B, Bradman A, Castorina R (1999) Exposures of children to organophosphate pesticides and their potential adverse health effects. Environ Health Perspect 107(Suppl 3):409–419

Eskenazi B, Marks AR, Bradman A et al. (2006) In utero exposure to dichlorodiphenyltrichloroethane (DDT) and dichlorodiphenyldichloroethylene (DDE) and neurodevelopment among young Mexican American children. Pediatrics 118:233–241

Eskenazi B, Marks AR, Bradman A et al. (2007) Organophosphate pesticide exposure and neurodevelopment in young Mexican-American children. Environ Health Perspect 115:792–798

Farr SL, Cooper GS, Cai J et al. (2004) Pesticide use and menstrual cycle characteristics among premenopausal women in the Agricultural Health Study. Am J Epidemiol 160:1194–1204

Farr SL, Cai J, Savitz DA et al. (2006) Pesticide exposure and timing of menopause: the Agricultural Health Study. Am J Epidemiol 163:731–742

Fenske RA, Lu C, Curl CL et al. (2005) Biologic monitoring to characterize organophosphorus pesticide exposure among children and workers: an analysis of recent studies in Washington State. Environ Health Perspect 113:1651–1657

Fenster L, Eskenazi B, Anderson M et al. (2007) In utero exposure to DDT and performance on the Brazelton neonatal behavioral assessment scale. Neurotoxicology 28:471–477

Flocks J, Clarke L, Albrecht S et al. (2001) Implementing a community-based social marketing project to improve agricultural worker health. Environ Health Perspect 109(Suppl 3):461–468

Flocks J, Monaghan P, Albrecht S et al. (2007) Florida farmworkers' perceptions and lay knowledge of occupational pesticides. J Community Health 32:181–194

Frisvold G, Mines R, Perloff JM (1988) The effects of job site sanitation and living conditions on the health and welfare of agricultural workers. Am J Agric Econ 70:875–885

General Accounting Office (2000) Pesticides: improvements needed to ensure the safety of farmworkers and their children. GAO/RCED-00-40. General Accounting Office, Washington, DC. http://www.gao.gov/archive/2000/rc00040.pdf. Cited 17 Jul 2008

Gentry AL, Grzywacz JG, Quandt SA et al. (2007) Housing quality among North Carolina farmworker families. J Agric Saf Health 13:323–337

Goldman L, Eskenazi B, Bradman A et al. (2004) Risk behaviors for pesticide exposure among pregnant women living in farmworker households in Salinas, California. Am J Ind Med 45:491–499

Grieshop JI, Stiles MC, Villaneuva N (1996) Prevention and resiliency: a cross cultural view of farmworkers' and farmers' beliefs about work safety. Hum Organ 55:25–32

Halfacre-Hitchcock A, McCarthy D, Burkett T et al. (2006) Latino migrant farmworkers in Lowcountry South Carolina: a demographic profile and an examination of pesticide risk perception and protection in two pilot case studies. Hum Organ 65:55–71

Hofmann JN, Carden A, Fenske RA et al. (2008) Evaluation of a clinic-based cholinesterase test kit for the Washington State cholinesterase monitoring program. Am J Ind Med 51:532–538

Holden C (2000) Abundant fields, meager shelter: findings from a survey of farmworker housing in the eastern migrant stream. Housing Assistance Council, Washington, DC

Hoppin JA, Adgate JL, Eberhart M et al. (2006a) Environmental exposure assessment of pesticides in farmworker homes. Environ Health Perspect 114:929–935

Hoppin JA, Umbach DM, London SJ et al. (2006b) Pesticides associated with Wheeze among commercial pesticide applicators in the Agricultural Health Study. Am J Epidemiol 163:1129–1137

Hoppin JA, Umbach DM, Kullman GJ et al. (2007a) Pesticides and other agricultural factors associated with self-reported farmer's lung among farm residents in the Agricultural Health Study. Occup Environ Med 64:334–342

Hoppin JA, Valcin M, Henneberger PK et al. (2007b) Pesticide use and chronic bronchitis among farmers in the Agricultural Health Study. Am J Ind Med 50:969–979

Hoppin JA, Umbach DM, London SJ et al. (2008) Pesticides and atopic and nonatopic asthma among farm women in the Agricultural Health Study. Am J Respir Crit Care Med 177:11–18

Hunt LM, Tinoco Ojanguren R, Schwartz N et al. (1999) Balancing risks and resources: applying pesticides without protective equipment in Southern Mexico. In: Hahn RA (ed). Anthropology in public health: bridging differences in culture and society. Oxford University Press, New York

Kamel F, Rowland AS, Park LP et al. (2003) Neurobehavioral performance and work experience in Florida farmworkers. Environ Health Perspect 111:1765–1772

Kamel F, Tanner CM, Umbach DM et al. (2007) Pesticide exposure and self-reported Parkinson's disease in the agricultural health study. Am J Epidemiol 165:364–374

Kamel F, Engel LS, Gladen BC et al. (2005) Neurologic symptoms in licensed private pesticide applicators in the agricultural health study. Environ Health Perspect 113:877–882

Kirrane EF, Hoppin JA, Kamel F et al. (2005) Retinal degeneration and other eye disorders in wives of farmer pesticide applicators enrolled in the agricultural health study. Am J Epidemiol 161:1020–1029

Lee WJ, Sandler DP, Blair A et al. (2007) Pesticide use and colorectal cancer risk in the Agricultural Health Study. Int J Cancer 121:339–346

Mahajan R, Blair A, Lynch CF (2006) Fonofos exposure and cancer incidence in the agricultural health study. Environ Health Perspect 114:1838–1842

McCauley LA, Anger WK, Keifer M et al. (2006) Studying health outcomes in farmworker populations exposed to pesticides. Environ Health Perspect 114:953–960

Occupational Safety and Health Administration (nd) Occupational safety and health standards for agriculture, 1928 subpart I – general environmental controls, 928.110. http://www.osha.gov/pls/oshaweb/owadisp.show_document?p_table = STANDARDS&p_id = 10959. Cited 6 Apr 2008

Perry MJ, Marbella A, Layde PM (1999) Association of pesticide safety beliefs and intentions with behaviors among farm pesticide applicators. Am J Health Promot 14:18–21

Purdue MP, Hoppin JA, Blair A et al. (2007) Occupational exposure to organochlorine insecticides and cancer incidence in the Agricultural Health Study. Int J Cancer 120:642–649

Quandt SA, Arcury TA, Austin CK et al. (1998) Farmworker and farmer perceptions of farmworker agricultural chemical exposure in North Carolina. Hum Organ 57:359–368

Quandt SA, Arcury TA, Mellen BG et al. (2002) Pesticides in wipes from farmworker residences in North Carolina. In: Levin H (ed). Proceedings of Indoor Air 2002, Santa Cruz, CA 4:900–905

Quandt SA, Arcury TA, Rao P et al. (2004a) Agricultural and residential pesticides in wipe samples from farmworker family residences in North Carolina and Virginia. Environ Health Perspect 112:382–387

Quandt SA, Doran AM, Rao P et al. (2004b) Reporting pesticide assessment results to farmworker families: development, implementation, and evaluation of a risk communication strategy. Environ Health Perspect 112:636–642

Quandt SA, Hernández-Valero MA, Grzywacz JG et al. (2006) Workplace, household, and personal predictors of pesticide exposure for farmworkers. Environ Health Perspect 114:943–952

Rao P, Arcury TA, Quandt SA et al. (2004) North Carolina growers' and extension agents' perceptions of Latino farmworker pesticide exposure. Hum Organ 63:151–161

Rao P, Gentry AL, Quandt SA et al. (2006) Pesticide safety behaviors in Latino farmworker family households. Am J Ind Med 49:271–280

Rao P, Quandt SA, Doran A et al. (2007) Pesticides in the homes of farmworker: Latino mothers' perceptions of risk to their children's health. Health Educ Behav 34:335–353

Reigart JR, Roberts JR (1999) Recognition and management of pesticide poisonings, 5th edn. Environmental Protection Agency, Washington, DC. http://www.epa.gov/oppfead1/safety/healthcare/handbook/handbook.htm. Cited 17 Jul 2008

Rohlman DS, Arcury TA, Quandt SA et al. (2005) Neurobehavioral performance in preschool children from agricultural and non-agricultural communities in Oregon and North Carolina. Neurotoxicology 26:589–598

Rubel AJ (1960) Concepts of disease in Mexican-American culture. Am Anthropol 62:795–814

Sakala C (1987) Migrant and seasonal farmworkers in the United Stated: a review of health hazards, status, and policy. Int Migr Rev 21:659–687

Salazar MK, Napolitano M, Scherer JA et al. (2004) Hispanic adolescent farmworkers' perceptions associated with pesticide exposure. West J Nurs Res 26:146–166

Saldana TM, Basso O, Hoppin JA et al. (2007) Pesticide exposure and self-reported gestational diabetes mellitus in the Agricultural Health Study. Diabetes Care 30:529–534

Sanborn M, Cole D, Kerr K et al. (2004) Pesticide literature review. Ontario College of Family Physicians, Toronto, Ontario. http://www.cfpc.ca/local/files/communications/current%20issues/pesticides/final%20paper%2023apr2004.pdf. Cited 17 Jul 2008

Shipp EM, Cooper SP, Burau KD et al. (2005) Pesticide safety training and access to field sanitation among migrant farmworker mothers from Starr County, Texas. J Agric Saf Health 11:51–60

US Environmental Protection Agency (US-EPA). Pesticide worker protection standard training 40CFR Part 170. http://www.epa.gov/oppfead1/safety/workers/PART170.htm. Cited 17 Jul 2008

Valcin M, Henneberger PK, Kullman GJ et al. (2007) Chronic bronchitis among non-smoking farm women in the agricultural health study. J Occup Environ Med 49:574–583

Vela-Acosta MS, Bigelow P, Buchan R (2002) Assessment of occupational health and safety risks of farmworkers in Colorado. Am J Ind Med 42(Suppl 2):19–27

Weller SC (1983) New data on intracultural variability: the hot-cold concept of medicine and illness. Hum Organ 42:249–257

Weyrauch KF, Boiko PE, Keifer M (2005) Building informed consent for cholinesterase monitoring among pesticide handlers in Washington State. Am J Ind Med 48:175–181

Zahm SH, Blair A (2001) Assessing the feasibility of epidemiologic research on migrant and seasonal farmworkers: an overview. Am J Ind Med 40:487–489

Zahm SH, Colt JS, Engel LS et al. (2001) Development of a life events/icon calendar questionnaire to ascertain occupational histories and other characteristics of migrant farmworkers. Am J Ind Med 40:490-501

Chapter 6
Tuberculosis, Sexually Transmitted Diseases, HIV, and Other Infections Among Farmworkers in the Eastern United States

Scott D. Rhodes

Abstract Farmworkers in the United States (US) have been disproportionately affected by the intersecting epidemics of tuberculosis (TB), sexually transmitted diseases (STDs), and HIV. Furthermore, farmworkers tend to be politically, socially, and economically disenfranchised, which contributes to their increased vulnerability to infectious diseases. This chapter examines the epidemiology of infectious diseases, specifically TB, STDs, and HIV, among farmworkers; explores the risks facing farmworkers; outlines existing and promising approaches for the prevention, care, and treatment among farmworkers; and recommends new areas for practice and research. Because data that document risk and infection rates among farmworkers are lacking and the current intervention arsenal is weak, focus must be placed on strengthening our understanding of needs and the development of effective multilevel strategies to intervene upon the health needs of this particularly vulnerable population. Nowhere is this more urgent than in the eastern US, an area in which little research has been done to understand and support farmworkers and a region that bears disproportionate burdens of TB, STDs, and HIV.

6.1 Introduction

Farmworkers in the United States (US) have been disproportionately affected by the intersecting epidemics of tuberculosis (TB), sexually transmitted diseases (STDs), and HIV. Although data describing current infection rates among farmworkers in the US are limited, farmworkers are estimated to be about six times more likely to develop TB compared to other employed adults in the US (Centers for Disease Control and Prevention 1992b; Institute of Medicine 2000). Given that most farmworkers in the US are Latino/Hispanic, STD infection rates among Latinos/Hispanics provide insight into the burden borne by farmworkers. In 2003, the rates of syphilis, gonorrhea, and chlamydia were two–four times higher among Latinos/Hispanics than among whites (Centers for Disease Control and Prevention 2004). Moreover, although the rates of syphilis are declining within some vulnerable

T.A. Arcury and S.A. Quandt (eds.), *Latino Farmworkers in Eastern United States*,
DOI: 10.1007/978-0-387-88347-2_6, © Springer Science+Business Media, LLC 2009

populations, including African Americans, rates continue to increase rapidly among US Latinos/Hispanics each year. Moreover, HIV infection rates among farmworkers in the eastern US range from 2.6% (Centers for Disease Control and Prevention 1992a) to 13% (Jones et al. 1991); these rates suggest that HIV infection rates among farmworkers are 5–22 times higher among farmworkers than within the general US adult population.

Farmworkers are susceptible to other types of infections, including impetigo, influenza, gastroenteritis, and Methicillin-resistant *Staphylococcus aureus* (MRSA). Often occurring in healthcare facilities such as hospitals, nursing homes, and dialysis centers, a second type of MRSA known as community-associated MRSA has emerged and may be of greater importance in terms of prevention and treatment for farmworkers. Community-associated MRSA occurs among otherwise healthy people in the wider community and is responsible for serious skin and soft tissue infections and pneumonia. Despite what is known about these infections in the general population and some specific subgroups, much less is known about prevalence of these various infections and their associated risks among farmworkers.

Farmworkers tend to be politically, socially, and economically disenfranchised, which contributes to their increased vulnerability to infectious diseases. This chapter examines the epidemiology of infectious diseases, specifically TB, STDs, and HIV, among farmworkers; explores the risks facing farmworkers; outlines existing and promising approaches for the prevention, care, and treatment among farmworkers; and recommends new areas for practice and research.

6.2   Tuberculosis (TB)

Tuberculosis (TB) is a disease caused by a bacterium called *Mycobacterium tuberculosis* that most often attacks the lungs. However, *M. tuberculosis* can attack any part of the body such as the kidney, spine, and brain. If not treated properly, active TB can be fatal. TB is spread through the air from one individual to another. TB is transmitted on small airborne droplets that are produced when an individual with TB of the lungs, throat, or larynx coughs, sneezes, or talks. These droplets can linger in the air for extended periods, and individuals who inhale them may become infected. About 10% of those initially infected will eventually develop active disease, and about half of those will develop active disease within two years following infection. The other 90% of untreated infected individuals will never develop active TB. Individuals who do not develop active TB have what is called latent TB infection (LTBI). Individuals who have LTBI do not feel sick, have no symptoms, and cannot spread TB to others. Some individuals with latent TB infection develop TB disease, thus appropriate completion of treatment of LTBI can considerably reduce lifetime risk of TB disease (Heymann 2004).

6.2.1 Epidemiology

Worldwide, tuberculosis is one of the top three infectious diseases in terms of mortality. Nearly a third of the world's population is infected with *M. tuberculosis*, the bacterium that causes TB, although active TB disease develops in only a fraction of these people. Each year, over 9 million people develop the disease and about two million die, mainly in developing countries. However, TB has reemerged in the US as well. This resurgence is attributable to a variety of factors including increased rates of HIV infection, the development of multidrug-resistant TB, increased immigration from countries where TB is endemic, and national and international neglect toward the elimination and treatment of the disease (Centers for Disease Control and Prevention 2008; Institute of Medicine 2000).

The exact rate of TB among farmworkers is not known, but the risk of TB among farmworkers is estimated to be at least six times greater than among the general US public (Centers for Disease Control and Prevention 1992b; Institute of Medicine 2000). Studies of farmworkers in the eastern US have uncovered rates of positive TB skin tests of 23–45% in New York (Much et al. 2000; Poss and Rangel 1997); 28.3% in Indiana (Garcia et al. 1996); 37% in the Delmarva peninsula (Jacobson et al. 1987); 41% in North Carolina (Ciesielski et al. 1991); 41–44% in Florida (Centers for Disease Control and Prevention 1992a; Much et al. 2000) and 48% in Virginia (Centers for Disease Control 1986). It should be noted, too, that most of these studies are older and thus outdated.

It has been suggested that skin tests using purified protein derivative (PPD) may result in false-positives among individuals who are from countries (e.g., Mexico) that use the Bacille Calmette-Guérin (BCG) vaccine against TB. However, most adults who received Bacille Calmette-Guérin before age 7 and who have a positive PPD skin test after age 21 are infected with *M. tuberculosis*. Thus, a positive PPD skin test is not likely due to receiving the Bacille Calmette-Guérin as a child (Ciesielski 1995).

6.3 Sexually Transmitted Diseases (STDs) and HIV

STDs remain a major public health challenge in the US and throughout the world. Although substantial progress has been made in preventing, diagnosing, and treating certain STDs within some populations and communities, it is estimated that approximately 19 million new infections occur each year in the US (Workowski and Berman 2006; Naughton and Rhodes 2009). More than 25 organisms cause infections that are transmitted through sexual contact. The causes of STDs are bacteria, parasites, and viruses. Many STDs go unnoticed and untreated because they are often asymptomatic. An extended lag time may occur between infection and the repercussions of an STD. Most STDs affect both men and women, but in many cases the health complications are more severe for women. For example, if a pregnant woman has an STD, it can cause serious health problems for the baby.

Although it can be transmitted through blood to blood contact through needle and/or syringe sharing, HIV is commonly sexually transmitted. Besides blood, HIV can be transmitted through semen, vaginal fluids, and breast milk of a person infected with HIV. Unfortunately, a vaccine or cure for HIV is several years, perhaps decades, away (Anonymous 2001). However, advances in medical treatments have improved the outcomes for some persons living with HIV/AIDS who have access to these advances. Dramatic improvements in HIV treatment came in 1996 when highly effective, but also very toxic, medications such as protease inhibitors and non-nucleoside reverse transcriptase inhibitors became available and were used as part of highly active antiretroviral therapy to suppress HIV viral replication and improve immune function. Although they do not work for everyone and access to them can be difficult because of reasons such as price, these medications have changed the lives of many of those living with HIV/AIDS in the US.

6.3.1   Epidemiology

STDs, including HIV infection, are major health problems among migrant workers in the US, but data that explore STD and HIV among farmworkers are extremely limited. Thus, it is necessary to explore STDs and HIV by ethnicity. Rates of reportable STDs and HIV are higher among Latinos/Hispanics than among whites. In 2003, the rates of syphilis, gonorrhea, and chlamydia were two to four times higher among Latinos/Hispanics than among whites (Centers for Disease Control and Prevention 2004, 2005). Syphilis rates increased by more than 20% among US Latinos/Hispanics each year between 2000 and 2003, while dramatically declining among African Americans (Centers for Disease Control and Prevention 2004). Another study in Decatur, Alabama, found a 5% positive syphilis rate within a door-to-door convenience sample of predominately Latino/Hispanic men (Paz-Bailey et al. 2004). Although little is known about the extent to which farmworker communities in the eastern US are affected by STDs, these studies illustrate what may be happening in eastern US farmworker communities.

Latinos/Hispanics in the US are disproportionately affected by HIV/AIDS. Nationally, the AIDS case rate among Latinos/Hispanics is 3.5 times higher than in whites and is only second to African Americans (Centers for Disease Control and Prevention 2007). The highest prevalence of HIV among Latinos/Hispanics is found in the eastern part of the US, particularly in the Northeast (Fernandez et al. 2004). HIV prevalence has been reported between 2.6% (Centers for Disease Control and Prevention 1988) and 13% (Jones et al. 1991) among farmworkers in the eastern US. The prevalence among farmworkers is much higher than that among the general US adult population, which is approximately 0.6% (Centers for Disease Control and Prevention 2007). Of course, the studies of HIV among farmworkers are extremely outdated; each of them is over 15 years old. Given the rise of HIV infection rates over time among minority populations, the rates may very well be higher.

Several studies have documented that farmworkers are behaviorally at high risk for HIV. Lifetime use of condoms has been identified as low while sex with multiple partners, sex with commercial sex workers, and with partners with histories of STD infection have been identified as common (Aranda-Naranjo and Gaskins 1998; Brammeier et al. 2008; Fernandez et al. 2004; Ford et al. 2001; Inciardi et al. 1999; Jones et al. 1991; McVea 1997; Organista et al. 1996, 1997; Sanchez et al. 2004).

6.4   Risks

The factors that affect risk for infectious diseases such as TB, STDs, and HIV can be organized into three domains, as presented in Fig. 6.1. These domains include intrapersonal factors that affect risk including knowledge of infectious diseases and available services; cultural and social factors including "sexual silence," gender role socialization and machismo, and the use of *curanderos* (traditional healers); and factors related to the immigration experience and being a farmworker including substandard housing, fears related to discovery and documentation, barriers to services, loneliness, and cultural conflicts.

6.4.1   Intrapersonal Factors

Intrapersonal factors influencing risk include the lack of a thorough understanding of transmission, prevention, and treatment strategies and of US healthcare services, even of those services for which they are eligible (Eng and Butler 1997; Rhodes et al. 2007; Sanchez et al. 2004). Studies have found that although some farmworkers have an understanding of how TB is transmitted, they also may hold misconceptions. While reporting that TB can be contracted by breathing in the air exhaled by an individual infected with the disease, farmworkers have reported TB to be transmitted by eating off the same plate or sleeping on infected bedcovers (Poss 2001).

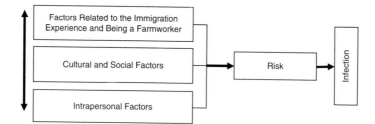

Fig. 6.1 Factors affecting infectious disease exposure among farmworkers in the eastern US

Some farmworkers have reported that TB can be contracted by smoking tobacco or being exposed to cold and hot temperatures (Chap. 2) (Poss 1999, 2000).

Besides having little knowledge of and misconceptions about TB, farmworkers also have information needs pertaining to the prevention, care, and treatment of STDs and HIV. During a focus group study to explore STD and HIV concerns among Latino men (Rhodes et al. 2007), a farmworker from Mexico asked, "AIDS? I don't know much about it to be honest. Can you get it from urine?" Although knowledge (e.g., knowing about TB, STD, or HIV or how to access treatment) does not imply behavior change, having a context in which to place prevention messages is required for those messages to be understood and given meaning.

Furthermore, farmworkers often lack information about how to access available services for proper screening, treatment, and follow-up of infectious diseases. Although there are a multitude of barriers to utilizing healthcare services (Arcury and Quandt 2007), a fundamental barrier is the lack of knowledge about where services are provided, what services are available, and how to access services (Martin et al. 1996; Rhodes et al. in press).

Often farmworkers come from countries where TB is highly prevalent or even endemic (Centers for Disease Control and Prevention 2006). A majority of farmworkers in the eastern US come from Mexico and Central America (Carroll et al. 2005). In 2005, Mexico had an estimated 27 TB cases per 100,000 people, while El Salvador, Guatemala, and Honduras each had an estimated 68, 110, and 99 cases per 100,000 people, respectively (World Health Organization 2007). These numbers substantially differ from case rates in the US which, in that same year, had just under five cases per 100,000 overall, with whites having an estimated 1.2 cases per 100,000 (Centers for Disease Control and Prevention 2006). Thus, farmworkers may become symptomatic after arriving in the US.

6.4.2 Cultural and Social Factors

Attitudes and beliefs held by farmworkers may not support safer sex as a method to prevent STD and HIV infection. These attitudes and beliefs may be culturally and socially prescribed. For example, some Latinos/Hispanics may consider the open discussion and "negotiation" of condom use inappropriate and the use of condoms as sacrificing sensitivity, sensation, and passion and interrupting sexual spontaneity (Organista et al. 2004). Furthermore, Latinos/Hispanics in general, and farmworkers in particular, may be constrained by "sexual silence" which is characterized by shying away from the open discussion of sex and sexuality. This discomfort with talking about sex and sexuality may lead to condom use not being discussed or initiated among partners. Sexual concerns may not be discussed even with healthcare providers (Solorio et al. 2004). When conversations do occur, messages expressed are often vague and/or inaccurate. For Latino/Hispanic male farmworkers who have sex with men, their orientation or behavior may further preclude discussions about sex (Somerville et al. 2006).

Besides the disinclination to discuss sex and sexuality, gender role socialization prescribes that Latino/Hispanic men must avoid "feminine behaviors," be perceived as powerful, be and appear dominant, and prove their manhood by taking risks. This often is called "machismo" (Chap. 2) (Falicov 1996; Rhodes et al. 2006, 2007; Rothenberg 1995). Engaging in risk may affirm one's masculinity; using condoms can be seen as weakness, and for some men seeking or utilizing healthcare services for screening, treatment, and follow-up also shows weakness (Rhodes et al. 2007). As a farmworker who was interviewed in a study exploring the influences on STD and HIV risk behaviors among Latino/Hispanic men (Rhodes et al. in press) reported, "Some men, some Latino men just like me, are going to do what it takes to show others that they are men. You know, how men are supposed to be: strong, in charge, macho." Thus, sexual risk behavior, which puts men at risk for STDs and HIV, may be a way to show others that one is still a man and conforms to cultural and social standards of what it means to be a man.

Although the data around sexual behavior and sexual risk are limited, the high prevalence of farmworkers' contact with commercial sex workers has been documented. Reported rates range from 18 to 28% among farmworkers in the eastern US (Parrado et al. 2004; Viadro and Earp 2000). This high prevalence of the use of commercial sex workers is associated with the environment in which farmworkers live and work.

Not technically farmworkers themselves, commercial sex workers in rural communities may have a client base comprised of farmworkers. Thus, they are similarly at increased risk for STD and HIV infection. In the eastern US, the commercial sex work industry has changed as the immigrant community has changed. Ten to fifteen years ago, commercial sex workers solicited male farmworkers at labor camps, bars, and other locations where they congregated, often on paydays and in areas in which farmworkers cash their paychecks. These commercial sex workers tended to be African American and white women. That demographic is changing in some areas. Often commercial sex workers are Latina/Hispanic women who were lured into their work through promises of employment. They did not realize that the help they had crossing the border into the US, for example, would have to be paid back through their sexual servitude. Many of them find themselves working at informal brothels in rural communities and may be traded or bought and sold across communities (Bletzer 2005; Knipper et al. 2007; Parrado et al. 2004; Paz-Bailey et al. 2004; Rhodes et al. 2007). STDs and HIV are a concern, but for commercial sex workers, human rights issues are clearly of fundamental importance.

Farmworkers also may rely on traditional medicine or informal over formal sources of health care. Sources of care include relatives or neighbors, herbalists, or *curanderos* (traditional healers) (McVea 1997; Suarez et al. 1996). In North Carolina, HIV-positive Latinos/Hispanics have reported using amulets that are sold by *curanderos* who claim that if worn during sexual intercourse they protect against STD and HIV infection, negating the need for condom use (Bowden et al. 2006).

6.4.3 Factors Related to the Immigration Experience and Being a Farmworker

The experience of coming to the US and living as a farmworker is rife with challenges that also may increase farmworker susceptibility to infectious diseases such as TB, STDs, and HIV. These risks include substandard and crowded housing, fears related to discovery and deportation, barriers related to accessing healthcare services, loneliness, and cultural conflicts.

Farmworkers tend to live in substandard, crowded, and poorly ventilated housing conditions (Chap. 3) (Bennett et al. 2008; Gentry et al. 2007; Much et al. 2000; Rust 1990). A national survey of farmworker housing conditions completed by the Housing Assistance Council (HAC), a nonprofit organization whose mission is to promote affordable housing in rural areas in the US, found that 52% of the 4,600 housing units assessed were "crowded," which was ten times the national average for household overcrowding. Federal standards classify crowding as more than one person per room, excluding kitchens and bathrooms; HAC excluded dormitories and other structures designed for high occupancy. A majority of housing units also were identified as being highly or moderately substandard, having holes in walls, being infested with rodents or insects, or having substantially damaged roofs (Holden 2002). This type of environment increases the risk for exposure to and infection with TB, for example. Although the risk is great for TB, these types of housing conditions also contribute to influenza, hepatitis, and gastroenteritis.

Fearing discovery and deportation, undocumented farmworkers often have been found to avoid formal systems of health care. This fear may lead to low levels of exposure to preventive education, as well as reluctance to seek screening and treatment for infectious diseases. This fear of formal systems of care has led some Latinos/Hispanics, for example, to rely on traditional approaches to health (Chap. 2) (Rhodes et al. 2007). Furthermore, farmworkers may avoid seeking care regardless of documentation status; a generalized distrust of formal systems has been found to dissuade some immigrant populations from accessing services (Rhodes et al. 2006).

Furthermore, rural communities, especially those in the eastern US that do not have a long history of large numbers of non-English speaking populations, frequently do not have the capacity to meet the healthcare needs of farmworker populations (Arcury and Quandt 2007). For example, healthcare staff may not speak Spanish or other languages spoken by farmworkers, and interpreters may be sparse or ill-equipped to provide quality and effective interpretive services (Rhodes et al. 2007). Hours of operation of healthcare organizations may not correspond with the availability of farmworkers, and the locations may not be conveniently located for those with limited transportation options. These barriers and others like them make it challenging for farmworkers to get the care and treatment they need (Aranda-Naranjo and Gaskins 1998; Rhodes et al. 2008; Solorio et al. 2004). Thus, not only are the morbidity and mortality rates related to infectious diseases increased, but the chances of transmission of these infectious diseases to those previously uninfected are greatly increased.

Loneliness associated with social isolation resulting from immigration also may contribute to risk behaviors, such as sexual risk as well as increased alcohol consumption and episodic binge drinking that may lead to sexual risk. Many farmworkers leave their families and support networks in order to come to the eastern US and work on farms. Missing their families and communities coupled with finding themselves in challenging living situations may lead to risk behavior as they attempt to deal with this loneliness (Kim-Godwin and Bechtel 2004; Rhodes et al. in press; Shedlin et al. 2005). Chapter 9 provides a thorough discussion of farmworker mental health.

Finally, increased poverty rates, harsh working conditions, and racial discrimination may challenge the self-image and traditional values of farmworkers (Amaro et al. 2001; Aranda-Naranjo and Gaskins 1998; Organista et al. 2004; Painter 2008). Immigrant farmworkers must cope with conflicting cultural and social norms and expectations while attempting to adjust to life in a new country (Takahashi 1997; Talashek et al. 2004; Viadro and Earp 2000). Norms and expectations, including those related to sexual behavior in particular and gender roles (whether "positive" or "negative," "healthy" or "unhealthy") may be challenged (Organista et al. 2000; Pulerwitz et al. 2002), and for some, the subsequent stress and depression may result in higher rates of risk behavior and increased rates of STD and HIV infection (Aranda-Naranjo and Gaskins 1998; Organista et al. 2004). As a 36-year-old former farmworker commented,

"You have no idea. I sold everything I had. I crossed the border illegally. I was scared. I had $70.00 in my pocket when I got here. I had to live with my sister-in-law. I hated it. In the beginning, I had to walk to the fields or get a ride. When I wasn't at work, I was getting drunk and looking for women. I missed my family. It wasn't easy. I didn't care about a condom."

6.5 Prevention, Care, and Treatment

Despite the needs for prevention, care, and treatment of infectious diseases among farmworkers in the eastern US, the existing intervention arsenal to meet these profound needs is extremely limited. Furthermore, what does exist is limited in scope and numbers of farmworkers who can be affected and may benefit from available interventions. This section highlights currently available interventions for TB, STD, and HIV prevention, care, and treatment.

6.5.1 TB Prevention, Care, and Treatment

In general, TB is a preventable disease. From a public health standpoint, the best way to control TB is to diagnose and treat individuals with TB infection before they develop active disease. However, reducing the risk factors of TB among farmworkers will reduce the need for treatment. Changes in farmworker housing standards, for example, would reduce the risks associated with overcrowding and poor ventilation, both of which are associated with TB infection.

The treatment protocol for TB presents special challenges for migrant farmworkers. The current typical treatment for latent TB infection consists of preventive drug therapy to destroy dormant bacteria that might become active in the future. Therapy usually consists of a daily dose of the TB medication isoniazid (INH). For treatment to be effective, it is necessary to take isoniazid for six to nine months, and long-term use can cause serious side effects, including hepatitis, a life-threatening liver disease. For these reasons, ongoing monitoring is necessary while an individual with latent TB infection takes isoniazid. Use of acetaminophen (e.g., Tylenol) and alcohol can greatly increase the risk of liver damage. For those with active TB disease, a multi-drug therapy is necessary. Depending on the severity of TB disease and whether there is drug resistance, the number of medications may be reduced after a few months; however, the combination therapy may be taken for up to 12 months.

The challenge with either therapy, for latent TB infection or active TB, is that many farmworkers in the eastern US are transitory. This makes treatment follow-up, ongoing access to medications and adherence, and management of side effects difficult. Often, farmworkers may move to another location before treatment is complete. They may be "lost" to providers who were treating them and they may not get back into the healthcare system for treatment. Adherence to medication protocols, particularly those that are long term such as TB, is not congruent with the migrant lifestyle.

Farmworkers also may feel better and thus think that continuation of their treatment is unnecessary. They may misunderstand disease progression, their TB treatment protocol, and/or the importance of adhering to a long-term regimen. These misunderstandings may result from language barriers, the costs of treatment (including financial as well as time and other resources), and distrust of evidence-based medicine (Briggs 2005; Centers for Disease Control 1986; Centers for Disease Control and Prevention 1992b). Risks of incomplete treatment include selection of increasingly resistant TB and infection of others with resistant TB.

6.5.1.1 TBNet

TBNet is a multinational tuberculosis patient tracking and referral project designed to work with mobile, underserved populations. Treatment of these populations is complicated by the fact that many farmworkers do not remain in a given location for sufficient lengths of time to complete the TB treatment regimen. TBNet was developed in the mid-1990s as a strategy to increase adherence to treatment through tracking and coordinating the care of TB patients who move between public health jurisdictions.

Staff from TBNet facilitate the completion of treatment among mobile TB patients such as migrant farmworkers through three programmatic components. First, TB clinics are supplied with wallet-sized Health Network cards for their patients. These cards can easily be carried by the patient wherever they go. The toll-free number on the card enables staff from TB clinics to call for a patient's medical records in order to continue the patient's treatment. Second, TBNet maintains a central storehouse of enrollee medical records. A patient's healthcare provider, whether in the US, Mexico, or Central America, can call TBNet on a toll-free line to request an up-to-date copy of the patient's medical record. Finally, mobile patients also can call TBNet on the toll-free line for help locating treatment facilities at their next destination. At the conclusion of treatment, TBNet notifies the enrolling clinic as well as the state or regional TB control personnel that the patient has completed treatment.

TBNet ensures coordination of continuous treatment of mobile TB patients. Data indicate that this approach to TB intervention among farmworkers may be effective. Patients who have been enrolled in the system have experienced a high TB drug regime completion rate. In 2005, for example, TBNet supported 402 patients, and 321 patients moved at least once during treatment. Some patients moved four or five times during treatment. The completion rate of the treatment regimen for those with active TB was 71.4% and for those with latent TB infection was 54.4%. TBNet was originally created for migrant farmworkers. Because of its success, it is expanding its patient base to include the homeless, immigration detainees, prison parolees, or anyone else who might be mobile during their treatment.

6.5.1.2   Directly Observed Therapy

Healthcare providers often are hesitant to initiate TB treatment unless they feel sure that a patient will complete the treatment protocol (Institue of Medicine 2000). Directly observed therapy for TB treatment is the delivery of every scheduled dose of medication by a healthcare provider. The provider directly administers, observes, and documents the patient's ingestion or injection of the tuberculosis medication. The purpose of directly observed therapy for TB treatment is to ensure patients receive the medication therapy required to prevent the spread of tuberculosis and to prevent multi-drug resistance (Volmink and Garner 2007). It can be difficult to follow farmworkers over time, but treatment and tracking systems that provide ongoing access to directly observed therapy services along with extended provider hours, off-site administration of therapy, and thorough recordkeeping and cross-jurisdiction coordination along farmworker migratory paths have proven to be successful in Florida, for example (Carter et al. 2008). The process of having to show up and present oneself to a healthcare provider for directly observed therapy may increase adherence because it reinforces the importance of the treatment regimen for some populations (Garner et al. 2007). This ongoing "checking in" may prove invaluable to ensure increased understanding of infectivity and disease progression, and trust of medicine among farmworkers.

6.5.1.3   Future Approaches to TB Treatment and Prevention

Increased multidrug-resistant TB argues for shorter, simpler, and less toxic regimes for the treatment. Treatment of TB requires a minimum of six to nine months of daily therapy for maximum effectiveness, depending on the drug combination. However, limited drug development research is currently being undertaken to develop alternatives to TB treatment due in part to the perceived limited market of patients with active TB in the US. Although investigators in academia and the bio-technology industry explore how to translate basic knowledge into pragmatic applications, industry decision-makers, who influence drug development efforts, base their priorities on the perceived economics of the potential market. The prevention, care, and treatment of TB are not viewed as profitable. Productivity is measured by patents and products that are ultimately marketed and the "bottom line." Thus, barring the development of new medications, new combinations of existing drugs and their regimens are being explored.

Although new combinations of drugs and drug regimens have been approved, data are limited. In combination with increasing rates of drug resistance, treatment of TB is particularly problematic because the new shorter-term protocols include drugs that are not as effective against TB because of drug resistance. Moreover, prospects for new drugs for the treatment of TB are hampered by the lack of techniques for the screening of drug activity against latent bacteria.

The only available vaccine against TB is Bacille Calmette Guérin (BCG). Bacille Calmette Guérin is a weakened version of a bacterium called *Mycobacterium bovis* which is closely related to *M. tuberculosis*, the agent responsible for TB. The efficacy rates of Bacille Calmette Guérin range from less than zero (i.e., vaccinated individuals were at higher risk) to 75–80%. The reasons for this variability may include differences in vaccine strains, differences in the rate of background infection with environmental mycobacteria, and other care and transport of the vaccine, differences related to patient level variables, such as age and socioeconomic status (Centers for Disease Control and Prevention 1996; Colditz et al. 1995; Rodrigues et al. 1993).

An ideal vaccine against TB must be safe, efficacious, easy to administer, long lasting, inexpensive, heat stable, not interfere with TB skin testing, and easily inte-grated into existing immunization schedules. Furthermore, there must be incentives for industry to focus on TB vaccine research. Currently, few biotechnology and pharmaceutical industries are investigating TB vaccination because the timeframe for full development, clinical testing, and final product marketing, if a successful vaccine were to be forthcoming, would be 10–20 years in the future. Thus, although vaccination research should be prioritized, it cannot replace behavioral and structural approaches (e.g., TBNet) that support initiation and completion of TB drug regimens.

6.5.2 Prevention, Care, and Treatment of STDs and HIV

The Dissemination of Effective Behavioral Interventions (DEBI) Project of the Division of HIV/AIDS Prevention, CDC, currently is diffusing science-based interventions to AIDS service organizations (ASOs), community-based organizations (CBOs), public health departments, and other prevention providers. These interventions are focused on reducing STD and HIV risks among populations and communities living in the US. One intervention entitled *VOICES/VOCES* targets urban nongay Hispanic men and women, predominantly from Puerto Rico, and African American men and women. The video-based, group-level intervention was tested in New York City STD clinics and found to increase condom use and decrease repeat STD infections (O'Donnell et al. 1998). Although this intervention provides insight for scientifically sound HIV prevention interventions with Latinos/Hispanics, it is less relevant for farmworkers, who tend to be less acculturated and have less real and perceived access to healthcare services. Over the next few years, eight additional interventions are expected to be diffused by the CDC. Only one targets Spanish speakers, but is designed for Puerto Ricans and aims to reduce drug use and injection-related HIV risk behaviors (Robles et al. 2004). Again, this intervention is not designed for the farmworker population that is found in the eastern US.

In a systematic review of the Latino/Hispanic HIV prevention intervention literature published in 2001, some evidence for influencing sexual risk behavior was found in 12 intervention studies; however, all studies had short follow-up (≤ 3 months), and often threats to contamination were high. The few studies that included diverse Latinos/Hispanics populations did not stratify results to examine differential effects for Latinos/Hispanics from Mexico and Central America. Because of the heterogeneity of these communities, strategies that were effective in some communities may not work in others without considerable adaptation, revision, and reconfiguration (Rothenberg 1995). Heterosexual Latinos/Hispanics were conspicuously absent from most studies (Darbes et al. 2002), and none of these studies were completed with farmworker populations.

However, a variety of lessons have been learned about STD and HIV prevention intervention efforts to date. Behaviorally focused interventions can be designed, delivered, and found effective to prevent STDs and HIV among communities considered to be at increased risk. These interventions tend to be founded on the lived experiences of community members; include multisessions; be theory based; teach condom use and problem-solving skills; and address barriers to condom use (Centers for Disease Control and Prevention & HIV/AIDS Prevention Research Synthesis Project 1999; Herbst et al. 2007; Rhodes et al. 2006).

With the gaps in the current arsenal to combat STDs and HIV, further research must be initiated and supported to meet the STD and HIV prevention needs of farmworkers. However, interventions based on individual behavior change may not be the only approach to STD and HIV prevention as they tend to reach limited numbers of people. Only those few who have access and choose to participate gain from such interventions. Moreover, STD and HIV prevention interventions are subject to the political will for funding and in terms of intervention content. For example, Stop AIDS Project in San Francisco was the target of a two-year investigation by the CDC and the US Department of Health and Human Services (HHS) based on allegations by conservative lawmakers that staff of Stop AIDS Project promoted and encouraged sexual activity. Innovative intervention activities within other distinct "hidden" and "high-risk" populations also have come under fire for the delivery of STD and HIV prevention interventions that were culturally appropriate for the populations for which they were designed. These interventions did not reflect the expectations of people with power for whom they were not designed (Block 2004).

The immediate social context of sexual or drug-injection behaviors can be influenced by changing the physical or normative environments within which they occur. An example might be working with brothel owners to require the use of condoms in brothels with commercial sex workers. Working with brothels to change practices and normalize condom use has been effective in international STD and HIV prevention efforts (Kumar 1998; Stadler and Delany 2006; Visrutaratna et al. 1995). Brothels with commercial sex workers are becoming increasingly common in rural communities in the eastern US, and to date the potential to partner with brothels in the US has remained largely unexplored.

Further, structural interventions also may include strategies to reduce or change sociocultural norms and expectations that influence behavior. For example, male farmworkers may struggle to reconcile their difficulties fulfilling traditionally masculine roles, and may use increased sexual behavior and sexual risk to salvage their gender selves. Besides focusing on the positive aspects of manhood and reframing the negative aspects to reduce risk, interventions that help male farmworkers effectively manage the incongruence between the practical realities of living in the US, such as taking on roles that may be less common for men and do not meet sociocultural norms and expectations and the culturally defined roles that are traditionally ascribed to men in their cultures, may be effective at reducing risk among farmworkers overall (Rhodes and Hergenrather 2007). What this might look like, however, requires further exploration and research.

One study of recently arrived immigrant Latino/Hispanic men in rural North Carolina used a lay health advisor approach within the social structure of a soccer league to reduce sexual risk. The intervention was known as *HoMBReS: Hombres Manteniendo Bienestar y Relaciones Saludables* (Men: Men Maintaining Wellbeing and Healthy Relationships). The intervention included imparting STD and HIV prevention knowledge and skills to male lay health advisors known as *Navegantes*, but it also taught the *Navegantes* how to serve as: (1) health advisors, provide referrals, and build condom use skills among other men, (2) opinion leaders to bolster the positive aspects and reframe negative aspects of what it means to be a man, and (3) community advocates to promote environmental change. The intervention was designed to address the sociocultural norms and expectations around what it means to be a man. Rather than focusing solely on individual behavior change, the intervention was developed to raise awareness, impart knowledge, and change norms and expectations (Rhodes et al. 2006, 2008). For example, formative data indicated that these men considered asking for help and seeking care as a sign of weakness (Rhodes et al. 2007; Rhodes and Hergenrather 2007). The intervention related asking for help and seeking care to other domains in which these behaviors were viewed as acceptable, such as finding housing or buying a car.

Because of the misconceptions about when and how to use a condom within a sample of immigrant Latino/Hispanic men, the majority of whom were male farmworkers (Rhodes et al. 2007), the *HoMBReS* intervention included activities to build condom use skills. A hands-on condom use activity that was included in the intervention

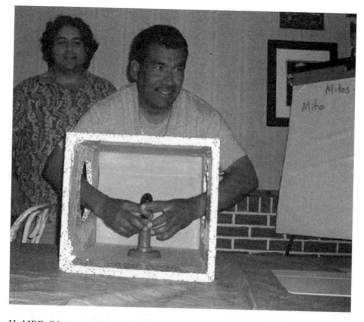

Fig. 6.2 *HoMBReS* intervention condom use night simulator

was developed to break down barriers around talking about condoms with other men and build practical experiences with condom use. Men practiced placing a condom on a penis model that they could not see. This activity was designed to break the ice around talking about sex and sexuality among Latino/Hispanic men and simulate the difficulty of putting on a condom in the dark. Figure 6.2 provides an illustration of an intervention participant, who was being trained to serve as a *Navegante*, practicing his condom use technique.

Because farmworker communities are diverse and their priorities and needs are distinct, *HoMBReS* also used community-specific materials to reach Latino/Hispanic men. Figure 6.3 provides an illustration of a condom tips brochure that was developed by a team of community and academic partners that included farmworkers in rural North Carolina for the *HoMBReS* intervention.

Discrimination and its effect on health and wellbeing of minority populations have been recognized as affecting health and wellbeing (Institute of Medicine 2003). Farmworkers report high levels of perceived discrimination and racism. However, to date, little intervention research has been developed to transform a community through some type of sociopolitical or cultural intervention (Guerin 2005; Smedley and Syme 2000).

For farmworkers living with HIV, access to therapeutic drugs, such as antiretroviral, may be limited because of their costs. Outpatient services and the necessary medications for HIV-positive farmworkers can be provided from sources such as those funded by the Ryan White HIV/AIDS Program. However, the AIDS Drug Assistance Program

a

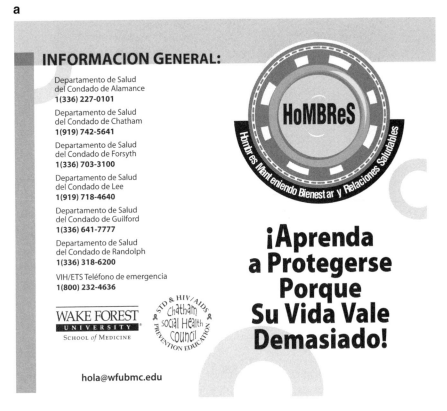

Fig. 6.3 *HoMBReS* intervention condom tips brochure

(ADAP) administered by each state may have varying requirements for documentation of residency status. Providers of care to farmworkers living with HIV/AIDS adhere to documentation standards to varying degrees and are often able to cobble together resources for care and treatment through these programs, the recycling of medications (although not legal), and the use of pharmaceutical assistance programs. Of course, it is challenging to ensure that farmworkers living with HIV get tested and receive the care and treatment they deserve due to other barriers as well, such as barriers inherent in their lifestyle and their frequent mobility.

6.6 Discussion

The disproportionately increased rates of TB, STD, and HIV transmission and infection among farmworkers in the eastern US illustrate the importance for strengthened and sustained effort to meet this vulnerable community's prevention

b

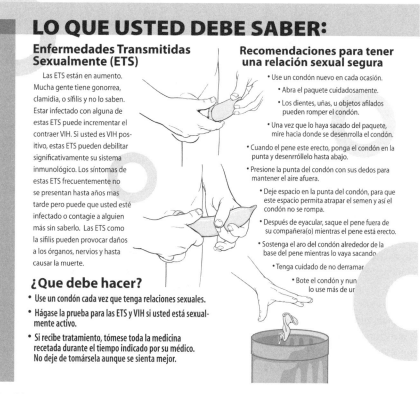

LO QUE USTED DEBE SABER:

Enfermedades Transmitidas Sexualmente (ETS)

Las ETS están en aumento. Mucha gente tiene gonorrea, clamidia, o sífilis y no lo saben. Estar infectado con alguna de estas ETS puede incrementar el contraer VIH. Si usted es VIH positivo, estas ETS pueden debilitar significativamente su sistema inmunológico. Los síntomas de estas ETS frecuentemente no se presentan hasta años mas tarde pero puede que usted esté infectado o contagie a alguien más sin saberlo. Las ETS como la sífilis pueden provocar daños a los órganos, nervios y hasta causar la muerte.

¿Que debe hacer?

* Use un condón cada vez que tenga relaciones sexuales.
* Hágase la prueba para las ETS y VIH si usted está sexualmente activo.
* Si recibe tratamiento, tómese toda la medicina recetada durante el tiempo indicado por su médico. No deje de tomársela aunque se sienta mejor.

Recomendaciones para tener una relación sexual segura

* Use un condón nuevo en cada ocasión.
* Abra el paquete cuidadosamente.
* Los dientes, uñas, u objetos afilados pueden romper el condón.
* Una vez que lo haya sacado del paquete, mire hacia donde se desenrolla el condón.
* Cuando el pene este erecto, ponga el condón en la punta y desenrróllelo hasta abajo.
* Presione la punta del condón con sus dedos para mantener el aire afuera.
* Deje espacio en la punta del condón, para que este espacio permita atrapar el semen y así el condón no se rompa.
* Después de eyacular, saque el pene fuera de su compañera(o) mientras el pene está erecto.
* Sostenga el aro del condón alrededor de la base del pene mientras lo vaya sacando.
* Tenga cuidado de no derramar
* Bote el condón y nun lo use más de ur

Fig. 6.3 (continued)

and treatment needs. Several steps must be taken to improve the health and wellbeing of farmworkers in the US.

First, further research is needed to explore the prevalence and incidence of infectious diseases, some of which are newly emerging (e.g., MRSA), among farmworkers in the eastern US. These studies should explore risk factors from an ecologic perspective, critically examining not only individual behavior but systems and policies that jeopardize this vulnerable community's health. This is a vital step and must be undertaken in order to prevent the spread of infectious diseases among farmworkers.

Second, intervention approaches and programs that are disease specific are needed to ensure that farmworkers have the basic knowledge and skills to promote and maintain their health. Research and practice must work together to develop interventions to meet the immediate infectious disease prevention needs of farmworkers. This effort should include the adaptation of existing programs that have been found effective in the prevention, care, and treatment of TB, STDs, and HIV. Furthermore, because of the unique circumstances of farmworkers, new programs must be developed, implemented, and evaluated. Currently, Federal STD and HIV prevention funding is linked to the use of a limited number of existing programs that have been found effective in preventing risk behaviors. However, none of these "approved" interventions were developed for or have been tested among Latinos/ Hispanics or farmworkers. Thus, to impact the epidemics of infectious diseases among farmworkers, much research and intervention development is still necessary.

It is important to note that some communities that have attracted farmworkers with jobs also have disproportionate rates of STDs and HIV. Thus, farmworkers in these communities are at increased risk; failure to act may lead to further infectious disease epidemics.

Third, providing culturally appropriate interventions that are disease and community specific is not sufficient. Creative and profound approaches that ensure the health and wellbeing of farmworkers are needed. These approaches may include policy changes to ensure the provision of better housing with less crowding, improved ventilation, and more toilet and shower facilities. These approaches may include improved social opportunities and mental health services that address gender socialization, loneliness, and cultural conflicts.

At a larger social level, these approaches may include increased farmworker wages and opportunities for professional and educational advancement. Rather than focusing on the individual, their presumed "choices," and a particular disease, a long-term approach to health promotion and disease prevention among farmworkers may include affecting a variety of health and wellbeing outcomes of communities and their members. Unfortunately, structural change is difficult, but it may be key to ensuring the health and wellbeing of a large group of workers who have such an important role in the US food production, and thus, economy.

Finally, although TBNet has been found effective, further expansion and thorough evaluation of it is clearly warranted. Although findings from TBNet look promising, the numbers of farmworkers who benefit from this type of intervention are shamefully small. Moreover, expanding TBNet to include HIV may prove effective to better track and treat farmworkers living with HIV.

As the TB, STD, and HIV epidemics have evolved over the years, a need exists to explore, understand, and intervene creatively upon factors associated with exposure and transmission. Nowhere is this more urgent than in the eastern US, an area in which little research has been done to understand and support farmworkers and a region that bears disproportionate burdens of TB, STDs, and HIV.

References

Amaro H, Vega RR, Valencia D (2001) Gender, context, and HIV prevention among Latinos. In Aguirre-Molina M, Molina CW, Zambrana RE (eds.) Health Issues in the Latino Community. Jossey-Bass, San Francisco, CA

Anonymous (2001) Future access to HIV vaccines. Report from a WHO-UNAIDS consultation, Geneva, 2–3 October 2000. AIDS 15(7):W27–W44

Aranda-Naranjo B, Gaskins S (1998) HIV/AIDS in migrant and seasonal farm workers. J Assoc Nurses AIDS Care 9:80–83

Arcury TA, Quandt SA (2007) Delivery of health services to migrant and seasonal farmworkers. Annu Rev Public Health 28:345–363

Bennett DE, Courval JM, Onorato I et al. (2008) Prevalence of tuberculosis infection in the United States population: the National Health and Nutrition Examination Survey, 1999–2000. Am J Respir Crit Care Med 177(3):348–355

Bletzer KV (2005) Sex workers in agricultural areas: their drugs, their children. Cult Health Sex 7:543–555

Block J (2004) Science gets sacked. Int J Health Serv 34:177–179

Bowden WP, Rhodes SD, Wilkin A et al. (2006) Sociocultural determinants of HIV/AIDS risk and service use among immigrant Latinos in North Carolina. Hisp J Behav Sci 28:546–562

Brammeier M, Chow JM, Samuel MC et al. (2008) Sexually transmitted diseases and risk behaviors among California farmworkers: results from a population-based survey. J Rural Health 24:279–284

Briggs CL (2005) Communicability, racial discourse, and disease. Annu Rev Anthropol 34: 269–291

Carroll D, Samardick RM, Bernard S et al. (2005) Findings from the National Agricultural Workers Survey (NAWS) 2001–2002: a demographic and employment profile of United States farm workers (No. 9). US Department of Labor. http://www.doleta.gov/agworker/report9/naws_rpt9.pdf

Carter RL, Lesneski C, Loor R et al. Adherence to directly observed therapy among Florida's migrant and seasonal farm workers. http://www.rwjf.org/reports/grr/023611.htm, Accessed 28 Feb 2008

Centers for Disease Control (1986) Tuberculosis among migrant farm workers - Virginia. MMWR Morb Mortal Wkly Rep 35:467–469

Centers for Disease Control (1988) HIV seroprevalence in migrant and seasonal farmworkers – North Carolina, 1987. MMWR Morb Mortal Wkly Rep 37(34):517–519

Centers for Disease Control (1992a) HIV infection, syphilis, and tuberculosis screening among migrant farm workers - Florida, 1992. MMWR Morb Mortal Wkly Rep 41:723–725

Centers for Disease Control (1992b) Prevention and control of tuberculosis in migrant farm workers; Recommendations of the Advisory Council for the Elimination of Tuberculosis. MMWR: Recomm Rep (RR-10):1–15

Centers for Disease Control and Prevention (1996) The role of BCG vaccine in the prevention and control of tuberculosis in the United States. A joint statement by the Advisory Council for the Elimination of Tuberculosis and the Advisory Committee on Immunization Practices. MMWR Recomm Rep 45(RR-4):1–18

Centers for Disease Control and Prevention (2004) Sexually transmitted disease surveillance, 2003. US Department of Health and Human Services, Atlanta, GA. http://www.cdc.gov/std/stats03/toc2003.htm

Centers for Disease Control and Prevention (2005) Cases of HIV infection and AIDS in the United States, 2003. HIV/AIDS surveillance report, 2003 (No. 15). US Department of Health and Human Services, Centers for Disease Control and Prevention Atlanta, GA. http://www.cdc.gov/hiv/topics/surveillance/resources/reports/2003report/pdf/2003SurveillanceReport.pdf

Centers for Disease Control and Prevention (2006) Reported tuberculosis in the United States, 2005. US Department of Health and Human Services, Atlanta, GA

Centers for Disease Control and Prevention (2007) Cases of HIV infection in the United States and dependent areas, 2005. HIV/AIDS surveillance report, 2005 (Vol. 17 Revised). US Department of Health and Human Services, Centers for Disease Control and Prevention, Atlanta. http://www.cdc.gov/hiv/topics/surveillance/resources/reports/2005report/pdf/2005SurveillanceReport.pdf

Centers for Disease Control and Prevention (CDC) (2008) Trends in tuberculosis – United States, 2007. MMWR Morb Mortal Wkly Rep 57(11):281–285

Centers for Disease Control HIV/AIDS Prevention Research Synthesis Project (1999) Compendium of HIV prevention interventions with evidence of effectiveness. Centers for Disease Control and Prevention, Atlanta, GA. http://www.cdc.gov/hiv/resources/reports/hiv_compendium/pdf/HIVcompendium.pdf

Ciesielski SD (1995) BCG vaccination and the PPD test: what the clinician needs to know. J Fam Pract 40:76–80

Ciesielski SD, Seed JR, Esposito DH et al. (1991) The epidemiology of tuberculosis among North Carolina migrant farm workers. JAMA 265:1715–1719

Colditz GA, Berkey CS, Mosteller F et al. (1995) The efficacy of bacillus Calmette-Guerin vaccination of newborns and infants in the prevention of tuberculosis: meta-analyses of the published literature. Pediatrics 96(1 Pt 1):29–35

Darbes LA, Kennedy GE, Peersman G et al. (2002) Systematic review of HIV behavioral prevention research in Latinos. Center for HIV Information, University of California, San Francisco

Eng TR, Butler WT (eds.) Committee on Prevention and Control of Sexually Transmitted Diseases, Institute of Medicine (1997) The Hidden Epidemic: Confronting Sexually Transmitted Diseases. National Academy Press, Washington, DC

Falicov CJ (1996) Mexican families. In: McGoldrick M, Giordano J, Pearce JK (eds.) Ethnicity and Family Therapy, 2nd edn. Guilford, New York

Fernández MI, Collazo JB, Hernández N et al. (2004) Predictors of HIV risk among Hispanic farm workers in South Florida: women are at higher risk than men. AIDS Behav 8:165–174

Ford K, King G, Nerenberg L et al. (2001) AIDS knowledge and risk behaviors among Midwest migrant farm workers. AIDS Educ Prev 13:551–560

Garcia JG, Matheny Dresser KS, Zerr AD (1996) Respiratory health of Hispanic migrant farm workers in Indiana. Am J Ind Med 29:23–32

Garner P, Smith H, Munro S et al. (2007) Promoting adherence to tuberculosis treatment. Bull World Health Organ 85:404–406

Gentry AL, Grzywacz JG, Quandt SA et al. (2007) Housing quality among North Carolina farmworker families. J Agric Saf Health 13:323–337

Guerin B (2005) Combating everyday racial discrimination without assuming racists or racism: new intervention ideas from a contextual analysis. Behav Soc Issues 14:46–70

Herbst JH, Kay LS, Passin WF et al. (2007) A systematic review and meta-analysis of behavioral interventions to reduce HIV risk behaviors of Hispanics in the United States and Puerto Rico. AIDS Behav 11:25–47

Heymann DL (2004) Control of Communicable Diseases Manual, 18th edn. APHA, Washington, DC

Holden C (2002) Bitter harvest: housing conditions of migrant and seasonal farmworkers. In Thompson CD, Wiggins MF (eds.) The Human Cost of Food: Farmworkers' Lives, Labor, and Advocacy. University of Texas Press, Austin, TX

Inciardi JA, Surratt HL, Colón HM et al. (1999) Drug use and HIV risks among migrant workers on the DelMarVa peninsula. Subst Use Misuse 34:653–666

Institute of Medicine (2000) Ending Neglect: The Elimination of Tuberculosis in the United States. National Academy Press, Washington, DC. http://www.iom.edu/object.file/master/4/119/TB8pagerfinal.pdf

Institute of Medicine (2003) Unequal Treatment: Confronting Racial and Ethnic Disparities in Health Care. National Academies Press, Washington, DC

Jacobson ML, Mercer MA, Miller LK et al. (1987) Tuberculosis risk among migrant farm workers on the Delmarva peninsula. Am J Public Health 77:29–32

Jones JL, Rion P, Hollis S et al. (1991) HIV-related characteristics of migrant workers in rural South Carolina. South Med J 84:1088–1090

Kim-Godwin YS, Bechtel GA (2004) Stress among migrant and seasonal farmworkers in rural southeast North Carolina. J Rural Health 20:271–278

Knipper E, Rhodes SD, Lindstrom K et al. (2007). Condom use among heterosexual immigrant Latino men in the southeastern United States. AIDS Educ Prev 19:436–447

Kumar S (1998) Model for sexual health found in India's West Bengal. Lancet 351(9095):46

Martin SL, Kupersmidt JB, Harter KS (1996) Children of farm laborers: utilization of services for mental health problems. Community Ment Health J 32:327–340

McVea KL (1997) Lay injection practices among migrant farmworkers in the age of AIDS: evolution of a biomedical folk practice. Soc Sci Med 45:91–98

Much DH, Martin J, Gepner I (2000) Tuberculosis among Pennsylvania migrant farm workers. J Immigr Health 2:53–56

Naughton MJ, Rhodes SD (2009). Adoption and maintenance of safer sex practices. In Shumaker SA, Ockene JK, Riekert K (eds.) The Handbook of Health Behavior Change, 3rd edn. Springer, New York, NY pp. 659–675

O'Donnell CR, O'Donnell L, San Doval A et al. (1998) Reductions in STD infections subsequent to an STD clinic visit. Using video-based patient education to supplement provider interactions. Sex Transm Dis 25:161–168

Organista KC, Organista PB, Garcia De Alba JE et al. (1996) AIDS and condom-related knowledge, beliefs, and behaviors in Mexican migrant laborers. Hisp J Behav Sci 18:392–406

Organista KC, Balls Organista P, Garcia de Alba JE et al. (1997) Survey of condom-related beliefs, behaviors, and perceived social norms in Mexican migrant laborers. J Community Health 22:185–198

Organista KC, Organista PB, Bola JR et al. (2000) Predictors of condom use in Mexican migrant laborers. Am J Community Psychol 28:245–265

Organista KC, Carrillo H, Ayala G (2004) HIV prevention with Mexican migrants: review, critique, and recommendations. J Acquir Immune Defic Syndr 37(Suppl 4):S227–S239

Painter TM (2008) Connecting the dots: when the risks of HIV/STD infection appear high but the burden of infection is not known-the case of male Latino migrants in the southern United States. AIDS Behav 12:213–226

Parrado EA, Flippen CA, McQuiston C (2004) Use of commercial sex workers among Hispanic migrants in North Carolina: implications for the spread of HIV. Perspect Sex Reprod Health 36:150–156

Paz-Bailey G, Teran S, Levine W et al. (2004) Syphilis outbreak among Hispanic immigrants in Decatur, Alabama: association with commercial sex. Sex Transm Dis 31:20–25

Poss JE (1999) Developing an instrument to study the tuberculosis screening behaviors of Mexican migrant farmworkers. J Transcult Nurs 10:306–319

Poss JE (2000) Factors associated with participation by Mexican migrant farmworkers in a tuberculosis screening program. Nurs Res 49:20–28

Poss JE (2001) Developing a new model for cross-cultural research: synthesizing the Health Belief Model and the Theory of Reasoned Action. ANS Adv Nurs Sci 23(4):1–15

Poss JE, Rangel R (1997) A tuberculosis screening and treatment program for migrant farmworker families. J Health Care Poor Underserved 8:133–140

Pulerwitz J, Amaro H, De Jong W et al. (2002) Relationship power, condom use and HIV risk among women in the USA. AIDS Care 14:789–800

Rhodes SD, Hergenrather KC (2007) Recently arrived immigrant Latino men identify community approaches to promote HIV prevention. Am J Public Health 97:984–985

Rhodes SD, Hergenrather KC, Montaño J et al. (2006) Using community-based participatory research to develop an intervention to reduce HIV and STD infections among Latino men. AIDS Educ Prev 18:375–389

Rhodes SD, Eng E, Hergenrather KC et al. (2007) Exploring Latino men's HIV risk using community-based participatory research. Am J Health Behav 31:146–158

Rhodes SD, Hergenrather KC, Griffith D et al. (in press). Sexual and alcohol use behaviours of Latino men in the southeastern USA. Cult Health Sexuality

Rhodes SD, Hergenrather KC, Zometa C et al. (2008) Characteristics of immigrant Latino men who utilize formal healthcare services in rural North Carolina: baseline findings from the HOMBRES study. J Natl Med Assoc 100:1177–1185

Robles RR, Reyes JC, Colón HM et al. (2004) Effects of combined counseling and case management to reduce HIV risk behaviors among Hispanic drug injectors in Puerto Rico: a randomized controlled study. J Subst Abuse Treat 27:145–152

Rodrigues LC, Diwan VK, Wheeler JG (1993) Protective effect of BCG against tuberculous meningitis and military tuberculosis: a meta-analysis. Int J Epidemiol 22:1154–1158

Rothenberg BA (1995) Understanding and Working with Parents and Children from Rural Mexico: What Professionals Need to Know About Child-Rearing Practices, the School Experience, and Health Concerns. Banster Press, Menlo Park

Rust GS (1990) Health status of migrant farmworkers: a literature review and commentary. Am J Public Health 80:1213–1217

Sanchez MA, Lemp GF, Magis-Rodriguez C et al. (2004) The epidemiology of HIV among Mexican migrants and recent immigrants in California and Mexico. J Acquir Immune Defic Syndr 37(Suppl 4):S204–S214

Shedlin MG, Decena CU, Oliver-Velez D (2005) Initial acculturation and HIV risk among new Hispanic immigrants. J Natl Med Assoc 97(7 Suppl):32S–37S

Smedley BD, Syme SL (eds.) (2000) Promoting Health: Intervention Strategies from Social and Behavioral Research. National Academy Press, Washington, DC. http://iom.edu/?id=16738

Solorio MR, Currier J, Cunningham W (2004) HIV health care services for Mexican migrants. J Acquir Immune Defic Syndr 37(Suppl 4):S240–S251

Somerville GG, Diaz S, Davis S et al. (2006) Adapting the popular opinion leader intervention for Latino young migrant men who have sex with men. AIDS Educ Prev 18(4 Suppl A):137–148

Stadler J, Delany S (2006) The 'healthy brothel': the context of clinical services for sex workers in Hillbrow, South Africa. Cult Health Sex 8:451–464

Suarez M, Raffaelli M, O'Leary A (1996) Use of folk healing practices by HIV-infected Hispanics living in the United States. AIDS Care 8:683–690

Takahashi LM (1997) Stigmatization, HIV/AIDS, and communities of color: exploring response to human service facilities. Health Place 3:187–199

Talashek ML, Peragallo N, Norr K et al. (2004) The context of risky behaviors for Latino youth. J Transcult Nurs 15:131–138

Viadro CI, Earp JA (2000) The sexual behavior of married Mexican immigrant men in North Carolina. Soc Sci Med 50:723–735

Visrutaratna S, Lindan CP, Sirhorachai A et al. (1995) 'Superstar' and 'model brothel': developing and evaluating a condom promotion program for sex establishments in Chiang Mai, Thailand. AIDS 9(Suppl 1):S69–S75

Volmink J, Garner P (2007) Directly observed therapy for treating tuberculosis. Cochrane Database Syst Rev (4) CD003343

Workowski KA, Berman SM (2006) Sexually transmitted diseases treatment guidelines, 2006. MMWR Recomm Rep 55(RR-11):1–94

World Health Organization (2007) Global tuberculosis control: surveillance, planning, financing: WHO report 2007. World Health Organization, Geneva. http://www.who.int/tb/publications/global_report/2007/en/

Chapter 7
Mental Health Among Farmworkers in the Eastern United States

Joseph G. Grzywacz

Abstract Farmworker mental health research is sparse, particularly in the eastern United States. Nevertheless, available evidence suggests that 20–50% of farmworkers have poor mental health as indicated by elevated symptoms of depression or anxiety, frequent heavy alcohol consumption, or recent experiences of lay-defined illnesses like susto or nervios. Farmworkers' poor mental health likely results from a variety of structural and social factors, including the absence of fixed-term permanent employment, poverty-level wages, separation from family and community for extended periods of time, and hostile attitudes toward immigrants. The challenge of poor mental health is exaggerated by the relative absence of mental health services for farmworkers and farmworker advocates' inability to initiate and sustain policy changes to better protect and treat mental health. Collectively, the available evidence suggests that farmworker mental health is a multifaceted social justice issue, especially in the eastern US.

7.1 Introduction

Farmworker mental health is a multifaceted social justice issue. Farmworkers, largely Latino/Hispanic immigrants, live and work on the margins of society where they are disproportionately exposed to hardships of poverty and discrimination, as well as monotonous and dangerous work. Farmworkers frequently lack social support resources because of physical separation from family and community. The emotional strain of their marginalized position in US society and their separation from kith and kin likely contribute to the development and perpetuation of a variety of mental health problems. Simultaneously, farmworkers have little access to specialized mental health care services, and they have little voice in changing the circumstances within which they live and work. The mental health threats confronted by farmworkers and the lack of mental health services and voice are particularly noteworthy in the eastern US where, prior to the 1990s, there were few Latino/Hispanic residents in the primarily rural areas where farm work is performed.

T.A. Arcury and S.A. Quandt (eds.), *Latino Farmworkers in Eastern United States*,   153
DOI: 10.1007/978-0-387-88347-2_7, © Springer Science + Business Media, LLC 2009

The goals of this chapter are to expose the social injustice of farmworker mental health and to promote mental health action for farmworkers. To achieve this goal, this chapter begins by describing the conceptual domain of mental health and presenting a simple model of the factors shaping mental health. Consistent with the guiding theme of this volume, this model emphasizes the social etiology of poor mental health. Then, existing epidemiological data are used to illustrate the burden of poor mental health borne by farmworkers, as well as the socially embedded factors that undermine farmworker mental health. An important element of this review is the sheer inadequacy of mental health services available to farmworkers and the relative powerlessness of farmworkers in initiating and sustaining changes to social circumstances that protect and treat poor mental health. We conclude the chapter with both a research agenda for better understanding farmworker mental health and an advocacy agenda for socially improving and protecting farmworker mental health.

7.2 Conceptual and Contextual Foundations

Before launching into a review of what is known about farmworker mental health and social justice, it is important to anchor the discussion by defining the key concepts and providing a basic conceptual framework. Social justice refers to a sense of fairness or equity in the distribution of social burdens and resources across distinct social groups. In subsequent sections, this chapter highlights four distinct domains of equity relevant to farmworker mental health: exposure to social risks for poor mental health, access to mental health services, and an active voice in improving the mental health of farmworkers.

7.2.1 Conceptualizing Mental Health

Mental health is a complex and multifaceted concept. As with other domains of health, mental health can be viewed along at least two discrete dimensions (Keyes 2002). The first dimension characterizes mental illness or the presence of symptoms and syndromes reflecting psychological hardship, such as chronic feelings of sadness, the loss of pleasure (anhedonia), or anxiety. The second dimension of mental health is typically referred to as mental well-being. It reflects the extent to which an individual shows signs of positive psychological functioning in terms of relationships with others, a sense of mastery over environmental conditions, and a strong sense of personal self worth. These two distinct domains of mental health are clearly evidenced in the Surgeon General's (US Department of Health and Human Services 1999) definition of mental health as "… a state of successful performance of mental function, resulting in productive activities, fulfilling relationships with people, and the ability to adapt to change and to cope with adversity" (p. 4).

Further complicating the mental health landscape for farmworkers is the presence of folk illnesses common in Latino/Hispanic culture, such as *susto* and *nervios* (see Sect. 2.6.2). Folk illnesses are part of culture-specific classifications and explanations for symptoms which frequently differ from biomedicine, the medicine of the twentieth century Western world which has gained widespread influence (Baer et al. 1998). *Susto* is a condition characterized by several symptoms including restless sleep, depressed affect, gastro-intestinal problems (nausea and diarrhea), and listlessness that are believed to be caused by a sudden fright that upsets or dislodges an individual's "immaterial substance or essence" (Rubel et al. 1984, p. 8). *Nervios* has been described as an idiom of distress (Lopez and Guarnaccia 2000) wherein individuals express culturally approved reactions to overwhelming stressful experiences (Baer et al. 2003). Guarnaccia et al. (2003) suggest that the timing of the stressful experience may contribute to different types of *nervios*. Although these and other folk illnesses common in Latino/Hispanic cultures overlap with psychiatric disorders and mental health states recognized by biomedicine, it is clear that they are also distinct and that they require different approaches to healing and treatment (Lopez and Guarnaccia 2000) because they are not viewed as "mental illness" per se by the Latino/Hispanics persons who suffer from them (Weller et al. 2002).

Conceptually, mental health is best viewed using a biopsychosocial model (Garcia-Toro and Aguirre 2007). There is little doubt that mental health has biological underpinnings. Evidence indicates, for example, that polymorphisms in the 5,10-methylenetetrahydrofolate reductase (MTHFR) gene are associated with several psychiatric disorders such as depression, schizophrenia, and bipolar disorder (Gilbody et al. 2007). Of primary importance to this chapter, though, is very clear evidence indicating that poor mental health including psychiatric disorder, compromised well-being and Latino/Hispanic folk illnesses like *susto* and *nervios* are intimately connected and shaped by circumstances and interactions in the social and cultural realm (Lopez and Guarnaccia 2000). Psychiatric disorder, for example, is elevated among the socioeconomically disadvantaged (Muntaner et al. 2004), and various indicators of psychiatric morbidity are elevated among individuals exposed to chronic interpersonal and social hardships such as recurrent exposure to acute life stressors (Monroe and Harkness 2005), chronic exposure to psychologically demanding jobs (Stansfeld and Candy 2006), and the burdens of caregiving (Pinquart and Sorensen 2003). Likewise, social circumstances such as high levels of job strain are believed to undermine mental health-related quality of life (Lerner et al. 1994) and exposure to life stress provides the very platform for mental health-related conditions such as *nervios* (Lopez and Guarnaccia 2000).

7.2.2 Specific Challenges to Farmworker Mental Health in the Eastern US

Several features differentiate the eastern US context from other regions where farmworkers live and work, and they present additional threats to farmworker mental health. Unlike farmworkers in the West where Latino/Hispanic workers have long been the primary source of labor, Latino/Hispanic workers are relatively new to the eastern US. Prior to 1990, most farmworkers in the eastern US were either African American or Haitian immigrants (see Sect. 2.5), but by 2004 estimates from the National Agricultural Workers Survey (NAWS) indicate that 72% of farmworkers in the eastern US claimed to be Latino/Hispanic. By contrast, trend data from the NAWS indicate that the proportion of farmworkers in the West who claim Latino/Hispanic ethnicity has been 80% or higher for the past 15 years. The rapid increase in the proportion of Latino/Hispanic farmworkers in the eastern US suggest that host communities were poorly equipped to deal with the large and rapid growth of Latino/Hispanics. Latino/Hispanic farmworkers arriving at the eastern US found, and continue to find, relatively few indicators of their culture and lifestyle, which likely creates a sense of disorientation and detachment. A large percentage of farmworkers in the eastern US are unaccompanied males, whereas farmworkers in other geographic regions tend to move in family groups (Trotter 1985). The absence of caring and supportive family members may exacerbate feelings of disorientation and loneliness, and it cuts deeply into the individuals' social support networks.

Differences between farmworkers in the eastern US and other regions of the country pose additional risk for poor mental health. A substantial proportion of farmworkers in the eastern US relative to the West and nationally were born in the US and claim English fluency (Fig. 7.1). Substantial evidence implicates greater acculturation, frequently measured in terms of nativity and English fluency or preference, with poorer mental health among Latino/Hispanics in general (Escobar et al. 2000) and Latino/Hispanic farmworkers in particular (Alderete et al. 2000). Less than half of the farmworkers in the eastern US are married, whereas approximately 60% of farmworkers nationally are married. Estimates from the 2004 NAWS indicate that 21% of farmworkers in the eastern US reside in living quarters provided by growers, whereas only 5% of farmworkers in the West live in grower-provided housing (Gabbard 2006). Although grower-provided housing may be financially compelling, the housing is frequently of low quality (see Chap. 3) and it creates a type of "total institution" because it is located in remote areas and few farmworkers

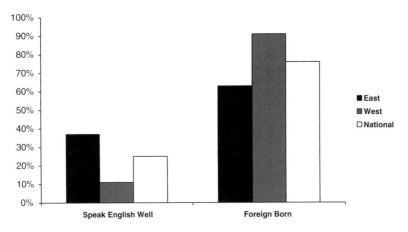

Fig. 7.1 Farmworker characteristics by geographic region

have their own transportation. Finally, although the eastern US has a similar number of settled farmworkers as other regions (see Fig. 2.1 in Chap. 2), it has a larger proportion of workers who follow the crops, creating a transient lifestyle and prolonged periods of separation from spouse and family that has been linked to poorer mental health (Grzywacz et al. 2005, 2006). Collectively, although farmworkers across the country are at risk of poor mental health, farmworkers in the eastern US confront several unique threats to their mental health.

7.3 The Mental Health of Latino/Hispanic Farmworkers

7.3.1 Psychiatric Epidemiology

Farmworker mental health research remains piecemeal and underdeveloped; nevertheless, available evidence suggests that poor mental health is common among farmworkers (Hansen and Donohoe 2003; Hovey and Seligman 2005). Alderete et al. (2000) reported that 20.6% of farmworkers in California met clinical criterion or "caseness" for lifetime incidence of one or more psychiatric disorders. These estimates were obtained using a modified version of the World Health Organization's Composite International Diagnostic Interview, one of the most sophisticated tools in psychiatric epidemiology (Kessler and Üstün 2004). The common classes of psychiatric disorder among farmworkers were anxiety disorder (12.5%), followed by substance abuse or dependence (8.7%) and mood disorder (5.7%). Prevalence statistics for the preceding 12 months are not available for farmworkers. However estimates from two separate psychiatric epidemiological studies suggest that 13% of foreign-born Latino/Hispanics met caseness for psychiatric disorder within the past 12 months (Alegria et al. 2007; Vega et al. 2004). Latino/Hispanic farmworkers report comparable levels of psychiatric disorder relative to recent immigrants not engaged in farm work and samples obtained from Mexico, and farmworkers report less psychiatric disorder than those who have been in the US for an extended period of time and US-born Latino/Hispanics (Alderete et al. 2000). No study has examined the epidemiology of psychiatric disorders among farmworkers in other regions of the country, including anywhere in the eastern US.

7.3.2 Mental Health Morbidity

Other region-specific studies suggest that poor mental health is prevalent among farmworkers. Vega et al. (1985a) were among the first to document that nearly 20% of California farmworkers reported levels of depressive symptoms suggesting clinically significant mental health problems. Alaniz (1994) reported that heavy drinking was common in farmworker camps in northern California, but more recent estimates suggest that only 10% of California farmworkers consume ten or more drinks per week (McCurdy et al. 2003). Approximately 20% of farmworkers traveling from Mexico through California report *nervios* (Mines et al. 2001). Turning to the central region of the country, researchers studying farmworkers along the US–Mexico border indicate that 41% of farmworkers report *nervios*, 37% report depression, and nearly one-fifth (17%) report *latidos* or heart palpitations attributed to anxiety (Weigel et al. 2007). An estimated 59% and 46% of Latino/Hispanics in a sample from a largely agricultural region of Texas reported personally experiencing *susto* and *nervios*, respectively. In the Midwest, researchers reported that 29% of farmworkers have potentially impairing levels of anxiety symptoms, and nearly four in ten farmworkers (37.8%) met caseness for depression using the Center for Epidemiologic Studies-Depression (CES-D) scale (Hovey and Magaña 2002b; Hovey and Magaña 2000). Additionally, in a small sample of 20 farmworker women in Michigan and Ohio, Hovey and Magaña (2003) reported that seven participants (35%) reported elevated levels of suicide ideation. Collectively, evidence suggests that 10–20% of farmworkers in the West and 30–60% of farmworkers in the Central region of the country manifest symptoms suggestive of mental health problems.

7.3.2.1 Mental Health Morbidity in the Eastern US

Mental health research among farmworkers in the eastern US is relatively recent. Trotter (1985) reported that drinking patterns were heavier in the eastern US relative to the Midwest and West. Subsequent research reported that nearly 25% of farmworkers in upstate New York, most of whom were Latino/Hispanic, reported frequent binge drinking (Chi and McClain 1992). Recent estimates of drinking behavior from farmworkers in North Carolina indicate that 27% of farmworkers reported frequent heavy drinking, or drinking five or more alcoholic beverages two or more times per month (Grzywacz et al. 2007). It was further estimated that over one third of farmworkers (39%) met screening criteria for alcohol dependence. Hiott et al. (2006) reported that 18.4% of farmworkers had impairing levels of anxiety, 37.6% met caseness for alcohol dependence, and 41.6% met caseness for depression. Consistent with the earlier point that the eastern US context presents added threats to farmworker mental health, levels of depressive symptoms in North Carolina are substantially higher than those reported by farmworkers in California (Alderete et al. 1999). However, despite high rates of potential depression, anxiety disorder, and alcohol dependence, farmworkers in North Carolina report levels of mental health-related quality of life similar to those reported by the general population (Grzywacz et al. 2008). An estimated 20% of farmworkers in Florida reported experiencing *susto* in response to pesticides (Baer and Penzell 1993).

Collectively, the literature on farmworker mental health suggests that indicators of poor mental health are common among farmworkers. Approximately one fifth of farmworkers have had at least one lifetime episode of psychiatric disorder. Although rates of psychiatric disorder are low compared to Latino/Hispanics in general and US born Latino/Hispanics specifically, they are disturbing. Heavy alcohol use and alcohol dependence is common among farmworkers, especially among those in the eastern US. Between 20 and 40% of farmworkers self-report symptoms potentially indicative of impairing mental health problems, and comparable percentages of farmworkers report experiencing folk illnesses like *susto* or *nervios*. No studies have put all of these indicators of mental health together into a single study, but when combined, the evidence suggests that up to 50% of farmworkers report some type of mental health condition.

7.4 The Social Injustice of Poor Mental Health Among Farmworkers

7.4.1 A Model of Social Justice

Social justice fundamentally refers to fairness or equity. Social justice applied to mental health includes at least four primary domains for considering fairness. The first primary domain draws attention to the burden of poor mental health and whether it is equally shared in the population. The second primary domain for considering social justice, which is intimately connected to the first, is one of exposure to demonstrated or presumed risk factors for poor mental health. As mentioned above, it is clear that social situations such as poverty, discrimination, and social marginalization are associated with increased risk of poor mental health. Ideally speaking, social justice advocates would argue for the absolute elimination of social factors that appear to contribute to poor mental health; however, more practical is equalization of the disparities between groups in the burden of social hardships. The third major domain of fairness relevant to mental health is equal access to high quality and affordable treatments for poor mental health. Finally, the fourth primary domain of fairness is that of social power and voice, meaning that all groups of individuals should have equal opportunity to raise issues about mental health, the causes of mental health, and access to mental health services without concern for sanction or social retaliation. Or put differently, the fourth domain focuses on fairness in individuals' abilities to effect changes in the social and structural circumstances underlying poor mental health.

7.4.2 Farmworkers' Unequal Burden and Threat of Poor Mental Health

The social injustice of poor mental health can be viewed in each of the domains suggested by the equity or fairness model of social justice. The sheer prevalence of poor mental health unfairly threatens farmworkers. While it is true that farmworkers actually have lower rates of psychiatric disorders than other Latino/Hispanic groups, as they are defined by conventional medicine (Alderete et al. 2000), the fact that one-third to one-half of farmworkers report elevated rates of impairing mental health symptoms and high levels of folk illnesses that are similar to mental health problems is concerning. The concern over farmworkers' elevated rates of mental health symptoms is further intensified when considered in the context of a dangerous occupation like farm work (Villarejo 2003; see Chap. 4). Evidence clearly implicates indicators of poor mental health, such as depression and alcohol abuse with elevated risk of occupational injury (Crandall et al. 1997). Similarly, recognizing high levels of suicide ideation in the only study of farmworkers (Hovey and Magaña 2003), the availability of potential agents for suicide is concerning. One review of the worldwide literature focused on pesticide poisoning indicated that for every one case of acute pesticide poisoning attributable to occupational exposure, there were 4.9 cases attributed to attempted suicide (London et al. 2005). The availability of pesticides as an agent of suicide is particularly concerning in the eastern US where farmworkers are detached from family, socially isolated, and where the absence of strict regulations for access to and storage of pesticides is underdeveloped. Figure 5.2 in Chap. 5 illustrates a common strategy for storing pesticides in farmworker camps in North Carolina, and it highlights how easy it would be for a distressed farmworker to obtain lethal doses of chemical. Collectively these data suggest that the burden of poor mental health and its consequences are unequally shouldered by farmworkers.

7.4.3 Farmworkers' Unequal Exposure to Mental Health Risks

Risk factors for poor mental health are woven into the structural basis of farmworker jobs, thereby creating unequal exposure to known threats to mental health. Migration itself is a risk factor for psychiatric disorder and other aspects of mental health (Cantor-Graae and Selten 2005), suggesting that the 42% of farmworkers who migrate, either domestically or internationally (Carroll et al. 2005), systematically place themselves at risk for mental health problems, simply to work. This is particularly the case in the eastern US where more farmworkers report following the crops (13% in the eastern US vs. 8% nationally, see Fig. 2.1 in Chap. 2). Poverty, a widely studied risk factor in psychiatric epidemiology, is endemic among farmworkers. Resulting in part from low pay, lack of overtime, and other components of the philosophy of agricultural exceptionalism (see Chap. 9), fully 25–60% of farmworkers live in poverty, depending on whether farmworkers are traveling alone or are accompanied by dependent family members (Carroll et al. 2005). The estimated number of farmworkers currently living in poverty does not consider the financial obligations farmworkers have for family members in their home communities and the remittances sent by these farmworkers (see Sect. 2.6.1). The chronic stress of financial hardship and subsequent devaluation of self worth resulting from being unable to financially support their families, frequently the primary reason for being in the US (Chavez 1992), takes a toll on farmworkers' mental health. Evidence indicates that individuals in work arrangements lacking a clear and explicit long-term employment relationship, sometimes referred to as contract or contingent workers, are at increased risk for poor mental health (Martens et al. 1999;

Virtanen et al. 2003). Recognizing that the majority of jobs in farm work (60%) are seasonal in nature (Carroll et al. 2005), results from studies examining the consequences of contract and contingent work arrangements highlight another threat to farmworker mental health. Collectively this evidence suggests that basic structural features of farm work, its labor market, its compensation system, and its inability to provide permanent jobs all present risks to farmworker mental health.

Farmworkers confront a variety of physical conditions in their work and daily lives that likely threaten mental health (Hansen and Donohoe 2003; Hovey and Seligman 2005). NAWS estimates indicate that 8% of farmworkers in the eastern US say that growers do not provide potable water or toilets in the fields, despite the fact that growers are required to provide these basic human rights (see Chap. 5). The absence of basic human rights is simultaneously a stressor and it likely undermines personal dignity and erodes individuals' sense of self worth. Farmworkers live in poor-quality housing and crowded conditions (see Chap. 3). Although there have been no studies linking these specific features of the physical work environment to farmworker mental health, studies do implicate poor-quality housing with depressive symptoms (Evans 2003). Indeed, indicators of poor housing quality and lack of access to toilets and potable water in the field are included in the Migrant Farmworker Stress Inventory and are believed to contribute to elevated symptoms of depression and anxiety (Hovey and Magaña 2002b). Thus, farmworkers' basic working and living conditions present several chronic stressors that likely undermine farmworker mental health.

The structure and basic organization of jobs in farm work pose risks to farmworker mental health. Farmworkers' jobs are highly routinized and require little skill, thereby creating another chronic stressor that likely undermines mental health (Karasek and Theorell 1990). Estimates obtained in 2002 from the NAWS indicate that only 17% of farmworkers nationally and 8% of farmworkers in the eastern US characterize their jobs as semiskilled or supervisory. Farmworkers in North Carolina who reported little opportunity to control their daily work tasks and little day-to-day variety in what is done had poorer mental health-related quality of life (Grzywacz et al. 2008). Farm work is among the most dangerous occupations (Frank et al. 2004; Villarejo 2003; see Chap. 4), and farmworkers confront a wide variety of hazards including pesticides (see Chap. 5) and physically demanding work conditions that require substantial physical exertion and working for long periods in awkward postures (Grzywacz et al. 2008; Vega et al. 1985; see Chap. 4). Pesticide exposure has been linked with *susto* (Baer and Penzell 1993) and associated with elevated depressive symptoms (Beseler and Stallones 2003). Researchers have suggested a potentially lethal cycle whereby pesticide exposure contributes to depressive symptoms which lead to the use of pesticides as means of suicide (London et al. 2005). Working for long periods in awkward postures has been associated with poorer mental health-related quality of life, particularly for farmworkers with little control over their jobs (Grzywacz et al. 2008).

The social circumstances surrounding migration and the farmworker lifestyle present significant stressors that pose additional risk to farmworker mental health (de Leon Siantz 1994; Hansen and Donohoe 2003; Hovey and Seligman 2005; Vega et al. 1985a). The forced choice to leave families and friends behind to earn a living working with crops in the US or different regions of the country creates ambivalence among farmworkers that has been linked to poorer mental health (Grzywacz et al. 2006). Then, the physical and emotional separation from family and friends and subsequent feelings of social isolation pose psychological stresses that have been associated with elevated depressive and anxiety symptoms (Grzywacz et al. 2005; Hiott et al. 2008; Hovey and Magaña 2002a; Lackey 2008). These stressors are likely to be particularly salient in the eastern US where a greater proportion of farmworkers are unaccompanied by family members. Food insecurity is another stressor believed to undermine mental health (Weigel et al. 2007): nearly one-half (47%) of farmworker households in North Carolina had low food security, 9.8% had experienced moderate hunger, and 5% severe hunger (Quandt et al. 2004).

Other stressors confronted by farmworkers are likely heightened in the eastern US. Social marginalization, concerns about immigration and possible deportation, and discrimination have all been implicated in farmworker mental health (Alderete et al. 1999; Hiott et al. 2006, 2008; Lackey 2008; Vega et al. 1985a). These stressors are intensified in the eastern US where entrance of immigrant Latino/Hispanics into local communities is relatively recent, and where there is a long history of racial discrimination. An illustration of the tension confronted by Latino/Hispanic farmworkers can be seen in Chatham County, a central North Carolina county with numerous Latino/Hispanic workers. In February 2000, non-Hispanic residents organized an anti-immigrant rally led by David Duke, a former Grand Dragon of the Ku Klux Klan (Glascock 2000). While not supported by the entire community, the rally exemplifies racism and tensions that characterize the social context of the largely rur al communities in the eastern US where farmworkers live and work to bring food and produce to the American table.

7.4.4 Farmworkers' Unequal Access to Mental Health Treatment

Farmworkers have few options for health care (Arcury and Quandt 2007; Villarejo 2003), including mental health treatment. Immigrant Latino/Hispanics in general do not use mental health services, but seek care from general practitioners and the public health clinic system (Vega et al. 1999). This general pattern has been documented among Latino/Hispanic farmworkers in California (Vega et al. 1985b); however, there have been no systematic studies of farmworkers' use of mental health services in the eastern US.

Multiple factors account for low rates of treatment seeking among Latino/Hispanics, but they can be categorized into two broad areas: barriers to treatment and culturally based mental health beliefs among Latino/Hispanics. The general lack of mental health resources is a significant barrier to mental health treatment in general, but the challenge is intensified for Latino/Hispanics and for farmworkers (Vega et al. 2007). Lack of money, transportation, and health insurance are also significant barriers to mental health treatment (Cabassa et al. 2006). Estimates obtained from the 2004 NAWS indicate that 25% of farmworkers in the eastern US have health insurance (Gabbard 2006), and it is unlikely that farmworkers' health insurance coverage includes specialized mental health services. Fear of potential deportation (Lackey 2008) and the possibility that seeking treatment jeopardizes ability to obtain permanent residency status also pose barriers to seeking treatment. Inability to understand English speakers or documents combined with a lack of understanding of the healthcare system further inhibit treatment seeking among Latino/Hispanics (Aviera 1996; Vega et al. 2007). Nearly one-quarter of farmworkers in the eastern US report that language is a major barrier to receiving care. Unacknowledged racism, cultural insensitivity, and stereotyping by health care providers in previous situations discourage Latino/Hispanics from seeking mental health treatment (Aviera 1996; Bohan 2006; Malgady et al. 1987; Rogler et al. 1987; Vega et al. 2007).

Trust of health care providers is a primary factor influencing treatment seeking among Latino/Hispanics. Latino/Hispanics place a greater emphasis on seeking help from family, folk healers, or other trusted community sources (Cabassa and Zayas 2007). Latino/Hispanics are also more likely to consider treatment alternatives such as nonmedical sources of prescription medications (Work 2005) or natural medicines (Mainous et al. 2005) obtained from a *curandero* (Applewhite 1995) or other trusted folk healer as opposed to prescriptions provided through conventional medicine (Lackey 2008). The stigma associated with mental health may also impede mental health treatment seeking among Latino/Hispanics. Alvidrez and Azocar (1999), for example, reported that Latina women were significantly more likely than Black or White women to endorse feeling embarrassed to talk about personal issues, afraid of what others might think, or believing that family members might disapprove or consider them to be *loco* (or crazy). The stigma associated with mental health is further exacerbated by the general lack of mental health professionals of Latino/Hispanic descent (Vega et al. 2007).

Expectations for treatment may also differ among Latino/Hispanics. For example, Latino/Hispanics are often more interested in immediate treatment rather than waiting on test results or long-term therapy. They are much more focused on the present problem rather than future prognoses, and may take a deferential rather than collaborative view of authorities such as doctors or therapists, all of which hinder the mental health treatment process (Alvidrez and Azocar 1999; Rosado and Elias 1993). The lack of understanding by non-Latino/Hispanic mental health providers of Latino/Hispanics beliefs regarding mental health issues further limits treatment seeking or culturally sensitive care. A greater understanding of the mental health needs and barriers to treatment among immigrant Latino/Hispanics is needed in order to inform the development of culturally sensitive treatments and systems of care for this growing population (Vega et al. 2007).

7.4.5 Farmworkers' Unequal Voice in Affecting Change

Farmworkers have relatively little say over the factors affecting their mental health or the availability of mental health services. The socially and legally imbedded issues undermining farmworkers' ability to effect changes in their living and working conditions are outlined in detail in Chap. 9, but generally reflect the fact that farmworkers have limited social power, in large part because many farmworkers are undocumented and therefore not eligible to vote in US elections. Even among those with appropriate documentation, concerns over basic human rights frequently go unmentioned as farmworkers are concerned about job loss or other forms of retaliation including perennial concerns about deportation. These concerns are exacerbated by public displays against immigrants such as those that have dotted the landscape across the Southeast, and have played out on national venues since 9/11 2001. When anti-immigration sentiments are high, farmworkers have little opportunity to secure improvements in basic aspects of everyday life, much less improvements in the availability of mental health services.

7.5   Research Solutions to the Social Injustice of Farmworker Mental Health

Several streams of mental health research are needed to begin resolving the social injustice of farmworker mental health. In this section we reiterate calls made by Vega et al. (2007) in describing research needs for Latino/Hispanic mental health; however, our recommendations focus more specifically on research needs for Latino/Hispanic farmworkers.

7.5.1   Systematic Documentation of Farmworker Mental Health

There is a desperate need for systematic research focused on documenting the mental health of the farmworker population. While this research will confront many of the "numerator" and "denominator" issues described for occupational health research among farmworkers (see Chap. 4), it is imperative that researchers accurately characterize the scope of the mental health problem among farmworkers. Ideally, this type of research would capture both broad and specific indicators of mental health to ensure adequate coverage of the mental health universe. Psychiatric epidemiology similar to that done by Alderete and colleagues in the West is needed across each of the major geographic regions in the country. Additionally, research considering other aspects of mental health, such as mental health-related quality of life, is needed to adequately describe farmworker mental health and their mental health needs. Incorporation of standardized mental health surveillance questions into the National Agricultural Workers' Survey would be invaluable for charting and monitoring farmworker mental health.

7.5.2   Prospective Studies of Change in Farmworker Mental Health

Prospective cohort studies of farmworker mental health are also needed. Studies that recruit and follow farmworkers over time (both short-term over the agricultural season and longer-term) are needed to clarify two main shortcomings in the farmworker mental health literature. First, prospective cohort studies would be invaluable for documenting patterns of farmworker mental health over time. Farmworker mental health research, much like studies of Latino/Hispanics in general (Alegria et al. 2007; Escobar and Vega 2000; Vega et al. 2004), suggests that mental health worsens with greater time spent in the US (Alderete et al. 2000). However, this conclusion must be interpreted cautiously as most of these studies are based on cross-sectional data and so researchers only know that individuals who have been in the US for longer periods have poorer mental health than those in the US for shorter periods: they have no idea whether lower values represent declines over time. Second, prospective cohort studies would offer needed insight into factors that may contribute to poorer mental health or mental health declines among farmworkers. Identifying "causes" of poor mental health among farmworkers is tenuous because the vast amount of evidence to date is based on cross-sectional study designs that collect data at one point in time and that rely on self-reported information in measuring both mental health and presumed "causes" of poor mental health. Studies that document the mental health trajectories of farmworkers over time and the factors that precede and potentially cause mental health declines would provide the foundation necessary for creating systematic strategies that protect and promote farmworker mental health.

7.5.3   Research Ensuring Valid Measurement of Farmworker Mental Health

Before rushing into wide-scale studies of farmworker mental health, research is needed to establish the properties of common instruments used in mental health research. Measurement is a key challenge impeding mental health research among farmworkers, particularly research that seeks to describe mental health patterns in the Latino/Hispanic farmworker population. Although high-quality measurement is always a challenge, it is particularly so among farmworkers who are disproportionately foreign-born, which raises questions about the cross-cultural equivalence of standard instruments and measures of mental health. Lackey (2008), for example, identified several colloquial symptoms used by immigrant Mexicans in the eastern US to describe "depression": several of these symptoms are not included in standard translated versions of instruments measuring mental health. Moreover, most farmworkers have little formal education: estimates from the most recent NAWS data indicate that the median and modal level of education among farmworkers is six years of education in Mexico. The lack of formal education undermines the ability to use self-administered questionnaires in surveillance research because many farmworkers are unable to read sufficiently well. Further, the relatively low literacy that may follow from the low levels of formal education raises questions about farmworkers' ability to understand and respond to questions asked in interviewer-administered questionnaires.

Measurement concerns are clearly illustrated by results of cognitive testing indicating that both the structure and content of the K-6 (Kessler et al. 2002), a validated instrument for measuring nonspecific mental distress in surveillance studies such as the National Health Interview Survey, were inappropriate for use with farmworkers (Grzywacz et al. 2008). The K-6 items were described by farmworkers as being too long, written using "upper class" language, and had content whose cultural connotation was viewed as inappropriate. These findings are concerning because the structure and content of items in the K-6 is highly similar to standard tools used in psychiatric epidemiology such as the Composite International Diagnostic Interview (Alderete et al. 2000; Alegria et al. 2007), or the Alcohol Use Disorder and Associated Disabilities Interview Schedule (Grant et al. 2004), thereby raising questions about the utility of those standard tools in farmworker research.

7.5.4   Research that Informs How to Strengthen the Delivery of Mental Health Services for Farmworkers

More research is needed to strengthen the infrastructure of the mental health care delivery system for Latino/Hispanic farmworkers. Studies are needed to evaluate the role of language and acculturation, both on the part of health care providers and patients, in accurate diagnosis and treatment of mental health problems. Research needs to evaluate training alternatives for better identification of mental health issues by health care providers in primary care settings like migrant clinics. Given the substantial variety in types of farmworkers, research is needed to identify ways to better track and maintain health care treatments among both seasonal farmworkers as well as various types of migrant farmworkers. Finally, research is needed to evaluate the effectiveness of various pharmacologic interventions with farmworkers, particularly the potential for drug–environment interactions given farmworkers' widespread exposure to pesticides (see Chap. 5).

Additionally, there is a need for research to explore various "soft touch" types of interventions. Soft touch interventions are based on the idea that many farmworkers do not need clinical treatments; rather, many need activities and strategies for adapting to and accommodating new experiences that frequently accompany immigration and separation from family and friends (Lackey 2008). Such interventions might focus on alternative ways of promoting communication between farmworkers and family and friends in their home communities via high-speed Internet connections or cellular telephones. Indeed, evidence from one study in the eastern US suggests that more frequent telephone contact may help lessen the anxiety that frequently accompanies farmworkers' separation from families (Grzywacz et al. 2006). Findings such as these coupled with the fact that telephones are a scarce commodity in some farmworker camps (see Fig. 7.2) suggest that enabling communication may protect farmworker mental health. Other interventions might focus on creating social networks within the farmworker community that build on culturally valued venues such as intercamp soccer leagues (Lackey 2008). Such soft-touch interventions, if demonstrated to be useful, have the value of being useful to large numbers of farmworkers at relatively low cost, which may promote sustainability.

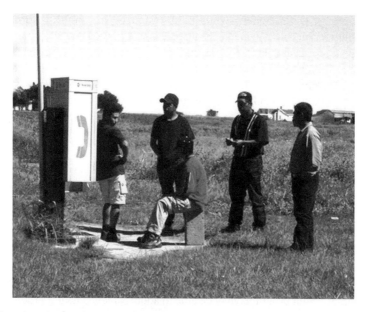

Fig. 7.2 Access to telephones or other forms of live communication with family members may protect farmworker mental health. Copyright, Thomas A. Arcury

7.6   Advocacy Solutions to the Social Injustice of Farmworker Mental Health

7.6.1   Creating Access and Availability to Mental Health Services for Farmworkers

There are several potential areas for advocacy to address the social injustice of farmworker mental health; however, two are particularly compelling. Advocacy initiatives that directly target access and availability of appropriate mental health care services are needed. The Migrant Clinicians' Network (MCN) provides a vehicle for delivering mental health services to farmworkers; however, it has insufficient resources to meet the comprehensive mental health needs of the diverse farmworker population. Farmworker advocates at the local, state, and national levels need to secure and channel financial resources for mental health services into the MCN. While resources are needed to support direct care within the network, resources also need to be allocated to ensure that clinicians receive ongoing training in the identification and either treatment or referral of mental health problems. An important component of the training is the creation of materials that are directly relevant to farmworkers, particularly migrant farmworkers who are accessing the MCN. Presently, the MCN is able to help clinicians locate mental health professionals in their area and provide general referrals to the agencies and centers that provide mental health information and resources (e.g., National Crisis Hotline, Substance Abuse and Mental Health Services

Administration). Unfortunately, while these resources are useful, they may have limited utility for meeting the mental health needs of farmworkers, given their distinct demographic profile and unique living and working conditions. Advocacy solutions are also needed for seasonal farmworkers, many of whom fall through the various safety net programs and end up uninsured and lacking access to even basic health services (Arcury and Quandt 2007), much less specialized mental health services.

7.6.2 Redesigning Farmworker Jobs

A second advocacy strategy for addressing the social injustice of farmworker mental health involves redesigning and upgrading farmworker jobs to ensure the provision of a livable wage and basic human rights. As outlined earlier in this chapter, there is considerable reason to believe that structural attributes of farm work, including its compensation system and its reliance on a contingent, largely foreign-born labor force present a persistent and undeniable threat to farmworker mental health. Thus, while migrant health programs may be able to address mental health problems after they occur, a more proactive approach requires a fundamental shift in the management and business processes in agriculture. Several of the strategies described in Chap. 9 for initiating change in the basic organization of farm work would likely prove to be invaluable in protecting farmworker mental health.

7.7 Conclusions

Available evidence on farmworker mental health is, admittedly, piecemeal and underdeveloped; nevertheless, it is clear that farmworker mental health reflects substantial social injustice. There is little doubt that mental health problems are prevalent among farmworkers, and that the burden of poor mental health is exacerbated by the fact that farm work is among the most dangerous occupations in the current economy. Evidence presented in this chapter, as well as other places throughout this volume, indicates that the very nature of farm work and the farmworker lifestyle presents manifold threats to mental health. Farmworkers have little access to basic services, much less specialized mental health services. Finally, farmworkers have little voice in shaping the circumstances confronted in their daily lives both on and off the job, including the types of services available for meeting mental health needs. Collectively these illustrations suggest that farmworker mental health is a pressing health issue that is fundamentally rooted in social injustice. It is clear that further research is needed to document the scope of the mental health problem among farmworkers and offer insight into viable routes for protecting and promoting farmworker mental health. However, it is also clear that advocacy strategies that expand mental health services to farmworkers and their families and that humanize the very nature of farm work are needed to minimize the unequal burden of poor mental health borne by farmworkers.

References

Alaniz ML (1994) Mexican farmworker women's perspectives on drinking in a migrant community. Int J Addict 29:1173–1188

Alderete E, Vega WA, Kolody B et al. (1999) Depressive symptomatology: prevalence and psychosocial risk factors among Mexican migrant farmworkers in California. J Community Psychol 27:457–471

Alderete E, Vega WA, Kolody B et al. (2000) Lifetime prevalence of and risk factors for psychiatric disorders among Mexican migrant farmworkers in California. Am J Public Health 90:608–614

Alegria M, Mulvaney-Day N, Torres M et al. (2007) Prevalence of psychiatric disorders across Latino subgroups in the United States. Am J Public Health 97:68–75

Alvidrez J, Azocar F (1999) Distressed women's clinic patients: preferences for mental health treatments and perceived obstacles. Gen Hosp Psychiatry 21:340–347

Applewhite SL (1995) Curanderismo: demystifying the health beliefs and practices of elderly Mexican Americans. Health Soc Work 20:247–253

Arcury TA, Quandt SA (2007) Delivery of health services to migrant and seasonal farmworkers. Annu Rev Public Health 28:345–363

Aviera A (1996) "Dichos" therapy group: a therapeutic use of Spanish language proverbs with hospitalized Spanish-speaking psychiatric patients. Cult Divers Ment Health 2:73–87

Baer RD, Penzell D (1993) Research report: susto and pesticide poisoning among Florida farmworkers. Cult Med Psychiatry 17:321–327

Baer RD, Clark L, Peterson C (1998) Folk illnesses. In: Love S (ed) Handbook of Immigrant Health. Plenum Press, New York

Baer RD, Weller SC, de Alba Garcia JG et al. (2003) A cross-cultural approach to the study of the folk illness nervios. Cul Med Psychiatry 27:315–337

Beseler C, Stallones L (2003) Safety practices, neurological symptoms, and pesticide poisoning. J Occup Environ Med 45:1079–1086

Bohan S (2006) Mental health without bias: experts seek better treatment for ethnic and racial minorities. In: Inside Bay Area. http://www.insidebayarea.com/

Cabassa LJ, Zayas LH (2007) Latino immigrants' intentions to seek depression care. Am J Orthopsychiatry 77:231–242

Cabassa LJ, Zayas LH, Hansen MC (2006) Latino adults' access to mental health care: a review of epidemiological studies. Adm Policy Ment Health 33:316–330

Cantor-Graae E, Selten JP (2005) Schizophrenia and migration: a meta-analysis and review. Am J Psychiatry 162:12–24

Carroll D, Samardick RM, Bernard S et al. (2005) Findings from the National Agricultural Workers Survey (NAWS) 2001–2002: a Demographic and Employment Profile of United States Farm Workers. US Department of Labor. http://www.doleta.gov/agworker/report9/naws_rpt9.pdf

Chavez LR (1992) Shadowed Lives: Undocumented Immigrants in American Society. Harcourt Brace, Fort Worth

Chi PSK, McClain J (1992) Drinking, farm and camp life: a study of drinking behavior in migrant camps in New York State. J Rural Health 8:41–51

Crandall CS, Fullerton L, Olson L et al. (1997) Farm-related injury mortality in New Mexico, 1980–91. Accid Anal Prev 29:257–261

de Leon Siantz ML (1994) The Mexican-American migrant farmworker family: mental health issues. Nurs Clin North Am 29:65–72

Escobar JI, Vega WA (2000) Mental health and immigration's AAAs: where are we and where do we go from here. J Nerv Ment Dis 188:736–740

Escobar JI, Hoyos Nervi C, Gara MA (2000) Immigration and mental health: Mexican Americans in the United States. Harv Rev Psychiatry 8:64–72

Evans GW (2003) The built environment and mental health. J Urban Health 80:536–555

Frank AL, McKnight R, Kirkhorn SR et al. (2004) Issues of agricultural safety and health. Annu Rev Public Health 25:225–245

Gabbard S (2006) Emerging trends in farmworker demographics: results from the National Agricultural Workers' Survey. Presentation at the NACHC National Farmworker Health Conference (May). San Antonio, TX

Garcia-Toro M, Aguirre I (2007) Biopsychosocial model in depression revisited. Med Hypotheses 68:683–691

Gilbody S, Lewis S, Lightfoot T (2007) Methylenetetrahydrofolate reductase (MTHFR) genetic polymorphisms and psychiatric disorders: a HuGE review. Am J Epidemiol 165:1–13

Glascock N (2000) Rally divides Silar City. In: The News & Observer. http://www.unc.edu/~hispana/nc05.html

Grant BF, Stinson FS, Hasin DS et al. (2004) Immigration and lifetime prevalence of DSM-IV psychiatric disorders among Mexican Americans and non-Hispanic whites in the United States: results from the National Epidemiologic Survey on Alcohol and Related Conditions. Arch Gen Psychiatry 61:1226–1233

Grzywacz JG, Quandt SA, Arcury TA et al. (2005) The work-family challenge and mental health: experiences of Mexican immigrants. Community Work Fam 8:271–279

Grzywacz JG, Quandt SA, Early J et al. (2006) Leaving family for work: ambivalence and mental health among Mexican migrant farmworker men. J Immigr Minor Health 8:85–97

Grzywacz JG, Quandt SA, Isom S et al. (2007) Alcohol use among immigrant Latino farmworkers in North Carolina. Am J Ind Med 50:617–625

Grzywacz JG, Quandt SA, Arcury TA (2008) Immigrant farmworkers' health-related quality of life: an application of the job demands-control model. J Agric Saf Health 14:79–92

Grzywacz JG, Alterman T, Muntaner C et al. (2008) Measuring job characteristics and mental health among Latino farmworkers: results of cognitive testing. J Immigr Minor Health. Epub ahead of print, August 9, 2008

Guarnaccia PJ, Lewis-Fernandez R, Marano MR (2003) Toward a Puerto Rican popular nosology: nervios and ataques de nervios. Cult Med Psychiatry 27:339–366

Hansen E, Donohoe M (2003) Health issues of migrant and seasonal farmworkers. J Health Care Poor Underserved 14:153–164

Hiott A, Grzywacz JG, Arcury TA et al. (2006) Gender differences in anxiety and depression among immigrant Latinos. Fam Syst Health 24:137–146

Hiott AE, Grzywacz JG, Davis SW et al. (2008) Migrant farmworker stress: mental health implications. J Rural Health 24:32–39

Hovey JD, Magaña C (2000) Acculturative stress, anxiety, and depression among Mexican immigrant farmworkers in the midwest United States. J Immigr Health 2:119–131

Hovey JD, Magaña CG (2002a) Psychosocial predictors of anxiety among immigrant Mexican migrant farmworkers: implications for prevention and treatment. Cultur Divers Ethnic Minor Psychol 8:274–289

Hovey JD, Magaña CG (2002b) Exploring the mental health of Mexican migrant farm workers in the Midwest: psychosocial predictors of psychological distress and suggestions for prevention and treatment. J Psychol 136:493–513

Hovey JD, Magaña CG (2003) Suicide risk factors among Mexican migrant farmworker women in the midwest United States. Arch Suicide Res 7:107–121

Hovey JD, Seligman LD (2005) The mental health of agricultural workers. In: Lessenger JE (ed) Agricultural Medicine: A Practical Guide. Springer-Verlag, New York

Karasek R, Theorell T (1990) Healthy Work: Stress, Productivity, and the Reconstruction of Working Life. Basic Books, New York

Kessler RC, Üstün TB (2004) The World Mental Health (WMH) Survey Initiative version of the World Health Organization (WHO) Composite International Diagnostic Interview (CIDI). Int J Methods Psychiatr Res 13:93–121

Kessler RC, Andrews G, Colpe LJ et al. (2002) Short screening scales to monitor population prevalences and trends in non-specific psychological distress. Psychol Med 32:959–976

Keyes CLM (2002) The mental health continuum: from languishing to flourishing in life. J Health Soc Behav 43:207–222

Lackey GF (2008) "Feeling blue" in Spanish: a qualitative inquiry of depression among Mexican immigrants. Soc Sci Med 67:228–237

Lerner DJ, Levine S, Malspeis S et al. (1994) Job strain and health-related quality of life in a national sample. Am J Public Health 84:1580–1585

London L, Flisher AJ, Wesseling C et al. (2005) Suicide and exposure to organophosphate insecticides: cause or effect. Am J Ind Med 47:308–321

Lopez SR, Guarnaccia PJ (2000) Cultural psychopathology: uncovering the social world of mental illness. Annu Rev Psychol 51:571–598

Mainous AG, Cheng AY, Garr RC et al. (2005) Nonprescribed antimicrobial drugs in Latino community, South Carolina. Emerg Infect Dis 11:883–888

Malgady RG, Rogler LH, Costantino G (1987) Ethnocultural and linguistic bias in mental health evaluation of Hispanics. Am Psychol 42:228–234

Martens MFJ, Nijhuis FJN, Van Boxtel MPJ et al. (1999) Flexible work schedules and mental and physical health. A study of a working population with non-traditional working hours. J Organ Behav 20:35–46

McCurdy SA, Samuels SJ, Carroll DJ et al. (2003) Agricultural injury in California migrant Hispanic farm workers. Am J Ind Med 44:225–235

Mines R, Mullenax N, Saca L (2001) The binational farmworker health survey. California Institute for Rural Studies, Davis. http://www.cirsinc.org/Documents/Pub1001.2.pdf

Monroe SM, Harkness KL (2005) Life stress, the "kindling" hypothesis, and the recurrence of depression: considerations from a life stress perspective. Psychol Rev 112:417–445

Muntaner C, Eaton WW, Miech R et al. (2004) Socioeconomic position and major mental disorders. Epidemiol Rev 26:53–62

Pinquart M, Sorensen S (2003) Differences between caregivers and noncaregivers in psychological health and physical health: a meta-analysis. Psychol Aging 18:250–267

Quandt SA, Arcury TA, Early J et al. (2004) Household food security among migrant and seasonal Latino farmworkers in North Carolina. Public Health Rep 119:568–576

Rogler LH, Malgady RG, Costantino G et al. (1987) What do culturally sensitive mental health services mean? The case of Hispanics. Am Psychol 42:565–570

Rosado JW, Elias MJ (1993) Ecological and psychocultural mediators in the delivery of services for urban, culturally diverse Hispanic clients. Prof Psychol Res Pr 24:450–459

Rubel AJ, O'Nell CW, Collado-Ardon R (1984) Susto, a Folk Illness. University of California Press, Berkley

Stansfeld S, Candy B (2006) Psychosocial work environment and mental health: a meta-analytic review. Scand J Work Environ Health 32:443–462

Trotter RT (1985) Mexican-American experience with alcohol: South Texas examples. In: Bennett LA, Ames GM (eds) The American Experience with Alcohol: Contrasting Cultural Perspectives. Plenum Press, New York

US Department of Health and Human Services (1999) Mental Health: A Report of the Surgeon General. Office of the Surgeon General, SAMHSA. http://mentalhealth.samhsa.gov/cmhs/surgeon-general/surgeongeneralrpt.asp

Vega W, Warheit G, Palacio R (1985a) Psychiatric symptomatology among Mexican American farmworkers. Soc Sci Med 20:39–45

Vega WA, Scutchfield FD, Karno M et al. (1985b) The mental health needs of Mexican-American agricultural workers. Am J Prev Med 1:47–55

Vega WA, Kolody B, Aguilar-Gaxiola S et al. (1999) Gaps in service utilization by Mexican Americans with mental health problems. Am J Psychiatry 156:928–934

Vega WA, Sribney WM, Aguilar-Gaxiola S et al. (2004) 12-month prevalence of DSM-III-R psychiatric disorders among Mexican Americans: nativity, social assimilation, and age determinants. J Nerv Ment Dis 192:532–541

Vega WA, Karno M, Alegria M et al. (2007) Research issues for improving treatment of U.S. Hispanics with persistent mental disorders. Psychiatr Serv 58:385–394

Villarejo D (2003) The health of U.S. hired farm workers. Annu Rev Public Health 24: 175–193

Virtanen M, Kivimaki M, Elovainio M et al. (2003) From insecure to secure employment: changes in work, health, health related behaviours, and sickness absence. Occup Environ Med 60:948–953

Weigel MM, Armijos RX, Hall YP et al. (2007) The household food insecurity and health outcomes of U.S.-Mexico border migrant and seasonal farmworkers. J Immigr Minor Health 9:157–169

Weller SC, Baer RD, de Alba Garcia JG et al. (2002) Regional variation in Latino descriptions of susto. Cult Med Psychiatry 26:449–472

Work DR (2005) Tiendas and contraband pharmaceuticals. North Carolina Medical Board Forum 10:16

Chapter 8
Health of Children and Women in the Farmworker Community in the Eastern United States

Sara A. Quandt

Abstract This chapter reviews research on health of women and children in farmworker communities in the eastern United States. Both women and children may be present in these communities as farmworkers themselves or as dependents. Both groups are at risk of health effects from farm work. Research indicates that children have limited access to care and significant unmet health needs. Obesity and food security are concerns. The environment poses significant risks, particularly from pesticides. Women lack access to reproductive health services. Exposure to pesticides is also a significant risk. Mental health and sexual harassment are important, but understudied problems. Overall, the research on health issues for women and children in farmworker communities in the eastern US is highly variable. Because access to linguistically and culturally appropriate services is limited, the needs of the population in this region and solutions to eliminate health disparities may be unique.

8.1 Introduction

As members of farmworker communities, women and children play multiple roles. They may be present as farmworkers themselves, or they may be dependents or family members of farmworkers. Nationwide, about one quarter of farmworkers are women. Estimates of children working for pay as farmworkers range from 290,000 15–17-year olds (by the Census Population Survey, which the General Accounting Office acknowledged to be an undercount) (GAO 1998) to 800,000 total child farmworkers (Human Rights Watch 2000). Even if they do not work as farmworkers, women and children in farmworker communities have health problems and health needs that set them apart from other women and children not living in farmworker communities. Figure 8.1 puts these factors into context.

Maternal and child health can be placed in the context of behaviors and exposures shaped by both the physical and social environments in which women and children live. In the case of members of farmworker families, both the community and family household environments have specific characteristics that ultimately affect health. At the community level, farmworker communities in the eastern US are often located in rural areas isolated spatially and culturally from surrounding population centers.

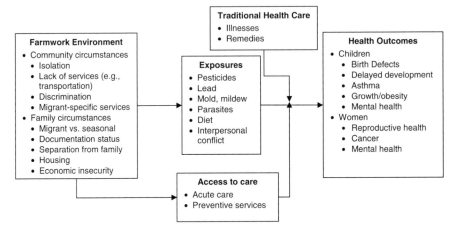

Fig. 8.1 Social ecology model of health for women and children in farmworker families

Until recently, most areas in the eastern US where farmworkers live have lacked services with Spanish-speaking staff (Florida is an exception), and discrimination against ethnic minorities is institutionalized. At the family level, the environment is shaped by whether or not the family migrates. Documentation status is also an important factor, affecting health from multiple perspectives: families without documents may not have access to governmental services including health care, or they may be reluctant to attempt to register for services, even if eligible, due to concerns about documentation status. Within families, some members may have documents (e.g., a child born in the US or a parent with a work visa) while others are undocumented.

The farmworker environment shapes the health-related exposures experienced by women and children. These include factors from agriculture (e.g., pesticides), as well as those resulting from substandard housing (e.g., lead and mold) and from low incomes (e.g., diet). The effect of these exposures on health is modified by access to care. When farmworker families have good access to care, the impact of exposures on health should be less than when access to care is more limited. The use of traditional health care, in terms of recognizing specific conditions and using culture-specific remedies and health care, can also affect the association of exposures and illnesses.

This chapter reviews research conducted on health and the determinants of health for women and children among farmworkers in the eastern US. As this research record is spotty and incomplete, the chapter also points out areas where research is needed.

8.1.1 Children in the Farmworker Community

Farmworkers in the US are relatively young. Most (63%) farmworker parents have one or two children, and 96% of these are under the age of 18 (Carroll et al. 2005). Children of farmworkers encounter a number of factors related to their parents' occupation that can lead to poor health outcomes. Because a majority of farmworkers are foreign-born and many lack legal immigration documents, their children are frequently in a precarious legal situation. When children are not citizens, their access to some programs is limited. If born in the US, the children are themselves US citizens, but their parents' legal status may restrict their opportunities to take part in all aspects of American society. For example, some parents without legal documents are reluctant to try to register their children for benefits such as food stamps for fear of calling attention to their own legal status.

Children whose parents are migrants may live with a single parent (usually the mother) while the other parent migrates. Or, if the entire family migrates, the child will migrate as well, a practice that can have negative consequences for school attendance and progress. Data from the National Agricultural Workers Survey (NAWS) (Mines 2000) show that children of farmworkers, on average, fall progressively behind their nonfarmworker peers throughout their school years. Many of the adolescent children of foreign-born workers are not enrolled in school. Those who are enrolled are more likely than other children to miss school, be tardy, sleep in class, and study less. They also report fewer hours of sleep at night, less time spent with friends, and more minor illnesses (Cooper et al. 2005b).

The fact that many farmworker parents have little formal education also accounts for some poor school performance. The extreme poverty of farmworker families further contributes to the diminished circumstances of farmworker children. Children of indigenous language-speaking parents are the most likely to live in poverty (Mines 2000).

The conditions in which these children live and the deficits they experience as children set them on a trajectory for additional problems. Comparing middle-school and high-school-enrolled children of migrant farmworkers with other children in the Texas border region, Cooper et al. (2005a) found that migrant children were more likely to report frequent substance use, to report not working for pay on weekends, but to report working for pay on weekday mornings before school.

A number of federally-funded services exist to try to address these problems. Migrant Head Start provides quality infant and preschool daycare and education. The Migrant Education Program helps children have educational continuity by providing school record exchanges and comprehensive assessment and support services. Although most of the programs offered were originally designed for children of migrant workers, some programs have been broadened to include children of seasonal, as well as migrant, workers.

8.1.2 Women in the Farmworker Community

Women comprise a minority of farmworkers nationwide. About 25% of all crop workers are women, according to the 2004 NAWS. In the eastern US, the proportion is lower, at 19%. Among newly arrived farmworkers, only 10% are women. Among women farmworkers, fewer are unauthorized (39% vs. 56% of male workers), and more are legal permanent residents (24% vs. 21%) or US-born citizens (33% vs. 20%) (Carroll et al. 2005).

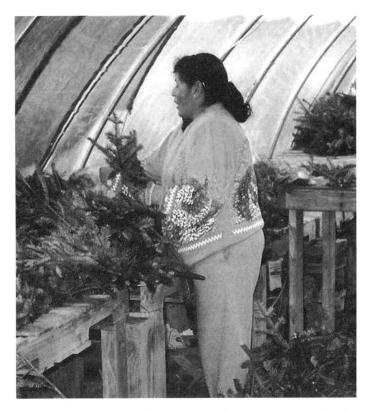

Fig. 8.2 Worker making wreaths and holiday roping from Christmas tree cuttings. Copyright, Thomas A. Arcury

Many women in farmworker communities in the eastern US are present as dependents of farmworkers. Some work part-time as farmworkers or in farming-related jobs. For example, women in Christmas tree-producing areas work seasonally making wreaths and roping from tree clippings (Fig. 8.2). Others work in packing houses during peak harvest. Such employees may experience health risks from doing unaccustomed work or from not receiving proper health and safety training.

8.2 Children's Health

8.2.1 Access to Medical Care

Children in the farmworker community have special needs for health services that set them apart from the general population (Gwyther and Jenkins 1998; American Academy of Pediatrics 2000). Yet their access to care, as indicated by insurance status, is lower than low-income children nationally (10% vs. 78% insured) (Rosenbaum and Shin 2005). In border areas (e.g., Texas and California), more than half of children's health care is obtained by returning to Mexico (Seid et al. 2003). For uninsured children, returning to Mexico leads to greater continuity of care. Because this option is not readily available to families in the eastern US, they are faced with significant challenges in accessing medical care.

Children of migrant workers have greater access to some federally funded migrant health services than children of seasonal (nonmigrant) workers. However, those who migrate are less likely than other children to have continuity of care. Because their parents work long hours with limited benefits, they cannot take children to receive medical care without losing work time. Parents may not have transportation to take children to clinics, may not know where the clinics are, and the clinics themselves may have limited hours and services. This type of care is likely to lead to inconsistencies in immunizations (Lee et al. 1990) and in evaluating developmental problems. Even apparently low-cost medications or treatments may be beyond a family's resources (Weathers and Garrison 2004).

Immigration status creates a barrier to medical care for children. Many lack health insurance or Medicaid coverage. Even those with Medicaid may have difficulties accessing care as they migrate because most states do not provide reciprocity of Medicaid. In mixed status families, parents without documentation may fear deportation if their children, even though qualified for services by US citizenship, access medical care.

A cross-sectional survey of migrant families in eastern North Carolina found that health services use by children less than 13 years of age was need-driven (Weathers et al. 2003). That is, children used health services when sick, rather than for well-child care. Younger children and girls were more likely to access care than older children and boys. Those visiting doctors were more likely to have insurance. Parents' documentation status did not predict whether or not children had insurance. Rather, parents who had been in the US for five or more years, having a family member with WIC benefits, a child of female gender, child's age less than 2 years, and able to leave work for child's medical care all predicted having insurance (Weathers et al. 2008b, c). It is likely that some of these factors describe children born in the US, thus enabling parents to have insurance for children. In a national sample of all children, children of foreign-born parents are more likely to lack a usual source of care than are those with US-born parents. Noncitizen children usually lack a regular source of care, regardless of parental nativity (Weathers et al. 2008a).

Unmet needs for care were explored in the North Carolina sample (Weathers et al. 2004). Over half of the children had an unmet need, defined as whether or not the child's caretaker reported a time in the past year when the caretaker felt the child needed medical care, but the child did not receive it. Reasons for the last episode of unmet needs were lack of transportation (80% of episodes), not knowing where to obtain care (32%), inconvenient clinic schedule (10%), no permission to leave work (9%), and difficulty in making appointments (9%). In multivariate analyses of factors enabling health care, unmet need was associated with "good," "fair," or "poor" health status (compared to "excellent" or "very good") and with depending on others for transportation. After adjustment for sociodemographic variables, unmet need was associated with ages 3–6 years and with high pressure for parents to work. Children aged 3–6 were more than twice as likely to have unmet needs than children over

6–12 years. Those whose parents reported very high pressure to work were almost six times more likely to have unmet needs.

Children receive medical care from alternative sources. A study in rural Alabama among Latino/Hispanic families found that parents mentioned use of home remedies, reliance on curanderos, and buying medications at tiendas as alternatives to taking a child to the doctor (Harrison and Scarinci 2007). Constraints on using doctors included cost, lack of insurance, communication barriers, and transportation. Parents noted mixed experiences with the healthcare system. While some perceived racism and noted a lack of respect, others had had more positive experiences (see Sect. 2.6.2).

The heterogeneity of experiences with care is evident in a study of two samples of farmworker families with children in different regions of North Carolina (Gentry et al. 2007). In this study, children tended to receive care from the same facility, though not see the same provider consistently. Children failed to receive care at the recommended frequency. In one region, 98% of parents were satisfied with the care received, while in the other, only 87% were satisfied. In the latter region, 64% reported that healthcare staff members were disrespectful to them or to their children, while the proportion perceiving disrespect was only 9% in the former.

8.2.1.1 Oral Health

Children in farmworker families generally have unmet needs for oral health care. Studies elsewhere in the country showed that children of farmworkers were more likely to have decayed tooth surfaces than other US school children and less likely to have filled surfaces (Woolfolk et al. 1984; Koday et al. 1990; Chaffin et al. 2003; Ramos-Gomez et al. 1999; Lukes et al. 2006). Adult farmworkers do not seek oral health care regularly (Lukes and Miller 2002; Lukes and Simon 2005; Entwistle and Swanson 1989).

In a recent study of self-reported family care among farmworkers in North Carolina, Quandt et al. (2007) found that children were the most likely of any family members to have received dental services in the previous year. However, 27% never received care and 13% only received emergency care. Most children did not pay a fee for dental services, indicating the availability of services in the area. Only 5% were rated by their mothers as having excellent oral health. Thirty-four percent were rated as fair or poor.

Lukes and Simon (2006) surveyed dental services available to migrant and seasonal farmworkers in community and migrant health centers across the US. They found that clinic hours varied from 1 to more than 40 h per week. Many clinics had no evening or weekend hours. Over half reported difficulty finding dentists to staff the clinics.

8.2.2 Nutritional Status

Overweight is a primary concern related to nutrition for children of farmworkers. Nationally, 41% of Hispanic boys and 32% of Hispanic girls aged 2–19 years are overweight (at or above the 95th sex-specific body mass index) or at risk for overweight (at or above the 85th percentile) (Ogden et al. 2006). While there are no comprehensive data on farmworker children, data from a multiyear study in the eastern US suggest that farmworker children do not differ from national reference data. Markowitz and Cosminsky (2005) analyzed growth data from 677 children aged 2–18 years of Mexican migrant farmworkers in southern New Jersey. Twenty percent were classified as "overweight," and 24.2% "at-risk-of-overweight." Stunting was diagnosed in 11.1% (less than the 5th percentile of height for sex for age). Stunting is often cited as an indicator of long-term undernutrition. There was a slight trend toward those overweight and at risk for overweight being born in the US, rather than in Latin America, and for the opposite trend for stunting.

8.2.2.1   Food Security

Considerable controversy currently exists on the relationship of low food security and overweight in children (Casey et al. 2006). Food security is an economic, household-level measure that represents an assured supply of nutritionally adequate and socially acceptable food (National Research Council 2006). Food security can be adequate, low, or very low. These latter categories mark the lack of an assured supply of food for the household. Populations with low food security are poor, and often have fluctuating income so that money with which to purchase food sometimes does not last from one payday to the next. This scenario describes many farmworkers well, as their income goes up with the abundance of a crop and down when there is no work because of drought, hurricane, or the end of a growing season. Drewnowski has argued that the high rates of obesity seen in households with low food security reflect the high cost of nutrient-dense foods like fruits and vegetables (Drewnowski and Darmon 2005). When families cannot afford these, they purchase lower cost foods, which tend to be energy dense and therefore lead to weight gain.

Food security is a problem for some farmworker families. In three studies of a total of 216 farmworker families with children in different regions of North Carolina and in different seasons, striking differences from the US reference population were found in food security (Quandt et al. 2006). Levels of adequate food security were significantly lower and levels of low food security were significantly higher in each of the surveys (Fig. 8.3). Levels of very low food security and very low food security among children were also higher, though the differences were not statistically significant, probably due to small sample sizes.

In-depth interviews conducted with farmworker mothers in the study areas provide insight into four components of the farmworker experience of low food security (Quandt et al. 2006). Low food security was experienced *quantitatively* and *qualitatively* (Table 8.1). Mothers attempted to keep the amount of food children were eating stable, but changed the quality of food. For example, more rice and beans were substituted for meat and fresh vegetables; kool-aid was substituted for fruit juice. *Psychologically*, low food security was difficult. Mothers experienced a range of emotions, from fear and loneliness to embarrassment and guilt. They reported reluctance

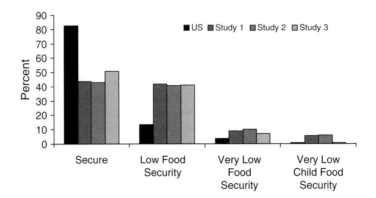

Fig. 8.3 Food insecurity levels compared with national data for 2004 for households with children (Nord et al. 2005). Values are proportions ± 95% confidence intervals. *Asterisks* indicate differences between Latino studies and national data (Quandt et al. 2006)

Table 8.1 Components of the food insecurity experience of Latino immigrants that emerged from in-depth interviews (Quandt et al. 2006)

Component	Description
Quantitative	Cycles of income result in cycles of food shortages
	Mild: try to keep the size of meals the same, regardless of their content
	Moderate: adults eat less to spare children
	Severe: having to go without food for a meal or day
Qualitative	Cyclic shortages affect types of food available
	Cut back on meat, fruit, and other expensive types of food when money is tight
	Substitute less expensive foods
	Try to feed children normal meals at the expense of adults
Psychological	Initial reaction: worry and stress about competing expenses and low earnings
	Initial reaction: fear of applying for help because of lack of documents
	Initial reaction: embarrassment at having persons from home know of food insecurity
	Initial reaction: loneliness, home-sickness
	Initial reaction: guilt because not able to support family left in country of origin
	Accommodation: get used to having less
	Accommodation: come to terms with situation and ask for help
	Empowerment: plan for shortages to take care of yourself
Socioeconomic	Lack of transportation to get to food pantries
	Treated with disrespect when applying for assistance
	Need to send money home
	Borrow money, but not food
	Boss gives garden land for home food production

to ask for help, particularly from acquaintances from their home communities, as they feared these persons would tell families at home that the immigrants were not able to provide for their families in the US. Over time, it appears that families learned to accommodate and take control of the situation, planting gardens, saving money, and storing food. *Socioeconomically*, they lacked transportation to get to food sources and experienced disrespect while applying for assistance. They struggled with the tension between needing to feed their families here and pressure to send money home to family members in their country of origin.

Similar results were obtained from a mixed method study of food security among farmworkers in southwestern Virginia (Essa 2001). Although few workers reported not eating or eating less than they wanted due to economic constraints, a large percentage of those with children reported that they often knew their children were hungry but could not afford enough food to feed them more.

An early study in Florida found that over 30% of families reported experiencing periods when they ran out of food or did not have enough to eat. Almost half reported seasonal food shortages (Shotland et al. 1989).

In contrast, research in five counties in Pennsylvania found much higher levels of food security (Cason et al. 2003). Ninety-two percent of the 401 workers interviewed reported being food secure. However, the authors do not report inclusion criteria or household status; and it appears that unaccompanied men as well as workers with children living with them were included. Despite the reported high food security, 24-h dietary recalls found high percentages reporting zero servings of fruits (18.9%), vegetables (37.6%), and dairy products (33.1%) in the previous day. While 24-h recall results must be interpreted with caution, they provide a good snapshot at the population level, suggesting that workers may have been making accommodations to restricted food availability. Focus group results in the same study supported this, with participants reporting problems in buying food (e.g., lack of income and transportation) and strategies to stretch their food dollars.

The patterns of accommodating food shortages are likely to promote overweight in children. Reducing food variety and increasing consumption of low-cost starchy and sugar-sweetened foods leads to greater caloric intake. Concern that food shortages will occur also leads families to eat more in times of plenty, and there may be physiological adaptations to feast/famine eating patterns that result in weight gain.

8.2.3   Mental Health

Children of farmworkers are at risk for mental health problems due to their living in poverty and, frequently, in impoverished environments. Adults with whom they interact often exhibit psychiatric problems (Alderete et al. 2000) and psychological issues such as depression and anxiety (Grzywacz et al. 2006a, b) (see Chap. 7). Rates of drug and alcohol abuse in farmworker camps and communities are sometimes high (Inciardi et al. 1999; Chi and McClain 1992; Grzywacz et al. 2007). Mistreatment of children has been found among farmworkers in the eastern US (Alvarez et al. 1988; Larson et al. 1990). The migrant lifestyle forces children to constantly leave behind friends and familiar surroundings, preventing them from becoming integrated into a community.

Research with 8–11-year-old children of farmworkers (85% Hispanic, 15% African American) in North Carolina found that 66% of the children met criteria for at least one psychiatric disorder (Martin et al. 1995; Kupersmidt and Martin 1997). Anxiety disorder was the most common (39%); affective disorders were diagnosed in 8% and attention deficit hyperactivity disorder (ADHD) and disruptive behavior in 4% each. These rates were higher than community comparison samples. Systematic observations of the housing environment of the children confirmed that there were few books and toys, crowding, and poor sanitation. Interviews with children and mothers indicated that exposure to violence was high among the children. Forty-six percent of the children had witnessed violence, with 39% witnessing someone being beaten or mugged, 20%, someone being shot at, and 11%, someone being murdered. Nineteen percent of the children had been the victims of violence themselves. Both psychiatric disorders and witnessing violence were somewhat more common among the African American farmworkers, but sample sizes were too small to make meaningful comparisons. Children found to have a psychiatric diagnosis were over five times more likely to have seen a health professional (usually a physician) about it than those without (Martin et al. 1996). However, less than half the children with a diagnosis saw a health professional.

Martin and Kupersmidt conclude that the elevated levels of psychiatric disorders found in this population are a normal response to the environment and lifestyle these children experience. Current programs for farmworker children such as Migrant Head Start and Migrant Education seek to address these mental health problems by maintaining programmatic consistency to provide children with continuity in educational settings as they move from place to place.

8.2.4 Children's Environmental Health

Latino/Hispanic children in the US experience environmental exposures contributing to their health disparities (Carter-Pokras et al. 2007). Often the double jeopardy of living in impoverished environments (including living in dilapidated housing and near industrial chemicals) as well as inadequate public information about detecting and preventing such exposures places these children at substantial risk. Current research on environmental health among farmworker children in the eastern US focuses on pesticides; older studies focused on lead exposure and parasites. Despite a national focus on asthma triggers in housing of low-income populations, no research was found on asthma among farmworkers' children.

8.2.4.1 Housing

Particularly for young children who spend most of their time indoors, housing is the primary source of health exposures. In general, farmworkers live in poor-quality housing (see Chap. 3). Housing Assistance Council data for the eastern US found that at least 80% of all types of housing, excluding dormitories and barracks, were crowded (more than one person per room, excluding bathrooms and kitchens) (Housing Assistance Council 2000). On average, 50% of all housing types had children present.

Although some states had lower levels of crowding, children still lived in more than half of the crowded units in some of these states (Florida, New Jersey, New York, South Carolina, and Virginia), and in over 40% in other states (Kentucky and Maryland). Florida was cited as having a greater number of housing problems compared to other areas in the eastern US (and the US as a whole) (Housing Assistance Council 2001). Florida led all other regions in the proportion of substandard housing units and crowded housing units. These substandard and crowded conditions subject children to high levels of stress as well as the possibility of infectious disease transmission.

8.2.4.2 Pesticides

Pesticide exposure of children in farmworker communities is of concern because of the potential for developing a number of life-threatening conditions after cumulative exposure (e.g., childhood leukemia, brain cancer, non-Hodgkins's lymphoma) (Infante-Rivard and Weichenthal 2007). An unambiguous cause and effect relationship has yet to be established linking pesticide exposure and childhood cancers, but the associations are strong enough for concern and caution.

Children in farmworker families are at risk for pesticide exposure through a variety of pathways (Fenske 1997) (see Chap. 5). Pesticide applications in nearby fields can result in drift into home and yards where children play. Family members who work in fields or apply pesticides can bring home residues on skin, clothing, shoes, tools, and farm products (Fig. 8.4). When family vehicles are used to transport workers, these are contaminated with pesticide residues (Curl et al. 2002). If children

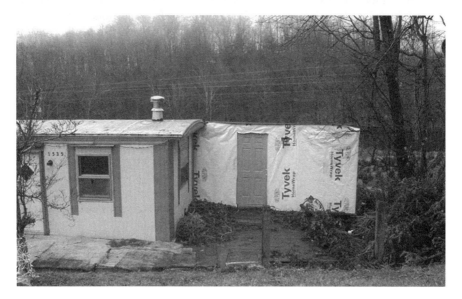

Fig. 8.4 Farmworker house showing Christmas tree clippings brought home for wreath-making by women. Copyright, Thomas A. Arcury

go into pesticide-treated fields to play, they come in contact with pesticide residues. Pesticide residues that get into houses are slow to break down, so they circulate in the air, contaminating toys, food, and other items children may put into their mouths (Quandt et al. 2004; Lewis et al. 2001).

Because of poor-quality housing, children may also come in contact with pesticides applied by landlords or family members to control pests in the home or yard (Lewis et al. 2001). Farmworker housing, like that of many economically disadvantaged families, is often in poor repair with leaky pipes and inadequate food storage and trash disposal facilities attracting pests. Holes in floors, walls, windows, and screens allow pests into homes.

Due to their large surface to volume ratios and slower metabolism of pesticides, children receive greater doses of pesticides and are at particular risk for the health consequences of exposure (Faustman et al. 2000; Weiss et al. 2004). The hand-to-mouth behaviors of young children promote greater exposure for children than for adults.

Studies on pesticide exposure of farmworker children in the eastern US demonstrate that they are exposed to a wide variety of pesticides. A study of urinary metabolites collected in summer 2004 from 60 Latino/Hispanic farmworker children aged 1–6 years in eastern North Carolina found metabolites of 13 of the 14 pesticides investigated (Arcury et al. 2007). These data were collected in eastern North Carolina. These included metabolites of seven organophosphorus pesticides, of which those from parathion, chlorpyrifos, diazinon, and malathion were the most frequently found (Fig. 8.5). Other commonly found pesticides included evidence of metabolites of pyrethroid insecticide 3PBA and the herbicides 2,4-D and acetochlor. The types of pesticides found demonstrate the role of drift or track-in as pathways in children's exposure. Chlorpyriphos was banned for indoor use in 2001. Parathion has no indoor use and is used in cotton, not in crops where farmworkers would work.

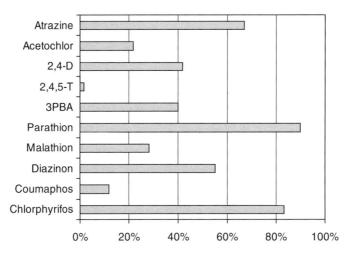

Fig. 8.5 Proportion of Latino/Hispanic farmworker children aged 1–6 years with metabolites for specific pesticides in urine; North Carolina, summer 2004 (Arcury et al. 2007)

Urinary metabolites from organophosphate pesticides were analyzed from 16 children from ten Latino/Hispanic farmworker families in western North Carolina (Arcury et al. 2005). In all cases, measurable dialkyl or dimethyl metabolites of organophosphorus pesticides were found. All but one child had at least one metabolite at or above the 50th percentile for total sample, age group, gender, or Mexican Americans of the 1999–2000 cycle of the National Health and Nutrition Examination Survey (NHANES) (CDC 2005; Barr et al. 2004). Ten of 16 children had at least one metabolite above the 90th percentile in comparisons with the NHANES reference data.

Environmental wipe samples were collected from the floors, toys, and children's hands in 41 farmworker houses in western North Carolina with a child less than seven years of age (Quandt et al. 2004). Samples were analyzed for eight pesticides known to be used in agriculture in the study area and 13 others commonly found in house dust throughout the US (Camann et al. 2000). The patterns of occurrence supported the idea of a pathway from floors to toys to children's hands. Pesticides were found in 95% of houses, with residential pesticides more common than agricultural.

All three studies tried to find predictors of exposure. In the western North Carolina studies (Quandt et al. 2004; Arcury et al. 2005), living adjacent to farm fields predicted the presence of agricultural pesticides and organophosphate metabolites; residing in a house judged hard to clean was a predictor of residential pesticides and organophosphate metabolites. In eastern North Carolina, boys, children in rental housing, and those with mothers working part-time had a greater number of pesticides detected (Arcury et al. 2007).

These studies suggest that pesticides are fairly ubiquitous in the environments where farmworker children live and play. Almost all have some exposure. Detecting the exact predictors of pesticide exposure may take much more fine detailed measurement, including timing of exposure relative to predictors. Health outcomes from pesticide exposure are equally inconclusive from studies in the eastern US. None of these studies – or any others – have attempted to measure health effects of pesticides in farmworker children, either immediate effects or long-term. Based on existing research, it is impossible to know whether the levels of exposure observed in these children are dangerous. Except in the case of poisoning with very high amounts of pesticides, health effects known from epidemiologic and animal studies are the result of cumulative exposure over long periods of time. Nonetheless, these findings suggest that farmworker children live in an environment where cumulative exposure is likely and should be minimized.

8.2.4.3   Lead

Because lead accumulates in the body, children are at risk from both current exposure and past exposure earlier in their lives. Those who were born or have lived outside the US experience additional lead exposure from the exhaust emissions of cars using leaded gasoline. This lead accumulates in soil and can be redeposited as dust on food, toys, or other items children put in their mouths.

Available studies on lead exposure among farmworker children are few and dated. A 1970 survey of housing in 117 farmworker camps in upstate New York found that almost 100% had interior and exterior evidence of lead-based paints (Osband and Tobin 1972). An average camp had about half the surfaces covered with lead-based paint and 40% of the paint was peeling and chipping. In those camps that had more than 50% children, an even higher percentage of surfaces were in poor condition. The researchers observed children left alone in the camp while parents worked. Pica, the practice of eating nonfood items such as dirt or paint chips, appeared to be common among the children. Evidence of elevated lead levels were found in western New York State during 1975–1977 from a survey of children in a healthcare practice (Perrin and Merkens 1979). Migrant children's blood level was significantly elevated compared to nonfarmworker children, whether on Medicaid (impoverished) or not. In an unpublished study of wipes taken in 55 North Carolina farmworker households with a child five years or younger for lead detection, 20% of homes had at least one sample with lead above the action levels (Arcury, unpublished data).

Since paint used in housing has been largely lead-free since around 1980, most farmworker children are no longer exposed to lead through housing. Other sources, though, include the use of lead-containing folk remedies, lead glazing on cooking pots brought from Mexico, and lead in candy and other foods brought from Mexico. For example, candy wrapped in printed cellophane wrappers which contain lead or foods containing chili which can accumulate dust from exhaust emissions during processing are consumed in higher proportion by children of farmworkers than by other children in the population (Carter-Pokras et al. 2007).

Children may also be exposed to lead through cultural practices. Folk remedies administered by their parents sometimes contain high amounts of lead. For example, an orange powder called Azarcón or a yellow powder called Greta are given in small doses for a number of illnesses. These are 85–95% lead, and can cause poisoning (CDC 2002). The folk illness empacho, which is manifest by gastrointestinal symptoms, is treated in Mexico as well as in the US with these remedies (Baer et al. 1998; Weller et al. 1993).

8.2.4.4 Parasites

The unsanitary and crowded living conditions that characterize some farmworker housing raise the potential for parasitic infections in farmworkers and their children. Three studies, spanning 1986 to 1998, describe screening results for parasites. A sample of farmworker children from the Delmarva Peninsula, aged 0–17 years, was tested for intestinal parasites (Ungar et al. 1986). Children 0–1 year had no parasites. Among those two years or older, 37% had evidence of intestinal parasites. Breakdown by ethnic group showed that children born in Haiti had higher prevalence of parasites than those of other ethnic groups born in the US or elsewhere.

A convenience sample of farmworkers in North Carolina of mixed ethnicity that included children found the highest prevalence of intestinal parasites to be among

Hispanics, all foreign-born (Ciesielski et al. 1992). Fifty-six percent of Mexican workers and 86% of Central American workers had parasites. These findings were confirmed in a later random sample of workers. Hookworm was the most common parasite, and was associated with significantly lower hematocrit.

A review of over 2,000 migrant health records in a Georgia migrant clinic found that about 14% of farmworkers or family members received treatment for parasites (Bechtel 1998). Of those treated, 60% were children, 29% women, and 11% men. Since these records only included those presenting for treatment, it is impossible to know the prevalence of parasites in the general population. Nonetheless, these data suggest that farmworker children are at significant risk for intestinal parasites.

8.2.5   Children as Farmworkers

Children working as farmworkers fall into two groups: those accompanying their parents and working, and unaccompanied youth working on farms. Gabbard et al. (1999) report that about 80% of child farmworkers are emancipated minors living on their own. The majority of these are male, foreign-born, aged 16–17 years, and recent and undocumented arrivals in the US. Under the law, children working in agriculture are provided fewer protections than those working in other industries or even other working places doing the same tasks (e.g., golf courses or landscaping). Children can work in agriculture starting at age 14 except during school hours. Some tasks (e.g., pesticide application) are deemed too hazardous and must be carried out by children who are at least 16 years old (Davis 2000).

The exact number of child farmworkers is uncertain. The NAWS excludes all children less than 14 years of age, and the Current Population Survey excludes children less than age 15. The former estimated youth farmworkers at 128,500 for the years 1993–1996; while the latter estimated 155,000 (USGAO 1998). Adding to the problem of counting children working in agriculture is the fact that parents may not consider them "working" if their productivity (e.g., baskets of vegetables or berries) is counted toward that of other adult family members.

Child and adolescent farmworkers are at special risk because their developing bodies are potentially more susceptible to hazards than are the more mature bodies of older workers. Because they are still growing, they experience the lack of coordination and decreased flexibility characteristic of youth during growth spurts, which can place them at risk for strains, sprains, and other injuries. They are more susceptible to heat stress than are older workers. Lack of experience may put them at greater risk of injury from equipment ranging from ladders to tractors. Like other children and adolescents, they may show unpredictable emotional behavior. All these factors place them at elevated risk for occupational injuries (Vela Acosta and Lee 2001).

Despite the special dangers that young farmworkers face, there have been few efforts to count their injuries. Existing data tally all farm injuries of children together, thus including nonworking children and those of the farm owners or operators (Davis and Leonard 2000).

There are no published reports of pesticide exposure among children working in the fields in the eastern US. Nevertheless, there is reason to believe that such children are at risk for pesticide exposure in the fields. For example, the EPA reentry intervals (time after pesticide application at which it is safe to return to work in the fields) are set using the model of a 154-pound male. Thus the dose children would receive in the fields upon reentry is higher than that for adults. In a survey of farmworker adolescents in Texas, Shipp et al. (2007) found that only 21% of students reported ever receiving pesticide safety training. Boys were almost twice as likely as girls to have been trained. Those working only outside of Texas and only for contractors or commercial growers/owners were also more likely to have been trained.

8.3 Women's Health

Although women make up a quarter of farmworkers and an unknown number are present in farmworker communities as dependents, the literature on their health is extremely sparse. For women in the eastern US, there is even less research. Many of these women experience considerable isolation while in the US. They usually live in rural communities, sometimes at considerable distance from other persons and, in particular, from other Latino/Hispanic women. This lack of contact can contribute to their lack of health knowledge, limited access to care, and mental health issues.

For those women who work as farmworkers, the level of occupational injuries is unknown. Women are more likely than men to work part-time when there is the greatest demand for workers. Quinlan et al.'s (2001) finding that part-time, temporary, and other contingent work arrangements are associated with greater hazard exposure and injury rates and with lower worker knowledge of occupational safety and health suggests that women may experience more injuries and receive less safety training than men.

Other health problems associated with gender undoubtedly affect women who work in the fields. Bechtel et al. (1995) found that urinary tract infections were the most common health problem among women in Georgia. They reported that they were unable to leave the fields due to work pressure or there were no facilities to urinate during the work day. In addition, if women are expected to do the same work as men, they may be at risk for musculoskeletal disorders due to their smaller body size.

8.3.1 Reproductive Health

Women in farmworker communities face a number of factors that can seriously compromise their reproductive health. These include exposure to pesticides in the home or workplace; inadequate prenatal, pregnancy, and postnatal diet; and inadequate medical care.

8.3.1.1 Pesticide Exposure

Among agricultural exposures, pesticide exposure has perhaps the greatest potential for harming the developing fetus. Pesticides cross the placenta and are found in amniotic fluid; many are also present in breast milk (Bradman et al. 2003; Pohl and Tylenda 2000; Shen et al. 2007). Epidemiological studies indicate that exposure as long as two years prior to pregnancy can result in an elevated risk of kidney cancer in offspring (Tsai et al. 2006). Exposure to pesticides in the critical first trimester of pregnancy results in increased risks for anencephaly and spontaneous abortion (Lacasaña et al. 2006; Arbuckle et al. 2001). Pregnancy exposure can affect child development, with effects not appearing until 24 months postnatally (Eskenazi et al. 2007).

In a study of farmworker families in western North Carolina, a Christmas tree-producing area, Arcury et al. (2005) found that women showed evidence of exposure to organophosphorus pesticides. Most of the women were not regularly employed in agriculture, though some made wreaths and other decorative items from Christmas tree clippings in the home. All women had organophosphorus pesticide metabolites in their urine. The levels were, in general, slightly lower than but consistent with those of their husbands. Many exceeded the National Health and Nutrition Examination Survey (NHANES) 50th percentile for their gender, age, and ethnicity.

Maternal pesticide exposure and its teratogenic effects were recently highlighted by the birth of three severely deformed infants to female farmworkers in Florida who had all worked before and during pregnancy on North Carolina and Florida farms owned by a single agribusiness (Calvert et al. 2007; Chelminski et al. 2006). A review of available exposure data indicated a plausible association between possible pesticide exposure during organogenesis and birth defects in all of the children, though familial inheritance may have been a factor in one case. Numerous issues with regulatory compliance by the company employing the women were found, suggesting that the women may have had excessive exposure to pesticides that would have put them at risk. However, no evidence could tie the cases to specific pesticides used during the pregnancies.

8.3.1.2 Cancer Screening

Studies of farmworker cancer risk do not show female reproductive cancers to be elevated compared to nonfarmworkers (Zahm and Blair 1993). However, Hispanic women as a whole in the US are at increased risk of invasive cervical cancer (14.2/100,000), compared to all women (8.8/100,000) (NCI 2005). Mortality rates for Hispanic women also exceed rates for non-Hispanic White women (3.4/100,000 vs. 2.4/100,000) (CDC 2004). These figures have led to a focus on promotion of cervical cancer screening and, more recently, of vaccination to prevent genital human papillomavirus (HPV), a risk factor for cervical cancer, among young Latina/Hispanic women.

Latina/Hispanic women are at lower risk for breast cancer than non-Hispanic White women. This may be due to a number of factors, including earlier first birth and greater parity (Sweeney et al. 2008). Despite this, breast cancer is the top cause of cancer deaths among Hispanic women (U.S. Cancer Statistics Working Group 2006), suggesting that greater participation in screening is necessary.

Nationally, Latina/Hispanic women are less likely then non-Hispanic women to report a Pap smear in the past three years and a mammogram in the past two years (Coughlin et al. 2008). Rural women were less likely than urban women to have been screened. Few studies have been conducted with farmworker women on breast or cervical cancer screening (Coughlin and Wilson 2002). Hooks et al. (1996) collected in-depth interviews and a survey with farmworkers on the Delmarva Peninsula. They found fairly low understanding of cervical cancer and Pap tests. Similar results were found among farmworkers in Wisconsin (Lantz et al. 1994; Lantz and Reding 1994), where farmworker women reported low levels of knowledge about cancer causes, early detection, and treatment. Fatalistic attitudes, as well as misconceptions (e.g., that bruising can cause cancer) were common. A strong aversion to examination by male clinicians, as well as structural barriers such as cost, lack of transportation, and lack of time due to long work hours also prevented screening. Studies in Washington State and California's Central Valley had similar findings (Skaer et al. 1996a, b). A high percentage of women had never had screening examinations, and fear, embarrassment, and structural barriers all impeded improving rates of care.

A number of interventions have been designed to try to improve rates of cancer screening among farmworker women. In Washington State, a controlled trial of education only or education plus a voucher for mammography found that the voucher increased the mammography compliance from 18 to 88% (Skaer 1996b). Lay health advisors have been used in California (Boucher 2000; Goldsmith and Sisneros 1996) to train farmworker women about cervical and breast cancer screening. Results indicate significant increases in knowledge and some increase in screenings. Using a video with an entertaining story line, Meade et al. (2002) sought to increase knowledge, comfort with screening, and intentions to screen among farmworkers in Florida. While the video was successful at increasing women's knowledge and more said they intend to be screened, their comfort level with having Pap tests or mammograms was unchanged. Actual behavior change was quite low: 50% of women eligible for a Pap test and 17% eligible for mammography completed the exams. Those who failed to be screened cited structural barriers: transportation, migrating north, cost, and family or work responsibilities. Meade and Calvo (2001) also reported community–academic partnership efforts to increase cancer screening among farmworker women. They found that providing a mobile unit at central, rural places was insufficient. The addition of Spanish language health promotion materials and then a local female outreach worker helped increase the number of farmworker women who were screened.

8.3.1.3 Reproductive Health Services and Practices

Birth outcomes for farmworker women show high rates of infant mortality and low birth weight. Early prenatal care and proper pregnancy weight gain have been targeted as means to improve birth outcomes. Recent data for farmworker women are not available. However, data compiled by CDC for 1989–1993 prenatal care and birth outcomes among migrant farmworkers indicate a failure to meet goals for programs such as WIC and Healthy People 2000 (MMWR 1997). Only 62% of women initiated prenatal care in the first trimester; 9% waited until the last trimester or received no care. Pregnancy weight gain was less than recommended for 52% of women and greater than recommended for 24%. A demonstration to coordinate perinatal care for farmworker women in North Carolina was able to increase first-trimester care and total number of prenatal visits (Larson et al. 1992). This program used bilingual staff, outreach services, lay health advisors, and a multistate tracking system to ensure continuity of care for migrating women.

There are virtually no published data related to contraception knowledge and use among farmworker women. Because of the dangers posed by pesticide exposure at work and at home, the ability to time pregnancies is especially important to these women. Among low-income women of reproductive age, immigrant Hispanic women have less knowledge of reproduction and contraception than do non-Hispanic women of comparable incomes (Garcés-Palacio et al. 2008), and they are less likely (47.8% vs. 77.9%) to report using any type of contraception. Compared with national data that do not distinguish immigrant and nonimmigrant Hispanic women (Mosher et al. 2004), immigrant women are less likely (47.8% vs. 59%) to use any contraception. These findings suggest that farmworker women, who are largely immigrants, may benefit from education about contraceptive use and greater access to health services.

Douching by Latina/Hispanic women is reported to be high, with 30–40% of women in some age groups reporting the practice (Abma et al. 1997). The practice has been related to a number of negative health outcomes, including vaginal and pelvic infections, herpes, ectopic pregnancy, and preterm birth (Martino and Vermund 2002; Sutton et al. 2007). Studies of the practice reveal that many women have no knowledge of the possible health consequences. There are strong cultural supports for douching, including beliefs that stress the cosmetic and hygienic benefits of douching (McKee et al. 2009). While there are no studies of this practice among farmworker women, it is likely that the lack of information found in the general Latino/Hispanic population is also present in the farmworker community.

Farmworkers are at increased risk of HIV infection because of a combination of behavioral and ecological factors, including poverty, low educational attainment, and isolation. Much of the early research on HIV among farmworkers concentrated on males (e.g., MMWR 1992). A study in south Florida including both men and women found that an unexpectedly high number of women (15%) had been paid for sex, while the number of men paying was comparable to studies of farmworkers elsewhere (Fernández et al. 2004). Knowledge of HIV transmission was low in both genders. Women were at four times higher risk of sexually acquired HIV than men. The study indicates that men and women have different patterns of risk behaviors and different interventions are probably needed. It also counters the impression that women's risk is due to their sex partners' behaviors, as women appear to be engaging in risky behaviors themselves (see Chap. 6).

Female partners of male migrant farmworkers are at risk for HIV/AIDS even if they remain in Mexico. Returning men who have used sex workers, engaged in sex with other men, or engaged in intravenous drug use spread HIV/AIDS to women who are unaware of their partners' exposure. The problem is fostered by Mexican women's commitment to an illusion of fidelity and the opportunities presented to men who may be separated from partners for long periods of time (Hirsch et al. 2002, 2007).

8.3.2 Mental Health

Women in farmworker communities are subject to a variety of stressors that may lead to poor mental health (see Chap. 7). Some are comparable to other low-income communities: poverty, poor housing, long work hours, and inadequate access to healthcare resources. Others are particular to this community: physical isolation due to rural living, social isolation due to language, mobile lifestyle, separation from family of origin, and reluctance to seek help due to documentation concerns. Much of the research on mental health in this population has been centered in the Midwest (e.g., Hovey and Magaña 2000; Magaña and Hovey 2003) or West (e.g., Alderete et al. 2000) or has failed to disentangle mental health issues for men and women (e.g., Kim-Godwin and Bechtel 2004).

Because of the recent arrival of immigrants to many communities in the eastern US, the relatively smaller number of Latino/Hispanic women, and the lack of older adults in these communities, mental health-related experiences of these women may differ in some respects from those elsewhere. In focus group discussions with Latina/Hispanic women in low-wage jobs in North Carolina, women identified stressors such as the need for women to work in the US and the different expenses for life in the US (e.g., need to maintain a car) (Easter et al. 2007). Women cited "double work" (working both in and outside the home) as a new and unaccustomed stressor. Discrimination and racism add to the stress at work, as do language barriers. Traditional gender roles exacerbate the tension women feel. They report that men are better able to deal with work-related stress because they can relax at home, a privilege women lack. The disruption of family life caused by leaving some family behind in the country of origin took an emotional toll as mothers worried about the welfare of children left behind. Beyond that, working mothers missed the reliable child care offered by the extended family.

Intimate partner violence is a concern for women in farmworker communities. Those in the eastern US are less likely to have advocacy groups focused on their particular needs and culturally and linguistically appropriate resources to respond. Immigrants in rural communities do not know about local resources and are unfamiliar with US legal practices (e.g., protective orders) (Moracco et al. 2005). While the experience of intimate partner violence is approximately the same as non-Latina/Hispanic women, Latina/Hispanic women are more likely to lack social support and more likely to have children in the home (Denham et al. 2007). Nationally, acculturative stress and alcohol use appear to be associated with intimate partner violence (Caetano et al. 2007). The changing gender roles of women with immigration (e.g., more are likely to engage in paid employment and have incomes in the US than in Mexico) may contribute to changes in relationships in couples that lead to intimate partner violence (Grzywacz, unpublished data).

8.3.3 Sexual Harassment

Young girls and women working as farmworkers are at special risk for sexual harassment and assault. Farm work is male-dominated. Most supervisors and coworkers are male. Women often work in isolated areas. They rarely know the legal protections of women in the US, and their documentation status and embarrassment make them reluctant to complain. They face retaliation, including assignment to undesirable tasks and firing if they do report the problems. Despite the recognition by advocates (Human Rights Watch 2000), there is no research on the extent of the problem.

The Southern Poverty Law Center's Esperanza (www.Splcenter.org/legal/ijp.jsp) is a project aimed at addressing sexual harassment and gender discrimination among immigrant women, including farmworkers. Project staff members have initiated successful lawsuits on behalf of farmworker women in the Southeast. They have also developed educational materials to inform women of their rights and how to report abuses.

8.4 Conclusions

Research on women and children who work as farmworkers or who are members of farmworker families in the eastern US is spotty, at best. There are no accurate figures nationally or in the region of how many women and children are in the population, or what they do. Geographic coverage is far from complete. This is significant because of the different crops and their associated hazards and the different health resources available from state to state.

Coverage is equally incomplete if one looks from the perspective of health conditions. Environmental health is the area in which the most is known about women and children, though only the pesticide research is current. Lead and infectious disease studies are largely outdated. Some of the sources of lead exposure have changed. While immunizations were formerly a concern for children, it now appears that systems are in place to ensure most children receive immunizations. However, new infectious health threats exist, such as MRSA and drug-resistant tuberculosis.

Few of the health issues that are current for children (e.g., obesity, prevention of chronic disease, mental health) have received significant attention. What little research exists suggests that children in farmworker families are at risk, but the research is limited and some is quite dated.

There is increasing attention to critical exposures such as pesticides during pregnancy for women. However, definitive studies would require monitoring exposures and outcomes in a large number of women. Because no state in the eastern

US currently requires applicators to report pesticides applied, linking exposures to birth outcomes is difficult.

For some women's issues, farmworker women may be extremely vulnerable. Some do not have documents to be in the US, but their husbands or partners do. This probably makes these women less likely to report issues such as intimate partner violence. It also places them in a dependent position when it comes to obtaining health care for themselves or their children. Research on women's health should take into account documentation status and its role in promoting health problems and in treatment seeking.

This review of women and children's health highlights issues of social justice. As members of farmworker families, women and children are exposed to health hazards where they live. Laws regarding work in agriculture (see Chaps. 2 and 9) create exceptions so that children work at younger ages in an occupation with significant hazards for growing children. Despite the greater susceptibility of women of reproductive age to pesticides and other agricultural exposures (see Chap. 5), there are no special protections provided by existing policies.

Many of the women and children on which this chapter focuses are in the eastern US as members of families. Much of the research and many of the services available focus on "migrant" families. Yet with more restrictive national immigration policies, many families are settling out of the migrant streams. In some cases, family members participate in agriculture as seasonal workers without changing place of residence to work. In others, one or more members may migrate for work, while the others do not. These changes in residence patterns can change eligibility for services, as well as exposures for health risks. Both policies and research need to acknowledge that the labels "migrant" and "seasonal" do not capture the complexities of farmworker families. Researchers need to be clear in describing the families or family members they study. Policy makers need to broaden criteria to make all farmworker families eligible for services intended to address their particular health, education, and social services needs.

References

Abma JC, Chandra A, Mosher WD et al. (1997) Fertility, family planning, and women's health: new data from the 1995 National Survey of Family Growth. Vital Health Stat 23(19):1–114

Alderete E, Vega WA, Kolody B et al. (2000) Lifetime prevalence of and risk factors for psychiatric disorders among Mexican migrant farmworkers in California. Am J Public Health 90:608–614

Alvarez WF, Doris J, Larson O 3rd (1988) Children of migrant farm work families are at high risk for maltreatment: New York State study. Am J Public Health 78:934–936

American Academy of Pediatrics (2000) Guidelines for the care of migrant farmworkers' children. American Academy of Pediatrics, Elk Grove Village, IL

Arbuckle TE, Lin Z, Mery LS (2001) An exploratory analysis of the effect of pesticide exposure on the risk of spontaneous abortion in an Ontario farm population. Environ Health Perspect 109:851–857

Arcury TA, Quandt SA, Rao P et al. (2005) Organophosphate pesticide exposure in farmworker family members in western North Carolina and Virginia: case comparisons. Hum Organ 64:40–51

Arcury TA, Grzywacz JG, Barr DB et al. (2007) Pesticide urinary metabolite levels of children in eastern North Carolina farmworker households. Environ Health Perspect 115:1254–1260

Baer RD, Garcia de Alba J, Leal RM et al. (1998) Mexican use of lead in the treatment of empacho: community, clinic, and longitudinal patterns. Soc Sci Med 47:1263–1266

Barr DB, Bravo R, Weerasekera G et al. (2004) Concentrations of dialkyl phosphate metabolites of organophosphorus pesticides in the US population. Environ Health Perspect 112:186–200

Bechtel GA (1998) Parasitic infections among migrant farm families. J Community Health Nurs 15:1–7

Bechtel GA, Shepherd MA, Rogers PW (1995) Family, culture, and health practices among migrant farmworkers. J Community Health Nurs 12:15–22

Boucher F (2000) Lay health advisors increase cervical cancer screening rates among Mexican farmworkers. In: Proceedings of the 15th National Conference on Chronic Disease Prevention and Control. Living Healthier, Living Longer: The Will and the Way. Washington, DC

Bradman A, Barr DB, Claus Henn BG et al. (2003) Measurement of pesticides and other toxicants in amniotic fluid as a potential biomarker of prenatal exposure: a validation study. Environ Health Perspect 111:1779–1782

Caetano R, Ramisetty-Mikler S, Caetano Vaeth PA et al. (2007) Acculturation stress, drinking, and intimate partner violence among Hispanic couples in the U.S. J Interpers Violence 22:1431–1447

Calvert GM, Alarcon WA, Chelminski A et al. (2007) Case report: three farmworkers who gave birth to infants with birth defects closely grouped in time and place – Florida and North Carolina, 2004–2005. Environ Health Perspect 115:787–791

Camann DE, Colt JS, Teitelbaum SL et al. (2000) Pesticide and PAH distributions in house dust from seven areas of USA. Society of Environmental Toxicology and Chemistry 21st Annual Meeting, paper 570, Nashville, TN

Carroll D, Samardick RM, Bernard S et al. (2005) Findings from the National Agricultural Workers Survey (NAWS) 2001–2002: A Demographic and Employment Profile of United States Farm Workers. US Department of Labor

Carter-Pokras O, Zambrana RE, Poppell CF et al. (2007) The environmental health of Latino children. J Pediatr Health Care 21:307–314

Casey PH, Simpson PM, Gossett JM et al. (2006) The association of child and household food insecurity with childhood overweight status. Pediatrics 118:e1406–e1413

Cason K, Nieto-Montenegro S, Chavez-Martinez A et al. (2003) Dietary intake and food security among migrant farm workers in Pennsylvania. Harris School Working Paper Series 04.2. http://harrisschool.uchicago.edu/About/publications/working-papers/pdf/wp_04_02.pdf

Centers for Disease Control and Prevention (1992) HIV infection, syphilis, and tuberculosis screening among migrant farm workers – Florida, 1992. MMWR 41:723–725

Centers for Disease Control and Prevention (1997) Pregnancy-related behaviors among migrant farm workers – four states, 1989–1993. MMWR 46:283–286

Centers for Disease Control and Prevention (2002) Managing elevated blood lead levels among young children: recommendations from the Advisory Committee on Childhood Lead Poisoning Prevention. CDC, Atlanta, GA

Centers for Disease Control and Prevention (2004) Behavioral risk factor surveillance system. National Center for Chronic Disease and Prevention and Health Promotion: Atlanta, GA

Centers for Disease Control and Pevention (2005) Third national report on human exposure to environmental chemicals. CDC, Atlanta, GA. Available: http://www.cdc.gov/exposurereport/report.htm

Chaffin JG, Pai SC, Bargamian RA (2003) Caries prevalence in northwest Michigan migrant children. J Dent Child 70:124–129

Chelminski AN, Higgins S, Meyer R et al. (2006) Assessment of maternal occupational pesticide exposures during pregnancy and three children with birth defects: North Carolina, 2004. Occupational and Environmental Epidemiology Branch, Division of Public Health, North Carolina Department of Health and Human Services, Raleigh, NC. Available: http://www.epi.state.nc.us/epi/oii/Agmartreleasereport.pdf

Chi PSK, McClain J (1992) Drinking, farm, and camp life: a study of drinking behavior in migrant camps in New York State. J Rural Health 8:41–51

Ciesielski SD, Seed JR, Ortiz JC et al. (1992) Intestinal parasites among North Carolina migrant farmworkers. Am J Public Health 82:1258–1262

Cooper SP, Weller NF, Fox EE et al. (2005a) Comparative description of migrant farmworkers versus other students attending rural south Texas schools: substance use, work, and injuries. J Rural Health 21:361–366

Cooper SP, Weller NF, Fox EE et al. (2005b) Comparative description of migrant farmworkers versus other students attending South Texas schools: demographic, academic, and health characteristics. Tex Med 101:58–62

Coughlin SS, Wilson KM (2002) Breast and cervical cancer screening among migrant and seasonal farmworkers: a review. Cancer Detect Prev 26:203–209

Coughlin SS, Leadbetter S, Richards T et al. (2008) Contextual analysis of breast and cervical cancer screening and factors associated with health care access among United States women, 2002. Soc Sci Med 66:260–275

Curl CL, Fenske RA, Kissel JC (2002) Evaluation of take-home organophosphorus pesticide exposure among agricultural workers and their children. Environ Health Perspect 110:A787–A792

Davis S, Leonard JB (2000) The ones the law forgot: children working in agriculture. Farmworker Justice Fund, Washington, DC. Available: http://www.fwjustice.org/images/CHILD%20 LABOR%20REPORT%20-%20FINAL.pdf

Denham AC, Frasier PY, Hooten EG et al. (2007) Intimate partner violence among Latinas in eastern North Carolina. Violence Against Women 13:123–140

Drewnowski A, Darmon N (2005) The economics of obesity: dietary energy density and energy cost. Am J Clin Nutr 82(1 Suppl):265S–273S

Easter MM, Linnan LA, Bentley ME et al. (2007) "Una mujer trabaja doble aquí": vignette-based focus groups on stress and work for Latina blue-collar women in eastern North Carolina. Health Promot Pract 8:41–49

Entwistle BA, Swanson TM (1989) Dental needs and perceptions of adult Hispanic migrant farmworkers in Colorado. J Dent Hyg 63:286–292

Eskenazi B, Marks AR, Bradman A et al. (2007) Organophosphate pesticide exposure and neurodevelopment in young Mexican-American children. Environ Health Perspect 115:792–798

Essa JS (2001) Nutrition, health, and food security practices, concerns, and perceived barriers of Latino farm/industry workers in Virginia. MS thesis, Virginia Polytechnic Institute and State University. Online: http://scholar.lib.vt.edu/theses/available/etd-08102001-133508/unrestricted/Thesis-Chapters.pdf

Faustman EM, Silbernagel SM, Fenske RA et al. (2000) Mechanisms underlying children's susceptibility to environmental toxicants. Environ Health Perspect 108(Suppl 1):13–21

Fenske RA (1997) Pesticide exposure assessment of workers and their families. Occup Med: State of the Art Reviews 12(2):221–237

Fernández MI, Collazo JB, Hernández N et al. (2004) Predictors of HIV risk among Hispanic farm workers in South Florida: women are at higher risk than men. AIDS Behav 8:165–174

Gabbard S, Carroll D, Baron S et al. (1999) Teens in crop agriculture. Paper prepared for the National Adolescent Farmworker Occupational Health and Safety Advisory Committee. US Department of Labor, Washington, DC

Garcés-Palacio IC, Altarac M, Scarinci IC (2008) Contraceptive knowledge and use among low-income Hispanic immigrant women and non-Hispanic women. Contraception 77:270–275

Gentry K, Quandt SA, Davis SW et al. (2007) Child healthcare in two farmworker populations. J Community Health 32:419–431

Goldsmith DF, Sisneros GC (1996) Cancer prevention strategies among California farmworkers: preliminary findings. J Rural Health 12(4 Suppl):343–348

Grzywacz JG, Quandt SA, Early J et al. (2006a) Leaving family for work: ambivalence and mental health among Mexican migrant farmworker men. J Immigr Minor Health 8:85–97

Grzywacz JG, Hovey JD, Seligman LD et al. (2006b) Evaluating short-form versions of the CES-D for measuring depressive symptoms among immigrants from Mexico. Hisp J Behav Sci 28:404–424

Grzywacz JG, Quandt SA, Isom S et al. (2007) Alcohol use among immigrant Latino farmworkers in North Carolina. Am J Ind Med 50:617–625

Gwyther ME, Jenkins M (1998) Migrant farmworker children: health status, barriers to care, and nursing innovations in health care delivery. J Pediatr Health Care 12:60–66

Harrison L, Scarinci I (2007) Child health needs of rural Alabama Latino families. J Community Health Nurs 24:31–47

Hirsch JS, Higgins J, Bentley ME et al. (2002) The social constructions of sexuality: marital infidelity and sexually transmitted disease-HIV risk in a Mexican migrant community. Am J Public Health 92:1227–1237.

Hirsch JS, Meneses S, Thompson B et al. (2007) The inevitability of infidelity: sexual reputation, social geographies, and marital HIV risk in rural Mexico. Am J Public Health 97:986–996

Hooks C, Ugarte C, Silsby J et al. (1996) Obstacles and opportunities in designing cancer control communication research for farmworkers on the Delmarva Peninsula. J Rural Health 12(4 Suppl):332–342

Housing Assistance Council (2000) Abundant fields, meager shelter: findings from a survey of farm-worker housing in the eastern migrant stream. Housing Assistance Council, Washington, DC.

Housing Assistance Council (2001) No refuge from the fields: findings from a survey of farmworker housing conditions in the United States. Housing Assistance Council, Washington, DC.

Hovey JD, Magaña C (2000) Acculturative stress, anxiety, and depression among Mexican immigrant farmworkers in the midwest United States. J Immigr Health 2:119–131

Human Rights Watch (2000) Fingers to the bone: Unites States failure to protect child farmworkers. Human Rights Watch, New York

Inciardi JA, Surratt HL, Colón HM et al. (1999) Drug use and HIV risks among migrant workers on the DelMarVa Peninsula. Subst Use Misuse 34:653–666

Infante-Rivard C, Weichenthal S (2007) Pesticides and childhood cancer: an update of Zahm and Ward's 1998 review. J Toxicol Environ Health B Crit Rev 10:81–99

Kim-Godwin YS, Bechtel GA (2004) Stress among migrant and seasonal farmworkers in rural southeast North Carolina. J Rural Health 20:271–278

Koday M, Rosenstein DI, Lopez GM (1990) Dental decay rates among children of migrant workers in Yakima, WA. Public Health Rep 105:530–533

Kupersmidt JB, Martin SL (1997) Mental health problems of children of migrant and seasonal farm workers: a pilot study. J Am Acad Child Adolesc Psychiatry 36:224–232

Lacasaña M, Vázquez-Grameix H, Borja-Aburto VH et al. (2006) Maternal and paternal occupational exposure to agricultural work and the risk of anencephaly. Occup Environ Med 63:649–656

Lantz PM, Reding D (1994) Cancer: beliefs and attitudes of migrant Latinos. J Am Med Assoc 272:31–32

Lantz PM, Dupuis L, Reding D et al. (1994) Peer discussions of cancer among Hispanic migrant farm workers. Public Health Rep 109:512–520

Larson OW 3rd, Doris J, Alvarez WF (1990) Migrants and maltreatment: comparative evidence from central register data. Child Abuse Negl 14:375–385

Larson K, McGuire J, Watkins E et al. (1992) Maternal care coordination for migrant farmworker women: program structure and evaluation of effects on use of prenatal care and birth outcome. J Rural Health 8:128–133

Lee CV, McDermott SW, Elliott C (1990) The delayed immunization of children of migrant farm workers in South Carolina. Public Health Rep 105:317–320

Lewis RG, Fortune CR, Blanchard FT et al. (2001) Movement and deposition of two organophosphorus pesticides within a residence after interior and exterior applications. J Air Waste Manag Assoc 51:339–351

Lukes SM, Miller FY (2002) Oral health issues among migrant farmworkers. J Dent Hyg 76:134–140

Lukes SM, Simon B (2005) Dental decay in southern Illinois migrant and seasonal farmworkers: an analysis of clinical data. J Rural Health 21:254–258

Lukes SM, Simon B (2006) Dental services for migrant and seasonal farmworkers in US community/migrant health centers. J Rural Health 22:269–272

Lukes SM, Wadhawan S, Lampiris LN (2006) Healthy smiles healthy growth 2004 – basic screening survey of migrant and seasonal farmworker children in Illinois. J Public Health Dent 66:216–218

Magaña CG, Hovey JD (2003) Psychosocial stressors associated with Mexican migrant farmworkers in the midwest United States. J Immigr Health 5:75–86

Markowitz DL, Cosminsky S (2005) Overweight and stunting in migrant Hispanic children in the USA. Econ Hum Biol 3:215–240.

Martin SL, Gordon TE, Kupersmidt JB (1995) Survey of exposure to violence among the children of migrant and seasonal farm workers. Public Health Rep 110:268–276

Martin SL, Kupersmidt JB, Harter KS (1996) Children of farm laborers: utilization of services for mental health problems. Community Ment Health J 32:327–340

Martino JL, Vermund SH (2002) Vaginal douching: evidence for risks or benefits to women's health. Epidemiol Rev 24:109–124

McKee MD, Baquero M, Anderson MR et al. (2009) Vaginal douching among Latinas: practices and meaning. Matern Child Health J 13:98–106

Meade CD, Calvo A (2001) Developing community-academic partnerships to enhance breast health among rural and Hispanic migrant and seasonal farmworker women. Oncol Nurs Forum 28:1577–1584

Meade CD, Calvo A, Cuthbertson D (2002) Impact of culturally, linguistically, and literacy relevant cancer information among Hispanic farmworker women. J Cancer Educ 17:50–54

Mines R (2000) Children in immigrant and nonimmigrant farmworker families: findings from the National Agricultural Workers Survey. In: Hernandez DJ (ed.) Children of Immigrants: Health, Adjustment, and Public Assistance. Committee on the Health and Adjustment of Immigrant Children and Families, National Research Council.(pp. 620–658) The National Academy Press, Washington, DC

Moracco KE, Hilton A, Hodges KG et al. (2005) Knowledge and attitudes about intimate partner violence among immigrant Latinos in rural North Carolina: baseline information and implications for outreach. Violence Against Women 11:337–352

Mosher WD, Martinez GM, Chandra A et al. (2004) Use of contraception and use of family planning services in the United States: 1982–2002. Adv Data 350:1–36

National Cancer Institute (2005) Surveillance, epidemiology, and end results. SEER cancer statistics. Incidence of cervix uteri cancer. http://seer.cancer.gov/

National Research Council (2006) Food insecurity and hunger in the United States: an assessment of the measure. Panel to review the US Department of Agriculture's Measurement of Food Insecurity and Hunger. In: Wunderlich GS and Norwood JL (eds.) Committee on National Statistics, Division of Behavioral and Social Sciences and Education. The National Academies Press, Washington, DC

Nord M, Andrews M, Carlson S (2005) Household food security in the United States, 2004. Food Assistance and Nutrition Research Program, Economic Research Services, USDA, Economic Research Report No.11, Washington, DC

Ogden DL, Carroll MD, Curtin LR et al. (2006) Prevalence of overweight and obesity in the United States, 1999–2004. JAMA 295:1549–1555

Osband ME, Tobin JR (1972) Lead paint exposure in migrant labor camps. Pediatrics 49:604–606.

Perrin JM, Merkens MJ (1979) Blood lead levels in a rural population: relative elevations among migrant farmworker children. Pediatrics 64:540–542

Pohl HR, Tylenda CA (2000) Breast-feeding exposure of infants to selected pesticides: a public health viewpoint. Toxicol Ind Health 16:65–77

Quandt SA, Arcury TA, Rao P et al. (2004) Agricultural and residential pesticides in wipe samples from farmworker family residences in North Carolina and Virginia. Environ Health Perspect 112(3):382–387

Quandt SA, Shoaf JI, Tapia J et al. (2006) Experiences of Latino immigrant families in North Carolina help explain elevated levels of food insecurity and hunger. J Nutr 136:2638–2644

Quandt SA, Clark HM, Rao P et al. (2007) Oral health of children and adults in Latino migrant and seasonal farmworker families. J Immigr Minor Health 9:229–235

Quinlan M, Mayhew C, Bohle P (2001) The global expansion of precarious employment, work disorganization, and consequences for occupational health: a review of recent research. Int J Health Serv 31:335–414

Ramos-Gomez FJ, Tomar SL, Ellison J et al. (1999) Assessment of early childhood caries and dietary habits in a population of migrant Hispanic children in Stockton, California ASDC. J Dent Child 66:395–403

Rosenbaum S, Shin P (2005) Migrant and seasonal farmworkers: health insurance coverage and access to care. Kaiser Commission on Medicaid and the Uninsured, Washington, DC. http://www.kff.org/uninsured/upload/Migrant-and-Seasonal-Farmworkers-Health-Insurance-Coverage-and-Access-to-Care-Report.pdf (accessed 5–26–08)

Seid M, Castañeda D, Mize R et al. (2003) Crossing the border for health care: access and primary care characteristics for young children of Latino farm workers along the US-Mexico border. Ambul Pediatr 3:121–130

Shen H, Main KM, Virtanen HE et al. (2007) From mother to child: investigation of prenatal and postnatal exposure to persistent bioaccumulating toxicants using breast milk and placenta biomonitoring. Chemosphere 67:S256–S262

Shipp EM, Cooper SP, del Junco DJ et al. (2007) Pesticide safety training among farmworker adolescents from Starr County, Texas. J Agric Saf Health 13:311–321

Shotland J, Loonin D, Haas E (1989) Full fields, empty cupboards: the nutritional status of migrant farmworkers in America. Public Voice for Food and Health Policy, Washington, DC

Skaer TL, Robison LM, Sclar DA et al. (1996a) Cancer-screening determinants among Hispanic women using migrant health clinics. J Health Care Poor Underserved 7:338–354

Skaer TL, Robison LM, Sclar DA et al. (1996b) Financial incentive and the use of mammography among Hispanic migrants to the US. Health Care Women Int 17:281–291

Sutton M, Sternberg M, Koumans EH et al. (2007) The prevalence of *Trichomonas vaginalis* infection among reproductive-age women in the United States, 2001–2004. Clin Infect Dis 45:1319–1326

Sweeney C, Baumgartner KB, Byers T et al. (2008) Reproductive history in relation to breast cancer risk among Hispanic and non-Hispanic white women. Cancer Causes Control 19:391–401

Tsai J, Kaye WE, Bove FJ (2006) Wilms' tumor and exposures to residential and occupational hazardous chemicals. Int J Hyg Environ Health 209:57–64

Ungar BLP, Iscoe E, Cutler J et al. (1986) Intestinal parasites in a migrant farmworker population. Arch Intern Med 146:513–515

U.S. Cancer Statistics Working Group (2006) United States cancer statistics: 2003 incidence and mortality. U.S. Department of Health and Human Services, Centers for Disease Control and Prevention and National Cancer Institute. http://www.cdc.gov/cancer/npcr/npcrpdfs/US_Cancer_Statistics_2003_Incidence_and_Mortality.pdf

US General Accounting Office (1998) Child labor in agriculture: changes needed to better protect health and educational opportunities. Report to Congressional Requesters (GAO HEHS-98-193). US General Accounting Office, Washington, DC

Vela Acosta M, Lee B (eds.) (2001) Migrant and Seasonal Hired Adolescent Farmworkers: A Plan to Improve Working Conditions. Marshfield Clinic, Marshfield, WI

Weathers AC, Garrison HG (2004) Children of migratory agricultural workers: the ecological context of acute care for a mobile population of immigrant children. Clin Pediatr Emerg Med 5:120–129

Weathers A, Minkovitz C, O'Campo P et al. (2003) Health services use by children of migratory agricultural workers: exploring the role of need for care. Pediatrics 111(5 Part 1):956–963

Weathers A, Minkovitz C, O'Campo P et al. (2004) Access to care for children of migratory agricultural workers: factors associated with unmet need for medical care. Pediatrics 113:e276–e282

Weathers AC, Novak SP, Sastry N et al. (2008a) Parental nativity is an important factor associated with where children usually go for health care. Matern Child Health J 12:499–508

Weathers AC, Minkovitz CS, Diener-West M et al. (2008b) The effect of parental immigration authorization on health insurance coverage for migrant Latino children. J Immigr Minor Health 10:247–254

Weathers AC, Novak SP, Sastry N et al. (2008c) Parental nativity affects children's health and access to care. J Immigr Minor Health 10:155–165

Weiss B, Amler S, Amler RW (2004) Pesticides. Pediatrics 113(4 Suppl):1030–1036

Weller SC, Pachter LM, Trotter RT 2nd et al. (1993) Empacho in four Latino groups: a study of intra- and inter-cultural variation in beliefs. Med Anthropol 15:109–136

Woolfolk M, Hamard M, Bagramian RA et al. (1984) Oral health of children of migrant farm workers in northwest Michigan. J Public Health Dent 44:101–105

Zahm SH, Blair A (1993) Cancer among migrant and seasonal farmworkers: an epidemiologic review and research agenda. Am J Ind Med 24:753–766

Chapter 9
Farm Labor and the Struggle for Justice in the Eastern United States

Melinda F. Wiggins

Abstract Farm work has historically been performed by people of color who suffer widespread labor abuses and lack the power to make systemic change in the agricultural system. This continues today. Farmworkers are consistently treated as different from other employees, and are governed by different labor standards. There has been little to no effort to include farmworkers in the major labor laws, partly because of the difficulties organizing a primarily migrant, undocumented and disenfranchised farmworker population and partly due to the strong opposition by agricultural employers. This chapter focuses on the general strategies, which farmworker groups in the eastern US use to advocate for justice for farmworkers including organizing, advocacy, and service. It highlights national and state organizations that are involved with advocacy, paying particular attention to the role of research in working for farmworker justice.

9.1 Introduction

"I have taken or helped to take beaten workers away from labor camps. I was a participant in the first anti-slavery trial where a crew leader was convicted of slavery in North Carolina. And I hoped, that after 20 something years of my involvement, things would be different, but all along I have known in my heart that they will never be different as long as those of us in the churches and in the health care system and other systems are working for farmers. We must come to a place where farmworkers' own voices are being heard and where they are working for themselves and for their families" – NC Council of Churches advocate Sr. Evelyn Mattern at a 1998 rally in support of the Farm Labor Organizing Committee (Mattern 1998).

"We want to be able to earn our living. Isn't that the great American work ethic – a fair day's pay for a fair day's work? And that's all we're asking for, it's all very simple" – Farm Labor Organizing Committee President Baldemar Velasquez at a 1998 rally in North Carolina (Velasquez 1998).

Due to the poor living and working conditions experienced by farmworkers, as well as agricultural workers' exemption from most federal and state labor laws, many historians and advocates argue that the overall situation of farmworkers has not improved much in the last 75 years. Several farmworker advocates have gone so far as to say that

T.A. Arcury and S.A. Quandt (eds.), *Latino Farmworkers in Eastern United States*,
DOI: 10.1007/978-0-387-88347-2_9, © Springer Science+Business Media, LLC 2009

because of the lack of protections for field workers under the law, as well as their lack of organization and an increasing number of easily exploitable undocumented workers, they are in no better place than were industrial workers before the New Deal (Schell 2002).

Farm work is one of the lowest paid, least protected, and most dangerous occupations in the US (Gray and Kreyche 2007). It has always been a job filled with hardships, by way of stagnant, subpoverty wages and dangerous working conditions. Farmworkers earn as little as the minimum hourly wage or 35 cents a bucket for piece-rate crops and do not receive overtime. Agricultural workers labor for long hours in severe weather conditions; are exposed to pesticides; are at risk of musculoskeletal injuries, tuberculosis, parasitic infections, and dermatitis; and live in unsafe and overcrowded housing. Most farmworkers do not have health insurance, Social Security pension, disability insurance, or workers' compensation, and thus have few resources to help when injured on the job. The lack of protections covering farmworkers is exacerbated by the poor enforcement of labor laws and opposition by agricultural lobbies when increased protections are proposed.

Historically, agricultural employers have relied on a disenfranchised and easily exploitable workforce. Today, the majority of farmworkers come from Mexico primarily to make money to support their families. "My parents had some fields, I think fifteen acres, and we dedicated our lives to planting cotton, corn, beans, watermelon, melons, different crops. But everything changed when the Mexican president gave people the opportunity to sell the fields. Everybody sold the fields, and agriculture came down. My parents don't have any more money without the fields….I never before thought about coming to the United States, because I was very comfortable in my town…I was very happy. I like to remember that. I dream sometimes, that I am still planting cotton in Mexico with my brothers and my father" (Galván 2008). When faced with not being able to feed their families or migration, millions of impoverished Mexican farmers must choose the latter.

Farmworkers have few avenues to change their conditions. Agricultural employers' recruitment of undocumented workers and guest workers has made it even more risky for workers to stand up against workplace abuses. Those who make an annual trek back and forth from Mexico to the US have few avenues to advocate for themselves. "I arrived here in 1999, in April of 1999, contracted by the H2A program. I returned to Mexico on October seventh of the same year. Since that year, each year is practically the same date of coming and the same date of going…. For necessity I came from Mexico to the United States to work" (Pérez 2006).

In addition to strong opposition from employers, lack of documentation status, and constant migration, a number of other obstacles make it difficult for workers to organize. Antiunion sentiment, isolation from each other, and turnover in the fields further impede workers from holding unscrupulous employers accountable. In addition, many advocates agree that farmworkers' need to take care of their families often takes precedence over their own personal welfare and safety. "My description about the housing conditions is very bad. But [the farmworkers] don't care very much, because, for them, it is very important to make the money to send to their families" (Galván 2008). Thus many workers often resist complaining about work conditions, joining a union, or even talking with advocates for fear of losing their job or being deported.

Although only a small percentage of farmworkers organize to improve their situation, there are a significant number of examples of individual workers speaking out about abuses. "It took me years to realize that the workers aren't going to give up,… even if…the workers appear crushed,…there's always something that comes out of it" (Payne 1998). While farmworker wages, living and working conditions, and general well-being are in constant decline, agricultural workers and their allies have continued to advocate for justice in the industry. Even when faced with arrest, deportation, job loss, replacement, repression, violence, and even death threats, some farmworkers continue to resist poor conditions, below poverty wages, and lack of dignity in the fields.

Poor conditions alone do not usually create the environment necessary for farm-workers to organize. Most farmworker advocates agree that a number of circum-stances, including a progressive and supportive political, religious, and consumer consciousness, are needed in order for agricultural conditions to improve. Most of these efforts are led by farm labor unions, community-based organizations, and advocacy groups across the country which rally people of faith, consumers, students, and researchers to their cause. While many advocates believe that the self-determination of workers is critical to change, a number of farmworker organi-zations work to strengthen labor laws covering farmworkers and increase workers' access to services as an alternative or complement to organizing. The farmworker support organizations that are presented in this chapter help to demonstrate the many tools that farmworkers and their allies use to bring about changes in the agricultural system.

9.2   Agricultural Employers' Resistance to Change

The current agricultural system in the US has a historical connection to the system of indentured servitude and slavery. Even after slavery was abolished, most African slaves remained in the fields as sharecroppers and tenant farmers due to a two-tiered legal system that treated whites and Blacks differently. Even today, agri-culture relies on a primarily disenfranchised and easily exploitable group of workers that have little power to determine the conditions of their work. As many landowners resisted paying workers for their labor at the end of slavery, today most agricultural employers and their lobbyists strongly resist any changes that would require more regulation in the fields and greater rights for farm laborers, particularly the right of farmworkers to strike when there are crops in the fields waiting to be harvested. The organization of farm employers, as well as agribusiness' partnership with government, has contributed to the lack of association of workers and the inability of advocates to make any real improvements for farmworkers. Here are a few significant examples that laid the groundwork for agribusiness' success in keeping conditions as they are.

One of the most notable attempts to thwart oppression in the fields, spearheaded by Socialist party members Henry Clay and H.L. Mitchell, was undermined by federal subsidies to large growers. As with many efforts for change, the Southern Tenant Farmers Union (STFU) came about in a particular political context. Tenant farmers were affected by the Depression to a deeper degree than farm owners, and were left out of programs designed to assist families during these difficult times. Laying the groundwork for many farm labor organizing efforts to follow, the STFU built partnerships with ally organizations, participated in marches and rallies, lobbied their elected officials, and utilized documentation of farmworker conditions to spur on their cause (Griffith 2004). In response to the organization of workers, large landowners used their government subsidies to purchase farm implements such as harvesters, thus putting many STFU members out of jobs (Ortiz 2002). Although in many cases the introduction of machines has not replaced workers, this continues to be a common threat used by agricultural employers when they are faced with an organized workforce advancing toward a more just workplace.

Another significant attempt by farmworkers in the eastern US to collectively organize that was weakened by employers was the struggle led by African American bean pickers in Florida in the 1940s. Historian Cindy Hahamovitch (2002) argues that this attempt to collectively change working conditions was different from previous labor organizing and had far reaching and negative impact for farmworkers for decades to come. While farmworkers were organizing, growers were lobbying the federal government to quash the struggle by replacing organized workers with those that had agreed to no-strike clauses. This eventually led to the government approving and providing for an endless supply of foreign-born agricultural workers through temporary guest-worker visa programs. "African American farmworkers' wartime struggle did not fail for lack of organization. It was the growers' ability to enlist the aid of federal authorities that crushed their promising but short-lived initiative. Yet the consequences of African American farmworkers' wartime defeat were profound – and not just for them, but for all farmworkers in the eastern United States. Because farm-workers were unsuccessful in their organizing efforts, their living and working conditions remained desperate" (Hahamovitch 2002:104). Many growers continue to rely on guest workers from other countries to harvest their crops, often denying these jobs to workers that are already in the US in lieu of this more vulnerable workforce. Because guest workers are tied to a single employer and must return to their home country each year, their ability to participate in long-term efforts for change is minimal.

9.2.1 Agricultural Exceptionalism

While the New Deal federal labor laws made significant and long-term changes to the industrial workplace, farmworkers were exempt from most of these changes and have thus been consistently governed by different labor standards and treated differently from other employees. Farmworkers suffer from "agricultural exceptionalism," an historic practice of excluding farmworkers from legal protections benefiting other workers. Most of these exceptions date back to the 1930s, when Southern legislators and other power holders did not want the nearly 65% of African Americans who were farmworkers or domestic workers to receive the same treatment as Whites (Triplett 2004).

Notably, farmworkers are excluded from the *National Labor Relations Act* (NLRA) passed in 1935, which governs worker organizing and collective bargaining. To date, no state in the eastern US has provided farmworkers the same labor organizing protections as other workers that are covered by the NLRA. Thus, most farmworkers who organize in the workplace are at risk of being fired and employers have no legal obligation to negotiate a contract with a group of workers. It is no surprise that states that have passed their own state labor relations acts, specifically California, have seen the most successful farm labor organizing in the US, with not only the first major farm labor union, but also with the largest number of organized agricultural workers.

Another major labor law that treats farmworkers differently is the *Fair Labor Standards Act* (FLSA), which covers the minimum wage, overtime provisions, and child labor laws, among other protections. Nationally, farmworkers do not receive overtime and those who labor on small farms (those using less than 500 person-days of labor in a quarter in the preceding year) are not guaranteed the minimum wage. In addition, children as young as 12 are allowed to work in the fields, compared to 16 in other industries (see Chap. 8). No state in the eastern US has passed a law granting farmworkers overtime or enforcing more strict standards on child labor.

Farmworkers' poor representation in government has affected their ability to lobby for better legal protections and has led to a piece-meal approach to legislative change. Instead of incorporating farmworkers fully into the two key labor laws mentioned above, a special *Migrant and Seasonal Agricultural Worker Protection Act* (AWPA or MSPA) was passed in 1983 to specify certain housing, employment, and transportation standards for farmworkers. Yet, farmworkers who are certified to work on US farms on H-2A guest-worker visas, over 75,000 in 2007, are exempt from this federal protection (US Department of Labor Employment & Training Administration 2007).

Though not originally included in the 1970 *Occupational Safety and Health Act* (OSHA), farmworkers were afforded some minimal health and safety protections through the Field Sanitation Standard in 1987 (see Chap. 5), 17 years after all other workers were covered under OSHA. Yet again, farmworkers that work on small farms are exempt from this law mandating water and hand-washing in the fields. It took even longer for the federal government to pass basic pesticide protections for field workers. It was not until the mid-1990s that the Environmental Protection Agency's Worker Protection Standard was implemented. These regulations also have shortcomings, primarily in that they do not include a system to track pesticide exposure (Oxfam America 2004).

The lack of federal protections of farmworkers has led some advocates to lobby for state laws benefiting these workers. Yet, gains on a state level can be equally if not more difficult to achieve than in Washington, DC. "On the federal level, farm interests represent only one of thousands of organized groups trying to press their agendas on

Congress.… [By contrast, in] major farm states, agricultural groups have few peers in terms of influence" (Schell 2002:152). For instance, from the late 1990s until 2003, half of Florida's House Committee on Agriculture was composed of agribusiness representatives who made significant ($35 million) contributions to political campaigns. In addition to being out-resourced by agribusiness, farmworker advocacy groups often face direct opposition by growers. In one case in New York, the Farm Bureau funded a Cornell research project about migrant life, which was used to fight a campaign calling for farmworkers to be covered the same as all other employees under New York labor laws. In North Carolina, some grower representatives resisted changes to the *North Carolina Migrant Housing Act* calling the demand for mattresses in migrant labor camps an embarrassment to farmers statewide.

Because of this resistance by agricultural interests, farmworkers remain in jobs with little state (or federal) protection. For instance, in half of the states, farmworkers do not receive the same workers' compensation coverage as do other employees, and in many states workers' compensation for farmworkers is optional (Schell 2002). In the eastern US, Florida appears to have the most progressive laws protecting farmworkers. Florida affords workers the "right" of self-organization and access to visitors in labor camps. Florida also requires farms that employ as few as five workers to abide by the Field Sanitation Standard. In the 1990s, New York passed more stringent laws covering farmworkers' wages, sanitation, and access to drinking water (Gray and Kreyche 2007). Several states in the eastern US, including North Carolina, Maryland, and New York, have slightly stronger migrant housing codes than the federal OSHA standard. Yet, for the most part, states in the eastern US have not passed stronger laws protecting farmworkers, but have simply adopted the few federal labor standards covering farmworkers as their ceiling.

9.2.2   Lack of Enforcement

Because of exemptions, exceptions, and underenforcement, agricultural labor is a largely unregulated workplace. Where legal protections do exist, the violations are rampant, many employers simply ignore the law, and workers are often unable or unwilling to make a formal complaint. Thus the laws protecting farmworkers are rarely enforced. For instance, in 1990, the US General Accounting Office (1992) found that a majority of growers were in violation of the Field Sanitation Standard. In recent years, there has actually been a decrease in the level of enforcement of federal laws by agencies. The US Department of Labor (DOL) showed a more than 50% decline in the number of annual *Agricultural Worker Protection Act* investigations from those conducted in the 1980s to the1990s (Oxfam America 2004). Under President George W. Bush, the DOL's Wage and Hour Division has decreased its number of investigators, increased its budget at a slower rate, and decreased the number of enforcement cases it completed (Triplett 2004). The Department of Labor's focus on crew leaders also leaves farmers with an easy way to avoid responsibility by hiring labor contractors who take the fall for labor violations.

Enforcement at a state level often mirrors poor federal enforcement. For instance, in North Carolina there are only seven OSHA individuals charged with inspecting the over 4,000 labor camps in the state. The reason for this inadequate enforcement is that government agencies charged with enforcement are understaffed, often have close ties with employers, rarely speak the language of the workers, and do not always provide information about how to file complaints to workers in a culturally appropriate manner.

Because the state and federal laws protecting farmworkers are so weak and poorly enforced, many advocates have begun looking to international laws and labor clauses imbedded in free trade agreements to hold international agribusiness companies accountable for upholding workers' rights. Even though the US is a member of the International Labor Organization (ILO), it has failed to adopt most of the standards that would improve farm labor conditions. Furthermore, the US has not ratified the ILO conventions protecting workers' right to organize or the convention on safety and health in agriculture (Oxfam America 2004). So again, advocates find themselves faced with the US government's accommodation of employer interests and thus refusal to protect the health and safety and labor rights of its agricultural workforce.

9.3   The Birth of a Movement

To make improvements to farmworkers' health, safety, and general well-being, many workers and advocates believe that the key is an empowered workforce. The United Farm Workers (UFW), which grew out of both the National Farmworkers of America and the Agricultural Workers Organizing Committee, developed the most significant early model of farm labor organizing in the 1960s. Combining union organizing strategies with civil rights tactics, founders Cesar Chavez and Dolores Huerta built a base of local workers, which was supported by allies across the country. While originating and building its strongest support in California, the UFW has expanded to many states throughout the country. They also have offices in Washington, Oregon, and Florida and nearly a dozen support organizations, including the Cesar Chavez Foundation, La Campesina Radio Network, and the National Farm Worker Ministry. At its height in 1970, the UFW had over 50,000 members and was not only busy negotiating contracts, but was also lobbying for legislative changes primarily at the state level.

Just as the Southern Tenant Farmers Union developed within a particular political climate, the UFW was born within a particular time in history that supported its development. Not only was there an overall general consciousness among North Americans about social issues, but also the Chicano Movement and Civil Rights Movement were developing within a fairly liberal political and religious context (Mariscal 2004). While the UFW was integral to the Mexican American movement, Chavez's focus on labor, partnerships with liberal politicians, use of religious traditions, and multiethnic organizing was often at odds with the more militaristic aims of *la raza*.

Chavez followed in the steps of Gandhi and Martin Luther King, Jr. as he led the farmworker movement with a commitment to "militant nonviolence," both a focus on change and empathy for the oppressor. Chavez combined Christian practices such as fasting and pilgrimages and use of religio-cultural symbols such as La Virgin de Guadalupe and Don Quijote, with references to Emiliano Zapata and the Mexican Revolution, to raise consciousness about "tensions" that existed in the day-to-day lives of many Mexicans living in the US. Chavez's public and political emphasis on the poor conditions experienced by farmworkers and workers' rights issues positioned him as the leader of the farmworkers (Mariscal 2004; Buss 1993; Ferriss and Sandoval 1997).

9.3.1 Organizing for Change

While there are a number of community and labor organizing models, many farm labor union leaders, including Cesar Chavez, studied and utilized strategies popularized by the late community organizer Saul Alinsky. The Alinsky model focuses on mass meetings, cumulative victories, direct confrontations with targets, and concrete wins. Its separation of professional organizers and community leaders often leads to a lack of leadership development of rank and file workers (Castelloe et al. 2002). Even though Chavez and many other farmworker union leaders are indigenous, they maintained their role as public spokespersons and leaders of their organizations without fully developing lay leaders as their peers in the movement. During the 1960s, the Chicano movement critiqued the UFW's Alinsky style of organizing by calling for the union to focus less on the wins and more on building, less on campaigns and more on the movement. Their prodding begged the question that still plagues farm labor organizing today, "Does winning campaigns build a social movement?" (VeneKlasen and Patel 2006).

Other farm labor unions, Oregon-based *Pineros y Campesinos Unidos del Noroeste/* Northwest Treeplanters and Farmworkers United (PCUN) and the Ohio-based Farm Labor Organizing Committee (FLOC), also rely on many Alinsky organizing strategies. They often initiate direct action campaigns targeted at growers or agricultural companies, which have the power to hand over concrete wins to agricultural workers. While these unions tend to focus on specific commodities in a state or region, they are also involved with legislative advocacy, health and safety training, housing reform, and immigrants' rights coalitions at the state and national levels. They have each led significant victories for farmworkers, including FLOC's successful contract with over 8,000 H2A guest workers in North Carolina in 2004. This campaign, which lasted over a decade and culminated with the end of a five-year boycott of Mt. Olive Pickle Company, Inc. relied heavily on mass events and marches, and rallying consumers to demand that the pickle company's CEO negotiate with the workers. This was the first contract with H2A guest workers in the country, and has been used as a model for subsequent collective bargaining agreements with guest workers. In addition to providing basic health and safety protections, a day of rest, and bereavement leave, the contract also provides workers a grievance procedure to redress workplace problems.

The Alinsky model is often juxtaposed with that of more process-oriented organizing models, which emphasize the building of relationships, consensus decision-making, and human interdependence. For instance, women-centered organizing models tend to focus on the ongoing leadership development and empowerment of community members (Castelloe et al. 2002). The multicultural model includes "work that is specifically anti-racist, anti-sexist, anti-homophobic, or has as its primary goal the development of equitable, multi-cultural communities" (Stall and Stoecker 1997). Many small, regional, and community-based organizations supporting farmworkers tend to be more aligned with these nontraditional organizing models.

A few organizations in the eastern US that emphasize the process-oriented model of organizing include *El Comité de Apoyo a Los Trabajadores Agrícolas/* The Farmworker Support Committee (CATA) in Kennett Square, Pennsylvania, the North Carolina Farmworkers' Project in eastern North Carolina, Student Action with Farmworkers (SAF) in North Carolina, the Farmworker Association of Florida in central and southern Florida, and the Coalition of Immokalee Workers (CIW) in Immokalee, Florida (http://www.ciw-online.org/about.html). These organizations pursue worker empowerment, leadership development, and addressing the root causes of problems faced by agricultural workers. Several of these organizations, such as CATA and the CIW, focus primarily on increasing wages for farmworkers through contracts or agreements with employers, while others, such as the Farmworkers' Project, SAF, and the Farmworker Association, focus more on leadership development and health and safety issues.

The Farmworker Association of Florida, Inc. is a good example of how organizations use a number of strategies to make change. In addition to organizing workers, the Farmworker Association uses lobbying, leadership development, research, and health education to advance their mission to "build power among farmworker and rural low-income communities to respond to and gain control over the social, political, workplace, economic, health, and environmental justice issues that impact their lives" (http://floridafarmworkers.org/). Since its inception in the early 1980s, this grassroots community-based organization has worked with thousands of Mexican, Haitian, African-American, Guatemalan, and Salvadoran farmworkers to address wage, immigration, health and safety, and housing issues.

Student Action with Farmworkers (SAF) is another organization epitomizing the process-oriented organizing model. One of SAF's key programs mobilizes, trains, and supports young people from across the country to advocate for improved farm labor conditions (Fig. 9.1). Since its inception in 1992, SAF's Into the Fields program has provided over 500 college students with internship opportunities working with nearly 100,000 farmworkers through support organizations in the Carolinas. Through this program, SAF stresses relationship-building among a diverse group of student activists, as well as leadership development of students from farmworker families.

The CIW also demonstrates their emphasis on the community-based model of organizing through its development of farmworker leaders: "We strive to build our strength as a community on a basis of reflection and analysis, constant attention to coalition building across ethnic divisions, and an ongoing investment in leadership development to help our members continually develop their skills in com-munity education and organization" (http://www.ciw-online.org/about.html).

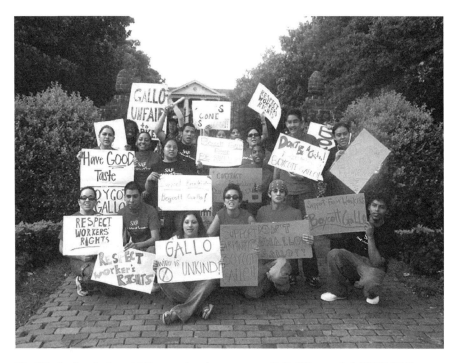

Fig. 9.1 Student Action with Farmworkers interns protest Gallo Wines at their 2005 Mid-Summer Retreat. Photograph by Carmela Meehan

At the same time, the CIW has successfully used mass rallies, general strikes, boycotts, and other direct action tactics to fight for fair wages and working conditions.

Thus, while it is important to note what distinguishes these models, what is clear is that more often than not, farmworker organizers and advocates utilize a combination of strategies and tactics found in each model. At times and places one model may be more appropriate than another, and they usually work in tandem. What remains a key challenge for community and labor organizing groups is how to facilitate meaningful participation by farmworkers, especially when professional staff employed by the organization have greater access to policy makers, employer groups, and other decision-makers (VeneKlasen and Patel 2006). In the end, developing a base of power that can sustain wins is as important as developing leaders for the sake of leadership development.

9.4 Policy Advocacy

"I was working with a crew leader from Michoacan, Mexico and he pay me in cash. I would ask for my receipts and he would get mad and then I went to some other place and there I did receive some receipts, and I already knew some of the laws here and I knew I was supposed to get some receipts for work you do…. The house and environment we lived in was very bad, in the state of Maryland, there was 25 people in one house and that was horrible because I didn't know what was happening. I knew that was wrong but at the time I didn't know there was a free legal service for farmworkers" (Frias 2007).

Though workers often have an understanding of basic human rights, most do not know what rights the US government or state governments afford them, nor do they have access to or knowledge of resources or support in their community. Based on research with farmworkers in New York, researcher and advocate Margaret Gray found that, "lack of knowledge of labor laws is critical because it contributes to workers' perceptions that labor rights in the US are associated with citizenship or residency and not with job tenure" (Gray 2007:7). While workers may fully understand that they are being taken advantage of, many may not know what support they will receive if they confront their employer or are not fully aware of the procedures for making a formal complaint to the government or advocating for policy changes.

Because of the many obstacles to farm labor organizing, there are a number of organizations that advocate for improved legal protections and litigate on behalf of farmworkers when laws that govern them are violated. Most notable are the organizations funded by the federal Legal Services Corporation, begun in the early 1970s to provide legal aid for low-income people throughout the country. The farmworker-specific programs provide agricultural workers with legal support to address workplace protections covered under the *Agricultural Worker Protection Act* and the few other laws covering farm laborers. Unfortunately, since 1996, legal aid money has been restricted from being used to lobby legislators, represent undocumented workers, or file class action lawsuits. Each of these restrictions severely limits the ability of organizations funded by Labor Services Corporation to advocate for the majority of farmworkers or to most efficiently represent farm labor crews experiencing workplace problems on a specific farm. While they can represent groups, each plaintiff has to be named individually instead of filing a class action, so it is not the best use of resources and it is often difficult to get each worker to agree to participate.

In response to the limitations placed on federally funded legal services, some states have independently funded nonprofit legal organizations that are able to file class action lawsuits and represent undocumented workers. Often these organizations work closely with legal aid offices to share information about common legal issues experienced by workers and share joint educational materials and strategies for reaching out to workers. In North Carolina, for instance, the North Carolina Justice Center is a nonprofit organization housed in the Legal Aid building that utilizes litigation, research, advocacy, and grassroots action to support improvements for low-wealth communities. The Justice Center has a strong immigrant rights program that includes education and litigation on behalf of farmworkers, as well as a statewide immigrants advocacy program.

There are few farmworker organizations primarily dedicated to policy advocacy. Washington, DC-based Farmworker Justice is the premier farmworker organization focused on administrative and legislative advocacy at the federal level. As is the case with many farmworker organizations that must meet many needs at once, Farmworker Justice uses education, coalition building, litigation, and support of organizing to improve farm labor conditions. For over 25 years, they have focused on monitoring legislative and policy issues affecting farmworkers. They work in collaboration with farmworker groups across the country to keep them informed of current regulations, proposed policy changes, and litigation efforts affecting farmworkers on the state, regional, and national level.

On a state level, a number of organizations that organize workers or mobilize advocates to support workers include policy advocacy as a part of their overall work. In a few cases, there are groups for which advocacy is a key strategy that supports their mission. For instance, in New York, advocates have identified farmworkers' exclusion from state labor laws as the leading reason that farmworkers are so vulnerable. The Justice for Farmworkers Coalition is a statewide effort that uses advocacy, organizing, and legal means to improve farmworker conditions. The coalition advocates for farmworkers to be treated equally under the law, stating that since "agribusiness is getting all of these tax breaks, why can't farmworkers just get a day of rest?" (Rev. Witt, personal communication May 8, 2008). The Rural and Migrant Ministry (RMM), a multifaith organization that has coordinated accompaniment, education, and youth empowerment programs for rural and migrant people in New York since 1981, helps facilitate the coalition (http://ruralmigrantministry.org/).

The Farmworker Advocacy Network (FAN) is the first and only network dedicated to government accountability and policy formation in support of farmworkers in North Carolina. Through this partnership, a diverse group of organizations identify problems and issues affecting the farmworker population in North Carolina, monitor government agencies that enforce housing, wage, and pesticide safety regulations affecting farmworkers, influence policies around these key issues, bring farmworkers' voices into the legislative process, and involve students and community activists in its campaigns. Since its inception in 2003, FAN has monitored farm labor legislation, participated in an international investigation of the H-2A program, supported litigation efforts, led a successful migrant housing campaign, and initiated a pesticide campaign. Each member of FAN brings unique expertise. Member organizations have access to current information about farmworker demographics and issues; are connected to the state and national student, religious, and environmental advocacy community; have the capacity to provide information on policies, laws, and the legislative process; and provide direct services to and organize farmworkers and their families (Fig. 9.2).

Unfortunately, instead of focusing on improvements in the laws that govern agricultural labor, most advocacy groups are often forced to work diligently to block policies that would have a negative impact on farmworkers. This is partly due to the lack of resources available to organizations dedicated to farm labor advocacy, the abundance of funds available to support corporate agribusiness interests, and the seeming lack of interest by elected officials in interfering in farm labor issues. Advocacy organizations are often met with strong opposition by grower associations that decry any government regulation of farms. Many farmworkers and their advocates believe that because legislators have not and may never prioritize farmworkers, advocates need to utilize more creative means for change. "The congress people in Raleigh, they don't want to listen. The field conditions and housing conditions for workers, they don't care…. [Some other activists] invited 2 congressmen to come to the fields. I picked 2 camps for them, 25 people in each

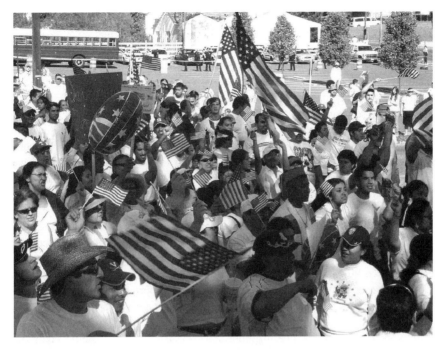

Fig. 9.2 Immigrants gather in Siler City, NC on 10 April 2006 to call for better treatment and a road to humane policy reform. Photograph by Lupe Huitron

camp. They said, 'No, we cannot go because we have a lot of work in the office.' I was very disappointed. We need to take other measures because the congressmen are ignoring everybody, ignoring the non-profit organizations" (Galván 2008).

9.4.1 Community-Based Research

While advocacy groups rely on a number of creative strategies to promote farmworker justice, many have found that credible research is needed to advance their campaigns, particularly in the policy arena. Research often provides community groups with the ability to document disparities and factors associated with them, which enable organizations to elevate a campaign and garner visibility and attention among policy makers, agricultural employers, and the larger public.

The research model that is most closely aligned with the philosophies of many advocacy organizations is that of community-based participatory research (CBPR). CBPR is "a collaborative and colearning process that stresses" (Vásquez et al. 2006:101) the "participation of the people being studied; use of the personal experiences and the perceptions of community members as data; a focus on 'empowerment'; and the final product, action by the community and community members to change the conditions causing the problems" (Arcury et al. 2001:429).

Some partnerships that have been successful at implementing CBPR projects have shared values, processes, and decision making, as well as standards that are more aligned with supporting the mission of the community-based organization. One successful partnership is that of the North Carolina Farmworkers' Project, SAF and Wake Forest University School of Medicine. This partnership is partially successful because Farm workers' Project staff members are involved with so many components of the research projects, from serving as coinvestigators, to collecting data, to copresenting the results and implementing the intervention. Another reason for the success is due to the involvement of farmworkers as interviewers. Often SAF interns from farmworker families conduct interviews and disseminate research findings to workers. This partnership has led to some innovative products and materials, as well as promotora-led interventions, that have increased knowledge about key health and safety issues among farmworkers and developed the leadership of individual farmworkers involved with the project.

While CBPR is touted as the most participatory model for community–academic partnerships, it has some challenges and shortcomings. In addition to common tensions between researchers and community members, there are particular challenges with regards to working with agricultural workers. These range from communication difficulties especially due to language differences, transportation challenges because many farmworkers lack their own modes of transportation, and the fact that few farmworker-led or community-based farmworker groups exist (Arcury et al. 2001). "Farmworker membership organizations have often struggled to build coalitions with potential allies…. While they often have supported legislative initiatives to improve farmworker conditions, labor and religious groups have not sustained their support for farmworker issues among the many other issues they address, in part because of the relative invisibility of farmworkers in society" (Schell 2002:144).

There are also a number of obstacles constructed by researchers, ranging from academics determining and driving a project to the involvement of growers in the project, which may impede farmworkers' participation in CBPR projects. For example, some farmworker-focused CBPR projects include all agricultural actors, including farmers or grower associations. Because of the power imbalance and often adversarial relationships between growers and workers, the involvement of employers may hinder farmworkers' ability to fully participate in the project. This may inhibit some advocacy and organizing groups from participating due to their interest in having farmworkers' voices heard over the more mainstream voices of agricultural employers. While CBPR uses a number of effective strategies to gain farmworkers' input, such as focus groups, interviews, and questionnaires, these methods usually focus on individual comments. This may run counter to the philosophies of many farmworker organizations that prefer to use consensus decision-making and speak with a collective voice.

Many advocates also note the difficulties in identifying the right researchers – those that are experienced with CBPR, committed to research with a marginalized farmworker population, and who do not have publishing or other academic pressures that would take away from the community organization's focus on bringing about change (Joan Flocks, personal communication April 20, 2008). Long-time Farmworker Association of Florida staff member Jeannie Economos stated that, "for advocacy sake, we really need that kind of scientific research and researchers willing to stick their necks out….

We need researchers that aren't afraid to be advocates for farmworker health" (personal communication April 18, 2008). Other organizations have expressed an interest in working with researchers who are interested in their perspective, connected to their work, and who want to be a part of the movement. The director of the Rural and Migrant Ministry in New York said that he is interested in having "someone to help strengthen efforts as an ally instead of outside expert – researchers who see themselves as allies" (Rev. Witt, personal communication May 8, 2008). According to Wake Forest University researcher Thomas Arcury and colleagues, this interest in wanting to be heard is common among advocates and is often in conflict with the primary interests of academics. "Community members expect community problems to be solved and their voices to be heard. Researchers expect their study procedures and results to reflect accepted standards of scientific practice" (Arcury et al. 1999:565).

Regardless of these limitations, CBPR that recognizes farmworkers' voices, honors community organizations' focus on collective action, and respects researchers' professional standards can be a powerful tool in the struggle for justice in the fields.

9.5 Service to Workers

While organizing, policy advocacy, and community-based research are important strategies to change conditions of farmworkers, advocating for a primarily undocumented and migrant workforce is a long-term commitment that yields slow change. Therefore, many advocacy and even most community organizing and farm labor unions often partner with service agencies to provide basic health, education, and social services to farmworkers, as an immediate amelioration. While advocacy and organizing groups are often critical of programs that may undermine systemic transformation, they often also support services for farmworkers. The Ohio-based labor union, the Farm Labor Organizing Committee, "takes the position that raising the wages of farmworkers and improving their working conditions will finally obviate the need for other social service programs." Yet, "the farm labor union, with its commitment to farm labor as viable work, must routinely overlook its own critical stance toward agencies and resources that buttress the farm labor system to seek help for workers when needed" (Morrissey 1999:100).

Some of the most significant services provided for mostly migrant farmworkers came about through policy changes enacted nearly 50 years ago. Consumer response to the CBS television documentary "Harvest of Shame" influenced the development of federal health, education, housing, and job training services for farmworkers nationwide. During this historic documentary shown on Thanksgiving Day in 1960, Edward R. Murrow interviewed Black and White farmworkers, as well as Mexican *Bracero* workers, about their poor living conditions, inadequate housing, and lack of protections under the law. As a result, federal funding programs such as the US Department of Education's migrant education program and Department of Health and Human Services' farmworker health program were created to address issues raised in the film. Since the development of these early federally funded services, a number of other farmworker agencies, such as the National Center for Farmworker Health, Farmworker Health Services, East Coast Migrant Head Start, and National High School Equivalency Program-College Assistance Migrant Program (HEP-CAMP) Association, have received federal funding or collaborate with federally funded programs to assist farmworkers and migrant workers in need.

A look at the nation's migrant health program shows the importance of these vital services. Through funding of local health centers, bilingual and bicultural health providers offer culturally appropriate health care to farmworkers and their families. They not only provide preventive care, but also address occupational safety and health needs. As a community that is low-income, uninsured, and has limited English proficiency, migrant and seasonal farmworkers qualify for care through this US Department Health and Human Services' special populations program. More than 807,000 farmworkers and their families received services through this program in 2006.

While it is hard to imagine farmworkers' lives without these critical services in the here and now, it is imperative to ask why a group of wage-earning people need government benefits in the form of housing, health care, and social services. If they work full time and contribute to the agricultural economy, they should by all rights earn a good living. If service agencies provide transportation, health care, and other basic services to workers for free, are they actually subsidizing agricultural employers who in turn pay workers less than a living wage? (Morrissey 1999). Some workers' rights and advocacy groups hold that direct service may actually sustain workers' below-poverty wages and undermine strategies addressing the systemic problems experienced by farmworkers. Social services sometimes act as a government subsidy to agribusiness by meeting basic needs not covered by low wages and few benefits provided by employers.

Another chasm between service approaches and worker organizing groups is the latter's commitment to improving conditions of farmworkers, instead of transitioning workers out of the fields. As was said of FLOC in the late 1990s, "The union is dedicated to farm work and convinced of its basic dignity…the union supports the migrant way of life" (Morrissey 1999). But several agencies, such as Telamon Corporation and Rural Opportunities, Inc. (ROI), offer services to farmworkers and provide skill development support so that they can be qualified for full-time year-round nonfarm jobs. A former Telamon staff member explained their programs this way: "Some want to be in training programs, some don't. Some just want supportive services and they move on. Those who want training and employment after we sit down and work up a plan and decide what employment or training they want to go in, then we proceed with that" (Ferguson 1998). This is quite different from the work of farm labor organizers who usually spend their time trying to improve the conditions of farm work. One former organizer with the United Farm Workers of Washington State said, "It's never positive to think about people getting out of farm labor, because there always needs to be people growing it, growing the food, working in the field, and if people keep recycling through, we're never going to be able to organize them" (Payne 1998). A farmworker from eastern North Carolina echoes this theme:

> "My biggest problem with farmworker advocates is that they try to take people off the migrant camps, because they think that everybody deserves a better life. Personally, I think that if that's what you want to do, that's what you want to do…. The first thing I would tell

anyone who wanted to be a farmworker advocate is, don't try to fix the farmworker. Don't try to take him or her out of farmworking. Fix up those camps and make the living conditions better. Raise the wages, and get rid of the middle-man; that includes the crew leader. If all this was done, you would have more people working the fields than in office jobs" (Adams 1998).

9.6 Conclusion

Throughout the history of commercial agriculture in the US, there has been a reliance on an easily exploited group of workers. The eastern US, and the South in particular, play a distinct role in this history because of the significant numbers of slaves, sharecroppers, tenant farmers, and farmworkers that lived and worked in this region. The failure of the US government to protect farmworkers, oppressive practices on many farms, and resistance by a highly organized agricultural industry have kept farmworkers in one of the most dangerous and lowest paid jobs in the country. Recent changes in global agriculture, including the consolidation of farms, increase of free trade agreements, and reliance on undocumented workers, have only added to an overwhelmingly dismal reality for agricultural workers and their families. The increased number of raids by Immigration and Customs Enforcement and a growing number of hate groups focused on Latino immigrants has created a climate of fear and repression for many farmworkers and their families.

The changes needed to improve farm labor conditions are both immediate and long-term. Service agencies need to continue providing free health, legal, and education services for farmworkers, while advocacy and organizing groups need increased resources to address the underlying causes of farmworkers' poverty and unsafe workplaces. Undocumented workers need protections in the workplace, workers' rights issues need to be at the forefront of community and labor organizing drives, and allies need to be active participants in the farmworker movement.

Farmworkers have always relied on students, academics, people of faith, and other advocates serving as allies in their struggle for change. Consumers have played a key role in collaboration with farmworkers beginning with the United Farm Worker's first successful grape boycott in the 1960s to the Coalition of Immokalee Workers' recent victories against Taco Bell, McDonald's, and Burger King (Fig. 9.3). Historian and farm labor activist Paul Ortiz goes so far as to claim that these student activists and their "counterparts stand in a long tradition of American abolitionism," continuing to fight to end oppression in the fields (Ortiz 2002).

In order for the rural agricultural workplace to be reformed, farmworkers deserve to be protected by the Universal Declaration of Human Rights, including having the right to freedom of movement, free choice of employment, just and favorable conditions of work, protection against unemployment, equal pay for equal work, the right to form and join trade unions, and a standard of living adequate for the health and well-being of themselves and their families (http://www.un.org/Overview/rights.html). In order to achieve justice, a number of specific changes need to be made:

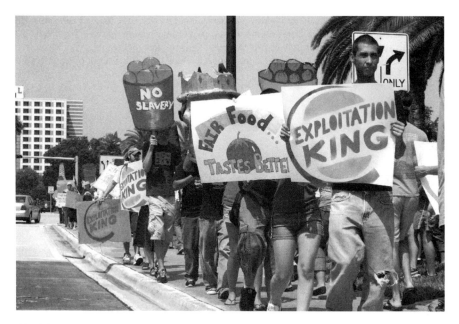

Fig. 9.3 Students and allies march at Burger King Headquarters in Miami, FL in support of the Coalition of Immokalee Workers Campaign for Fair Food. Photograph by Tony Macias

- Additional public and private resources should be provided for organizations supporting farmworkers.
- Farmworker agencies, advocacy organizations, and labor unions should form stronger collaborations.
- More academic–community alliances should be established to collaborate on farmworker-focused research.
- Farmworkers should be included fully in the *National Labor Relations Act* and the *Fair Labor Standards Act.*
- The Worker Protection Standard (WPS) should be strengthened, and enforcement of the WPS and the Field Sanitation Standards needs to be increased.
- Farmworkers should be covered the same as other employees by state labor and health and safety laws, including workers' compensation and minimum wage laws.
- Enforcement of laws covering farmworkers should be improved through greater resource allocation to enforcement agencies, collaboration among agencies, and less compliance with agricultural employers.
- Undocumented workers need to be protected on the job and be able to labor free from fear of deportation.
- There needs to be a guest-worker program that is worker-friendly, which allows workers to choose when and how often they cross the border and for whom they work.
- Farmworkers should be paid a living wage; provided benefits such as health insurance, sick days, and paid vacation; and have access to grievance procedures for addressing workplace problems.

References

Adams K (1998) Oral history of Vanessa. In: Manly L, Okie A, Wiggins M (eds) Fields Without Borders/Campos sin Fronteras: An Anthology of Documentary Writing and Photography by Student Action with Farmworkers' Interns. Student Action with Farmworkers, Durham

Arcury TA, Austin CK, Quandt SA et al. (1999) Enhancing community participation in a public health project: farmworkers and agricultural chemicals in North Carolina. Health Educ Behav 26(4):563–578

Arcury TA, Quandt SA, Dearry A (2001) Farmworker pesticide exposure and community-based participatory research: rationale and practical applications. Environ Health Perspect 109(Suppl 3):429–434

Buss F (ed) (1993) Forged Under the Sun/Forjada bajo el sol. The University of Michigan Press, Ann Arbor

Castelloe P, Watson T, White C (2002) Participatory change: an integrative approach to community practice. J Community Pract 10(4):7–31

Fair Labor Standards Act. Code of Federal Regulations Pertaining to ESA Title 29 Labor Chapter V Wage and Hour Division, Department of Labor. http://www.dol.gov/esa/whd/flsa/

Ferguson C (1998) Oral history of Clarence Ferguson by Lian E. In: Living the American Dream: Economic Justice for Farmworkers. A compilation of documentary works by 1998 Student Action with Farmworkers interns. Student Action with Farmworkers, Durham

Ferriss S, Sandoval R (1997) The Fight in the Fields: Cesar Chavez and the Farmworkers Movement. Harcourt Brace & Company, New York

Frias J (2007) Unpublished interview. Deposited in Duke University Libraries, Rare Book, Manuscript and Special Collections Library

Galván L (2008) Interview with Leonardo by Kleist P and Resor A. In: Nuestras Historias, Nuestros Sueños: Immigrantes Latinos en las Carolinas/Our Stories, Our Dreams: Latino Immigrants in the Carolinas. Edited by Blair A. Published by the Center for Documentary Studies at Duke University in association with Student Action with Farmworkers, Durham, p. 47

Gray M, Kreyche E (2007) The Hudson Valley farmworker report: understanding the needs and aspirations of a voiceless population. Bard College Migrant Labor Project: Annandale-on-Hudson, New York. http://mlp.bard.edu/index.edu. Cited 17 Jul 2008

Griffith D (2004) Challenges to farmworker organizing in the south: from the Southern Tenant Farmers Union to the Farm Labor Organizing Committee's Mt. Olive campaign. Cult Agric 26:25–37

Hahamovitch C (2002) Standing idly by: "organized" farmworkers in South Florida during the Depression and World Work II. In: Thomas C, Wiggins M (ed) The Human Cost of Food: Farmworkers' Lives, Labor & Advocacy. University of Texas Press, Austin

Mariscal J (2004) Negotiating César: César Chávez in the Chicano movement. Aztlán 29(1):21–50

Mattern E (1998) Speech from FLOC rally at Mt. Olive park transcribed by Hicks J. In: Living the American Dream: Economic Justice for Farmworkers. A compilation of documentary works by 1998 Student Action with Farmworkers interns. Student Action with Farmworkers, Durham

Morrissey M (1999) Serving farm workers, serving farmers: migrant social services in Northwest Ohio. Aztlán 24(2):95–118

Ortiz P (2002) From slavery to Cesar Chavez and beyond: farmworker organizing in the United States. In: Thomas C, Wiggins M (eds) The Human Cost of Food: Farmworkers' Lives, Labor & Advocacy. University of Texas Press, Austin

Oxfam America (2004) Like machines in the fields: workers without rights in American agriculture. An Oxfam America Report. http://www.oxfamamerica.org/newsandpublications/publications/research_reports/art7011.html/OA-Like_Machines_in_the_Fields.pdf. Cited 8 Aug 2008

Payne S (1998) Oral history of Sheila Payne by Steele M. In: Living the American Dream: Economic Justice for Farmworkers. A compilation of documentary works by 1998 Student Action with Farmworkers interns. Student Action with Farmworkers, Durham

Pérez L (2006) Unpublished interview. Deposited in Duke University Libraries, Rare Book, Manuscript and Special Collections Library

Schell G (2002) Farmworker exceptionalism under the law: how the legal system contributes to farmworker poverty and powerlessness. In: Thomas C, Wiggins M (eds) The Human Cost of Food: Farmworkers' Lives, Labor & Advocacy. University of Texas Press, Austin

Stall S, Stoecker R (1997) Community organizing or organizing community? Gender and the crafts of empowerment. COMM-ORG Working Paper, Volume 2. http://comm-org.wisc.edu/papers96/gender2.html. Cited 17 Jul 2008

Triplett W (2004) Migrant farmworkers. Congressional Quarterly Inc 1435:831–849

US Department of Labor Employment & Training Administration. http://www.foreignlaborcert.doleta.gov/h-2a_region2007.cfm

US General Accounting Office (1992) Hired farmworkers: health and well-being at risk. Report no. GAO/HRD-92–46. US Government Printing Office, Washington, DC

Vásquez VB, Minkler M, Shepard P (2006) Promoting environmental health policy through community based participatory research: a case study from Harlem, New York. J Urban Health 83:101–110

Velasquez B (1998) Speech from FLOC rally at Mt. Olive Park transcribed by Hicks J. In: Living the American Dream: Economic Justice for Farmworkers. A compilation of documentary works by 1998 Student Action with Farmworkers interns. Student Action with Farmworkers, Durham

VeneKlasen L, Patel D (2006) Citizen action, knowledge and global economic power: intersections of popular education, organizing, and advocacy. Just Associates. COMM-ORG Papers Volume 12. http://comm-org.wisc.edu/papers2006/darshana.htm

Chapter 10
Conclusions: An Agenda for Farmworker Social Justice in the Eastern United States

Thomas A. Arcury, Melinda F. Wiggins, and Sara A. Quandt

Abstract Improving the health, safety, and justice of farmworkers in the eastern United States will require advocacy to effect changes in labor, health, occupational, and environmental policy. This chapter summarizes three common themes on the health and justice of farmworkers that emerge from the chapters in this volume: (1) information to document farmworker health and safety is incomplete; (2) the limited information that is available provokes grave concerns about farmworker health and justice; and (3) deficits in farmworker health and farm labor justice result from current agricultural policy. Positive trends in farmworker health, safety, and justice in the eastern US are also documented in the chapters, including the efforts of advocacy organizations, victories by farmworker labor organizations, and the expansion of community-based participatory research. Finally, an agenda for farmworker social justice is outlined. Achieving farmworker social justice will require changing expectations of the US consumer to include fair treatment for those who labor to grow their food, research that documents the conditions of farm work, and changes in policy.

10.1 Introduction

Improving the health, safety, and justice of farmworkers in the eastern United States (US) will require advocacy to effect changes in labor policy, health policy, and occupational and environmental policy. Major obstacles to policy change exist. In this chapter we delineate common themes about farmworker health and safety for farmworker advocacy, review positive trends in farmworker advocacy, and present an agenda for farmworker social justice.

10.2 Common Themes

The chapters in this volume summarize different components of health, safety, and justice for farmworkers and their families in the eastern US. Although the chapters address diverse aspects of exposure to health risks and the prevalence of injury or illness, three common themes about farmworker emerge: (1) information needed to document farmworker health and safety is incomplete; (2) the limited information that is available provokes grave concerns about farmworker health and justice; and (3) deficits in farmworker health and achieving farm labor justice result largely from agricultural labor policy.

10.2.1   Lack of Information About Farmworkers

Each chapter demonstrates and laments the very limited data documenting the current status of health and safety for farmworkers in the eastern US. Although federal, state, and local agencies and programs provide services to farmworkers, these governmental entities seldom collect or publish information about farmworkers. The definitions of who is a farmworker differ among agencies and programs, making it extremely difficult to compare or combine the limited information that they do publish. Therefore, the characteristics of the populations served by these programs are not known. Academic and institute-based investigators have produced little peer-reviewed research on the health of farmworkers in the eastern US. Multiple studies on diverse health, safety, and justice themes have been conducted in only a few states (e.g., North Carolina) and areas (the Northeast and New England). Few or no studies focused on farmworker health and safety have been conducted in many states (e.g., Alabama, Kentucky, Maryland, Ohio, and Tennessee). The lack of attention to the health of farmworkers and their families by three of the four Centers for Agricultural Disease and Injury Research, Education, and Prevention in the eastern US supported by the National Institute for Occupational Safety and Health is telling of the lack of importance placed on addressing farmworker health and safety issues within a social justice framework by important sectors within the federal government and universities.

The lack of data is important. The scope and magnitude of health problems faced by farmworkers cannot be understood without data. Without data, appropriate programs to address farmworker health cannot be developed. Without data, legislators and government officials can ignore farmworker problems and claim there are no problems to be addressed. For example, some members of the 2008 North Carolina Governor's Taskforce on Pesticides argued that no changes in pesticide policy were needed because no data documented that farmworkers were actually exposed to pesticides, and no studies proved pesticide exposure had caused farmworker illness.

10.2.2   Grave Concerns for Farmworker Health and Justice

The second theme is that although information is limited, the information that is available documents grave concerns for the health and justice of farmworkers and their families. The housing available to farmworkers is largely substandard and exposes workers and their family members to environmental health risks. The ubiquitous nature of pesticide application in agriculture and in farmworker dwellings compounds the environmental health risks experienced by farmworker communities. In the eastern US, environmental and occupational regulations provide little protection to farmworkers from pesticide exposure, and the limited enforcement of these regulations further amplifies the potential for pesticide exposure among farmworkers.

Most farmworkers are young and physically fit. Yet, farmworkers experience high rates of musculoskeletal, dermatological, vision and auditory injury and illness, infectious disease, and poor mental health. Farmworker injury and illness reflect the nature of agriculture and the limited regulations applied to this industry. Although farmworkers experience high rates of occupational and environmental injury and illness, few programs and regulations have been designed to help reduce these outcomes. Farmworkers and their families in the eastern US seldom have health insurance, and many of them have limited access to health care. The few efforts to reduce farmworker injury and illness seldom consider the culture and educational attainment of farmworkers or the effects of a migratory lifestyle. Long-term consequences of occupational and environmental exposures are virtually unknown.

Farmworkers are not all men. Many women and children are also employed as farmworkers and experience the same or greater occupational health risks. The women and children who are not employed as farmworkers but who live with a farmworker are also exposed to the poor housing, pesticides, limited access to health care and other services, and poverty and food insecurity of farmworkers.

10.2.3 The Consequences of Agricultural Labor Policy

The third common theme for farmworker health and justice in the eastern US is that agricultural labor policy supports the exploitation of farmworkers, increases the risk of injury and illness, and denies justice. The concept of agricultural exceptionalism has been cited in several chapters. Although some states, notably the western states of California and Washington, have changed the status of agricultural labor to go beyond the minimum standards set by federal law, current agriculture labor policy in most states and in federal statute limits the ability of farmworkers to organize and be represented by a union. Current agricultural labor policy makes it acceptable for farmworkers to live in housing that does not meet standards that are minimal for other US residents. Current agricultural labor policy makes it acceptable for child farmworkers to work in hazardous conditions that are not acceptable for any other children in the US. Current agricultural labor policy makes it acceptable for farmworkers to work long hours without the right to overtime pay. Current agricultural labor policy makes it acceptable for farmworkers to work without a health safety net (workers' compensation), should they be injured. While limited health and safety regulations are imposed in agriculture, regulatory agencies responsible for enforcing these limited regulations in the eastern US are not provided with sufficient funding to review workplace safety standards or living standards.

Agriculture has been exempted from many federal and state labor laws, partly in an effort to protect "the family farm." However, much of contemporary agriculture, particularly agriculture that employs migrant and seasonal farmworkers, is agribusiness. While the family farm has nostalgic connotations, perpetuating the notion has serious consequences for farmworkers and their families.

10.3   Positive Trends

Positive trends to improve farmworker health and safety in the eastern US are also documented in the chapters. These positive trends include the efforts of national and state advocacy organizations, victories by farmworker labor organizations, and the expansion of community-based participatory research.

10.3.1   Efforts of Advocacy Organizations

Several state and national advocacy groups are working for policy changes to benefit farmworkers. Coalitions of health, ministry, and organizing groups have come together to improve laws and regulations. Several state coalitions have experienced recent policy victories, putting farmworker issues on their state legislative agendas for the first time. For example, the Farmworker Advocacy Network in North Carolina has been organizing for nearly five years to advance a policy agenda addressing farmworker wages, housing quality, and pesticide safety. Farmworker Advocacy Network members worked with North Carolina legislators to get bills passed in 2007 and 2008 that strengthen laws governing migrant housing and pesticide regulation enforcement. These new laws require mattresses in migrant housing, require employers to provide alternative housing if their current housing is uninhabitable, protect farmworkers from retaliation if they make pesticide complaints, and increase enforcement efforts by state agencies. While these bills are compromises, they have been enacted in a state where the agribusiness lobby is strong. They are important steps in the legislative battle to ensure that farmworkers are treated equitably under the law.

Other examples of successful farmworker advocacy in the eastern US are the recent victories of the Coalition of Immokalee Workers. Starting in 2001 with a boycott of Taco Bell, the Coalition of Immokalee Workers' tomato workers campaign has had success with fast food giants like Taco Bell, McDonald's, and Burger King. The campaign succeeded in getting farmworkers a penny more per pound of tomatoes picked. These historic victories have gleaned international attention to the struggles of farmworkers, including raising awareness of several slavery cases in Florida fields and of the role that third-party corporations play in keeping farmworker wages below poverty. The Coalition has successfully garnered the support of student activists across the US who have connected the exploitation of tomato workers in Immokalee,

Florida, with their own exploitation by fast food chains that market heavily to young people on college campuses. The approach used by the Coalition of Immokalee Workers allows them to make important incremental changes for farmworkers by focusing on one fast food chain after another.

10.3.2 Victories by Farmworker Labor Organizations

While the number of farm labor unions has not changed in recent years, these unions have used creative efforts to win important victories for farmworkers. In 2004, after nearly a decade of organizing consumers and cucumber workers in North Carolina, the Farm Labor Organizing Committee signed the first union contract with H2A guest workers in the history of the US. The victory came after years of a boycott of the Mt. Olive Pickle Company and numerous lawsuits by Legal Aid of North Carolina against the North Carolina Growers Association. The North Carolina Growers Association brings the majority of H2A workers to the fields of North Carolina. At the time of the signing of the contract, over 8,000 farmworkers were included in the collective bargaining agreement with the North Carolina Growers Association, Mt. Olive Pickle Company, and growers. The initial three-year contract was renewed for one additional year until the end of 2008. The United Farm Workers of America has joined the Farm Labor Organizing Committee to organize guest workers and to work multinationally in addressing effects of international trade and policy on local farmworker struggles.

10.3.3 Expansion of Community-Based Participatory Research

The expansion of community-based participatory research based on collaborations of farmworkers, farmworker organizations, health care providers, and academic scientists has improved the health and justice of farmworkers. The definition of community-based participatory research includes the need for action to change the conditions and improve justice (Arcury et al. 1999, 2001a). Several successes using community-based participatory research that improve the health of farmworkers in the eastern US have been documented. Community-based collaborations in Maine and New York have produced the ergonomic design of apple and blueberry harvest tools that reduce farmworker musculoskeletal injuries (Earle-Richardson et al. 2005; May et al. 2008) (see Chap. 4). Community-based collaborations in Florida and Illinois have developed education programs and selected occupationally and culturally appropriate eye-protection gear that reduces farmworker eye injuries (Luque et al. 2007; Forst et al. 2004) (see Chap. 4). A community-based collaboration in North Carolina is testing a culturally and educationally appropriate HIV education program that will reduce the incidence of farmworker infectious disease (Rhodes et al. 2006) (see Chap. 6). Community-based collaborations in North Carolina and Florida have designed culturally and educationally appropriate safety education programs to reduce pesticide exposure at work and at home (Arcury et al. 2008; Flocks et al. 2001, 2007; Quandt et al. 2001a, b) (see Chap. 5). Finally, a community-based collaboration in North Carolina has developed a culturally and educationally appropriate education program to teach farmworkers about nutrition (Quandt 2007). It is significant that all of these efforts have used members of the farmworker community as lay health advisors in program implementation.

Another component of community-based participatory research has been the effort to improve the knowledge of health care providers for the treatment of injuries and illnesses experienced by farmworkers. For example, collaborators in North Carolina have developed health care provider education programs addressing recognition, treatment, and prevention of green tobacco sickness and pesticide exposure among farmworkers (Arcury et al. 2001b; Hiott et al. 2005).

10.4   An Agenda for Farmworker Social Justice

Farmworkers perform tasks essential to agricultural production in the eastern US. The performance of these tasks places farmworkers and the members of their families at substantial risk for injury and illness. Farmworkers in the eastern US are provided limited protection and receive minimal compensation for their work. Farmworkers have little control over safety in their workplace or living environments. Due to the combination of these circumstances, farmworkers in the eastern US experience social injustices. An agenda for social justice for farmworkers must include three domains: (1) an altered perspective of the US consumer; (2) research that documents the conditions of farm work; and (3) changes in policy and regulation.

10.4.1   Changing the Perspective of the US Consumer

A fundamental component in improving the health and safety, and achieving social justice for farmworkers is changing the perspective of the US consumer. US consumers need to understand where their food is grown, they need to know whose labor is used to grow that food, and they need to know how their demands for inexpensive food result in injury and illness for those providing the labor to grow their food.

Agriculture is an industry fueled by consumer demand. Some dimensions of consumer demand have led to the situation of farmworkers described in this book: exposure to pesticides due to overuse of chemicals to produce blemish-free produce that will withstand storage and long-distance shipping to give supermarkets a season-less supply of foods, or hand-picking of tobacco to produce a leaf not damaged by machinery so it will fetch top dollar from transnational tobacco companies.

Consumer demand can be modified. Examples are the recent movement toward organic foods free from pesticides, hormones, and other chemicals, changes that are seen by consumers as promoting both health of the consumer and health of the environment. In a relatively short period, organic food has progressed from being food purchased only by well-heeled elites to being sold in Walmart, the nation's top food retailer. If consumer demand can be modified to protect the environment, why not create similar awareness of the human cost of food production itself with the goal of having consumers care as much about the people producing their food as they do about bugs?

To achieve this, US consumers need to have a better idea of the source of their food. They also need to understand that the demand for inexpensive food results in social injustice for the people – farmworkers – who plant, cultivate, and harvest the fresh fruits and vegetables that they eat. Stories of kindergartners visiting farms and being amazed at where milk really comes from are cute, but they are, unfortunately the tip of the iceberg for consumer ignorance. Multinational agribusiness has done a good job convincing consumers that their food is produced by modern methods used by a farmer in the air-conditioned comfort of a million-dollar tractor looking out over his amber waves of grain. Most consumers have little idea of the living and working conditions of farmworkers or of the low wages that farmworkers are paid.

Several trends have begun to change the perspective of the US consumer. Writers, such as Wendell Berry (1977, 2005), have had substantial influence on the thinking of Americans about agriculture and food. Berry argues for an obligation to community and environmental stewardship and for the interconnectedness of life: of people who consume food connected to the places and people who produce it and to the environment in which it is produced. The Slow Food International movement encourages consumers NOT to take their food for granted: to eat locally produced, unprocessed, and traditional foods. International Fair Trade Certification has worked to make consumers aware of the source of their food by providing guarantees about products such as coffee, tea, and chocolate. Among the components of Fair Trade Certification is the guarantee that the labor conditions on certified farms include freedom of association, safe working conditions, living wages, and no forced child labor. Like Fair Trade Certification, farmworker advocates are pushing for agricultural products in the US to have a Fair Labor Practices Certification (Henderson et al. 2006; Scientific Certification Systems 2007). Agricultural products with Fair Labor Practices Certification indicate that they were produced by workers provided with equitable hiring and employment practices, provided with safe workplace conditions, and provided with access to health, education, and transportation services.

10.4.2 Research Documenting the Conditions of Farm Work

The struggle for farm labor justice will be served by the availability of data documenting the social and demographic characteristics of farmworkers and their families. Data documenting the health and safety hazards that farmworkers experience and how these hazards are distributed among farmworkers are also needed, as are data documenting farmworker health status and the health care that farmworkers receive.

These are essential for understanding the scope of health problems and health resources available to farmworkers. Several research initiatives would improve information about farmworkers and the conditions of farm work.

One research initiative that would improve information about farmworkers and the conditions of farm work is having governmental agencies and service provider organizations systematically compile information about the farmworker communities that they serve. Agencies and provider organizations need to agree on a common definition of farmworker or to describe the characteristics of individuals in populations that they do serve so that comparisons can be made and information can be combined. Each of these administrative data sources will have common shortcomings, such as missed cases and incorrect data entry. However, the combination of sources will illuminate the characteristics of this vulnerable population. It will allow comparisons of farmworker communities across the eastern US and with farmworker communities in other regions.

A corresponding research initiative that would improve information about farmworkers and the conditions of farm work is the development of a farmworker database. Such a database has been proposed (Mull et al. 2001) but has not been implemented. A farmworker database would compile data from governmental agencies and service provider organizations and include data from independent research projects. Such a large, single database would provide the potential for sufficient statistical power to examine the prevalence and risk factors for infrequent injuries and illnesses that farmworkers experience. Analysis of this database would point to gaps in our knowledge that need to be included in revised administrative data systems and in new research projects. Analysis of the database would also point to needed programs, or revisions in existing programs, to meet health and safety needs of the farmworker community. A national farmworker database would further facilitate comparisons of farmworker communities across the US. A farmworker database that includes data from Canada and Mexico would be an extremely powerful tool.

Another research initiative that would help better document the conditions of health and safety among farmworkers in the eastern US is the establishment of a farmworker longitudinal cohort study. Such a study, the Agricultural Health Study, has been implemented for licensed pesticide applicators in Iowa and North Carolina, most of whom are farmers (Alavanja et al. 1996). The Agricultural Health Study began data collection in 1995 and has produced a large set of papers documenting the health of farmers. A longitudinal cohort study for farmworkers would allow analysis of causal pathways for injury and illness that could feed back into safety and health policy changes.

Finally, study of farmworkers must more often collect data that will allow measurement of health outcomes as well as the measurement of potential exposures. For example, research on farmworker housing has described the often abysmal conditions of such housing; research on agricultural pesticides has documented factors that might cause pesticide exposure. However, no farmworker housing research has collected data that measure health outcomes, such as asthma, mental health, or infectious disease, that are related to housing conditions. Little farmworker pesticide exposure research has measured the potential health effects of this exposure. Until health outcomes as well as exposure are measured, it will be difficult to argue for the need to limit exposure.

10.4.3 Advocacy for Policy Change

Social justice for farmworkers requires systemic changes in policy and regulation for labor, housing, pesticide safety, health care, wages, and immigration. Each of the individual chapters in this volume has made recommendations for specific changes in policy and regulations. Here we outline major policy and regulation changes that will improve the health, safety, and justice for farmworkers in the eastern US and in the nation.

Advocacy groups are working to effect change in policy and regulation in states as well as nationally. These advocacy groups need training, designated staff, and partnerships with a number of organizations to be effective at policy advocacy work. The few farm labor unions and community organizing groups that support agricultural workers need additional financial resources, staff members, and public support in order to advance their agendas. Because the majority of farmworkers today are recent immigrants, partnerships between farmworker organizations and immigrant rights groups could lead to strong and diverse coalitions working on common campaigns and progressive farm labor policy agendas at the state and federal level.

10.4.3.1 Labor Policy

In individual states and nationally, policies exempting agriculture from labor regulations need to be changed. On a federal level, farmworkers should be treated the same as other workers under the Fair Labor Standards Act and National Labor Relations Act. All farmworkers need to be provided with overtime pay and covered by minimum wage laws. Child labor needs to be removed from the fields. Farmworkers must have the same right to organize into unions without fear of retaliation or lack of redress as do other workers. Farmworkers' lives could be most improved if they were paid a living wage and provided with benefits, such as paid sick leave, holidays, and a grievance procedure. In addition, workers' compensation and environmental protection provided to workers in other industries must be provided to all agricultural workers. Advocates can look to international labor standards, as these tend to be much stronger than state or federal laws in the protections they provide to migrant workers.

10.4.3.2 Housing Policy

Regulations governing migrant farmworker housing, as well as the housing of most low-income families in rural communities, such as seasonal farmworkers, need to be revised. For migrant farmworker housing, regulations provide the bare minimum in sanitation and facilities. For the rental housing in which seasonal farmworkers live in most rural communities, often no regulations exist at all. Little enforcement is available for the housing regulations that do exist.

Regulations that provide farmworkers with safe and sanitary housing that includes facilities for food preparation, bathing, and laundry must be established. The housing provided to farmworkers must include security and privacy needed for mental as well as physical health. Sufficient staff must be provided to the agencies charged with enforcing these regulations.

10.4.3.3   Pesticide Policy

Pesticide exposure is a major concern for farmworkers and their families in the eastern US. The potential health effects of pesticides are insidious because they may not be apparent for years, and because they do greater harm to children than to adults. At a minimum, policy changes are needed to ensure the enforcement of existing pesticide safety regulations. These existing pesticide safety regulations, such as the US Environmental Protection Agency's Worker Protection Standard, need to be expanded to address the multiple pathways of pesticide exposure experienced by farmworkers and their families.

An environmental policy that can potentially improve the health and safety for farmworkers is improving the documentation of pesticide application. Current policy based on the US Environmental Protection Agency's Worker Protection Standard requires that pesticide applicators maintain a record of the pesticides they apply to specific fields. However, this information cannot be accessed to document the geographic distribution or level of pesticide application in areas in which farmworkers live. California has enacted regulations that require pesticide applicators to report monthly the types and amounts of pesticides they apply, and the location where the pesticides are applied (California Department of Pesticide Regulation 2000; Nuckols et al. 2007). The implementation of this reporting system nationally would show the level of pesticide exposure for farmworkers and other residents of agricultural communities.

Policy for active monitoring of the pesticide dose experienced by farmworkers would improve workers' health and safety. Washington State has a program in which cholinesterase levels for pesticide handlers are monitored (Weyrauch et al. 2005; Hofmann et al. 2008). Workers with a substantial decline in cholinesterase are removed from work. Policies requiring that workers be tested for cholinesterase depression or specific pesticide metabolites would identify individual workers who should be removed from specific tasks due to high exposure; policies requiring that at least a sample of workers be tested for cholinesterase depression or specific pesticide metabolites would indicate when changes in work practices causing high exposure need to be changed.

10.4.3.4   Health Care Policy

Few farmworkers in the eastern US are provided with health insurance. Many of the farmworkers in the eastern US cannot access some health services because they lack proper immigration documents. The current system of community and migrant clinics is insufficient to provide the health care needed by farmworkers and their families. For example, North Carolina provides state, in addition to federal, support for the 13–15 community and migrant clinics that operate across the state's 100 counties. However, several of these clinics operate on a limited schedule, and even if they operated on a full-time schedule, they would not be able to provide the care needed by the over 100,000 farmworkers in the state, as well as to the families of these farmworkers. This system of clinics needs to be expanded and funded to provide the needed care, and farmworkers need to be provided with health insurance. Further, policy changes are needed to assure adequate resources to federal and state agencies for development of interventions demonstrated to reduce effectively occupational injury and illness in farmworkers.

10.4.3.5 Immigration Policy

One of the most significant policy changes that would advance social justice for farmworkers is immigrant reform. Immigration and Customs Enforcement, "La Migra," causes fear for farmworkers, whether or not they have proper immigration documents. Although immigration reform is needed across the US, it would be a particularly important step for improving social justice for farmworkers. Current legislation such as *The Agricultural Job Opportunities, Benefits and Security Act*, "AgJOBS," is one approach to addressing immigration for farmworkers that is supported by most farmworker advocates and major agricultural employers. It would revise the current H2A temporary foreign agricultural worker program, and allow for "earned legalization" for many undocumented farmworkers and workers with H2A visas. Many farmworkers and their allies also advocate for comprehensive immigration reform, calling for substantial changes to our current immigration laws and enforcement.

10.4.3.6 Enforcement of Regulations

Finally, in addition to improved policy, there is a great need for increased enforcement of regulations. Fines must be increased and regulatory agencies must have real power to exact tangible consequences on noncompliant employers.

10.5 Conclusion

Health and safety for farmworkers and their families in the eastern US are inextricably tied to social justice. Farmworkers in the eastern US, as well as in other regions of the US, across North America, and around the world have become entangled in a global economy and a global agricultural system. Farmworkers and their allies must build equitable and long-term relationships with advocacy groups, academic scientists, and other organizations focused on improving the lives of farmworkers nationally and internationally. Globalization has had a tremendous impact on farmworkers, and it is important for advocates to think about global solutions to their work. Advocates and the labor movement must promote international labor standards that protect all agricultural workers.

Social justice for farmworkers can only be achieved through systematic changes in the way society understands its connection to food. Consumers need to know the sources of their food, and the working and living conditions of those who produce their food. Consumers must be willing to accept the costs of the food they consume. Documentation of the conditions of farm labor will help educate consumers and justify policy changes needed to provide safe working and living conditions for farm labor. Social justice in agriculture must be a commitment of a just society.

References

Arcury TA, Austin CK, Quandt SA et al. (1999) Enhancing community participation in a public health project: farmworkers and agricultural chemicals in North Carolina. Health Educ Behav 26(4):563–578

Arcury TA, Quandt SA, Dearry A (2001a) Farmworker pesticide exposure and community-based participatory research: rationale and practical applications. Environ Health Perspect 109(Suppl 3):429–434

Arcury TA, Quandt SA, Norton D (2001b) Green tobacco sickness among farmworkers in North Carolina. Netw Pract: J Primary Care Providers Community Health Centers. Autumn/Winter: 7–9

Arcury TA, Marín A, Snively BM et al. (2008) Reducing farmworker residential pesticide exposure: evaluation of a lay health advisor intervention. Health Promot Pract: e-pub 2008

Berry W (1977) The Unsettling of America: Culture & Agriculture. Avon Books, New York

Berry W (2005) The Way of Ignorance and Other Essays. Shoemaker & Hoard, Berkeley

California Department of Pesticide Regulation (2000) Pesticide use reporting: an overview of California's unique full reporting system. California Department of Pesticide Regulation, Sacramento

Earle-Richardson G, Jenkins P, Fulmer S et al. (2005) An ergonomic intervention to reduce back strain among apple harvest workers in New York State. Appl Ergon 36:327–334

Flocks J, Clarke L, Albrecht S et al. (2001) Implementing a community-based social marketing project to improve agricultural worker health. Environ Health Perspect 109(Suppl 3):461–468

Flocks J, Monaghan P, Albrecht S et al. (2007) Florida farmworkers' perceptions and lay knowledge of occupational pesticides. J Community Health 32(3):181–194

Forst L, Lacey S, Chen H et al. (2004) Effectiveness of community health workers for promoting use of safety eyewear by Latino farm workers. Am J Ind Med 46:607–613

Henderson E, Mandelbaum R, Mendieta O et al. (2006) Toward social justice and economic equity in the food system: a call for social stewardship standards in sustainable and organic agriculture. Peacework Organic Farm, Newark, NY; Comité de Apoyo a las Trabajadores Agrícolas/Farmworker Support Committee (CATA); Fundación RENACE, Bolivia; and Rural Advancement Foundation International-USA (RAFI-USA). http://www.cata-farmworkers.org/english%20 pages/AJPStandardsAug06.pdf. Cited 4 Aug 2008

Hiott A, Arcury TA, Quandt SA (2005) Pesticide recognition, treatment, and prevention in farmworkers. [Continuing Medical Education workshop on CD]. Department of Family and Community Medicine, Wake Forest University School of Medicine, Winston-Salem

Hofmann JN, Carden A, Fenske RA et al. (2008) Evaluation of a clinic-based cholinesterase test kit for the Washington State cholinesterase monitoring program. Am J Ind Med 51:532–538

Luque JS, Monaghan P, Contreras RB et al. (2007) Implementation evaluation of culturally competent eye injury prevention program for citrus workers in a Florida migrant community. Prog Community Health Partnersh 1(4):359–369

May J, Hawkes L, Jones A et al. (2008) Evaluation of a community-based effort to reduce blueberry harvesting injury. Am J Ind Med 51(4):307–315

Mull LD, Engel LS, Outterson B et al. (2001) National farmworker database: establishing a farmworker cohort for epidemiologic research. Am J Ind Med 40(5):612–618

Nuckols JR, Gunier RB, Riggs P et al. (2007) Linkage of the California pesticide use reporting database with spatial land use data for exposure assessment. Environ Health Perspect 115:684–689

Quandt SA (2007) Nutrition curriculum for promotora programs. Migr Health Newsline 24(4):3

Quandt SA, Arcury TA, Austin CK et al. (2001a) Preventing occupational exposure to pesticides: using participatory research with Latino farmworkers to develop an intervention. J Immigr Health 3:85–96

Quandt SA, Arcury TA, Pell AI (2001b) Something for everyone? A community and academic partnership to address farmworker pesticide exposure in North Carolina. Environ Health Perspect 109(Suppl 3):435–441

Rhodes SD, Hergenrather KC, Montaño J et al. (2006) Using community-based participatory research to develop an intervention to reduce HIV and STD infections among Latino men. AIDS Educ Prev 18:375–389

Scientific Certification Systems (2007) Fair labor practices & community benefits. SCS Sustainable Agriculture Department, Emeryville

Weyrauch KF, Boiko PE, Keifer M (2005) Building informed consent for cholinesterase monitoring among pesticide handlers in Washington State. Am J Ind Med 48:175–181

Index